AF614728

Dyslipidemias in Kidney Disease

Adrian Covic • Mehmet Kanbay
Edgar V. Lerma
Editors

Dyslipidemias in Kidney Disease

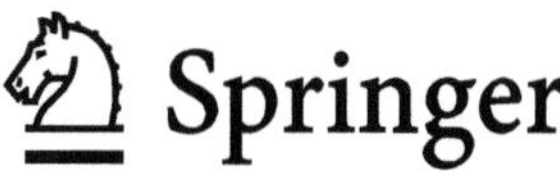

Editors
Adrian Covic
"C.I. Parhon" University Hospital
Iasi, Romania

Edgar V. Lerma
Department of Medicine
University of Illinois
at Chicago College of Medicine
Chicago, IL, USA

Mehmet Kanbay
Department of Medicine
Istanbul Medeniyet University
School of Medicine
Istanbul, Turkey

ISBN 978-1-4939-0514-0 ISBN 978-1-4939-0515-7 (eBook)
DOI 10.1007/978-1-4939-0515-7
Springer New York Heidelberg Dordrecht London

Library of Congress Control Number: 2014935372

Printed on acid-free paper

Springer is part of Springer Science+Business Media (www.springer.com)

To my father, who taught me the rigors of writing.

To my wife and daughters, who supported me in my life through good and bad times.

To my team, a second family.

Adrian Covic

To all my mentors and friends at Fatih University School of Medicine and Istanbul Medeniyet University School of Medicine, who encouraged me to become a medical doctor and to eventually decide to pursue nephrology as a career.

To my parents, my two lovely children, Sude and Murat, and my very loving and understanding wife, Asiye, who supported and encouraged me in all steps of my life.

Mehmet Kanbay

To all my mentors and friends at the University of Santo Tomas Faculty of Medicine and Surgery in Manila, Philippines, and Northwestern University Feinberg School of Medicine in Chicago, Illinois, who have, in one way or another, influenced and guided me to become the physician that I am.

To all the medical students, interns, and residents at Advocate Christ Medical Center whom I have taught or learned from, especially those who eventually decided to pursue nephrology as a career.

To my parents and my brothers, without whose unwavering love and support through the good and bad times, I would not have persevered and reached my goals in life.

Most especially, to my two lovely and precious daughters, Anastasia Zofia and Isabella Ann, whose smiles and laughter constantly provide me unparalleled joy and happiness, and my very loving and understanding wife, Michelle, who has always been supportive of my endeavors, both personally and professionally, and who sacrificed a lot of time and exhibited unwavering patience as I devoted a significant amount of time and effort to this project. Truly, they provide me with motivation and inspiration.

Edgar V. Lerma

Foreword

There is an increasing understanding of the pathophysiological relationship between the cardiovascular system and the kidneys; for many years, chronic kidney disease (CKD) has been accepted as an independent predictor of mortality and adverse cardiovascular events in patients with and without established cardiovascular disease (CVD).

CVD is the leading cause of death amongst patients with end-stage renal disease (ESRD), but even patients with the so-called mild renal insufficiency (approximate to stage 2–3 CKD) exhibit up to a 40 % increased risk of cardiac death as compared to those with normal renal function. Nephrologists very well know that patients with moderate renal impairment are far more likely to suffer cardiovascular death than progress to ESRD, information that is not universally known in non-nephrological circles. Furthermore, over the last years, nephrologists learned that the pattern of cardiovascular death changes as the glomerular filtration rate (GFR) falls. In 2008, the United States Renal Data System (USRDS) annual data report showed that approximately 40 % of deaths amongst dialysis patients were due to cardiovascular causes. Of these, 66 % were sudden deaths versus only 14 % secondary to acute myocardial infarction. Whereas in the general population, sudden death is most commonly due to coronary artery disease, the mechanism of sudden death in severe CKD and dialysis patients is less clear.

There is both a high prevalence of "traditional" cardiovascular risk factors in patients with CKD and a combination of other vascular pathophysiologies largely unique to renal disease.

Dyslipidemia is one of the well-established traditional risk factors for CVD development and progression in the general population. Although dyslipidemia is also common amongst patients with CKD, the pattern differs from that seen in the general population. Chronic CKD is a status of specific lipid disturbances, i.e., dyslipidemia with increased levels of triglycerides, small dense and oxidized LDL (oxLDL), and lower HDL cholesterol levels. In the particular setting of the nephrotic syndrome, total cholesterol and LDL levels also are elevated.

Randomized controlled trial (RCT) evidence shows that lipid-lowering therapy is effective as both primary and secondary prevention against CVD in the general population. Until recently there has been uncertainty as to whether lipid-lowering therapy, and in particular statin use, would also be beneficial in reducing cardiovascular events in CKD.

Apart from their lipid-lowering effects, it became clear over the last years that statins provide a number of additional, the so-called pleiotropic effects that may specifically protect the diseased kidney, by a number of anti-inflammatory, antioxidant, antiproliferative, proapoptotic, and anti-fibrotic effects as well as by exerting beneficial effects on renal hemodynamics. These potentially "renoprotective" effects of statins are based on their possible interference with the pathophysiological mechanisms of renal damage and progression, i.e., renal inflammation, mesangial cell proliferation and matrix synthesis, interstitial fibrosis, and impaired renal blood flow. In addition, specific effects of statins on glomerular endothelial cells and podocytes are also likely.

The recent explosion in knowledge and understanding of lipid metabolic derangements and their impact on kidney function, on the one hand, and on the cardiovascular complications suffered by CKD patients, on the other, has been amply described and discussed in vast scientific literature. However, this quite widespread knowledge was until now not yet condensed and summarized for the clinician in a digestible, one-volume format.

Dyslipidemias in Chronic Kidney Disease has quite successfully attempted to do just that. Under the capable editorship of Drs. Covic, Kanbay, and Lerma, the most recent data on several aspects of lipidology focusing on their relevance for the patient with kidney disease are discussed in 16, mostly stand-alone chapters, all authored by experts in the field. Most of the authors have been involved in either basic research or have been amongst the principal investigators in major RCTs devoted to the treatment of dyslipidemia in kidney patients.

The first chapter summarizes the epidemiology of dyslipidemia in the general population and the population with CKD and describes the overall beneficial effects of lipid-lowering drugs, mainly statins, on CVD in patients without and with mild to moderate renal insufficiency.

The second chapter focuses on modifications of the original hypothesis on lipid-mediated renal and vascular injury by describing how inflammatory stress accompanying CKD fundamentally modifies cholesterol homeostasis, causing lipid redistribution and renal vascular injury, as well as statin resistance.

Chapter 3 tempers the initial expectations based on interesting experimental animal data that statins may slow down the progression of CKD in patients. Despite a number of promising clinical studies, a thorough analysis of the literature reveals that at present there is no strong clinical evidence indicating that statins postpone a decline in renal function or, alternatively, reduce proteinuria. The authors correctly point out that large and well-designed prospective RCTs, specifically in CKD populations, are needed to clarify this potentially interesting aspect of lipid-lowering therapy.

Chapter 4 describes the pharmacological mechanisms involved in the lipid-lowering effects of this class of drugs. Statins inhibit HMG-CoA reductase and thereby reduce the hepatocyte cholesterol content, leading to an increased expression of LDL receptors. The final result is a pronounced reduction in serum LDL cholesterol. Although all statins show similar function by binding to the active site of HMG-CoA reductase, structural differences in statins explain differences in potency of enzyme inhibition and in pharmacokinetic behavior.

Chapter 5 discusses further some of the most relevant epidemiological and pathophysiological links between CVD and CKD, focusing on the multiple lipoprotein abnormalities present in CKD patients caused by a profound dysregulation of their metabolism. This chapter also discusses the role of the elevated plasma levels of Lp(a), which is now recognized as a risk factor for CV morbidity and mortality in hemodialysis patients, and disorders of VLDL, chylomicron, and HDL metabolism in CKD.

Chapter 6 describes the peculiar quantitative and qualitative abnormalities observed in patients with CKD from the early manifestations of disease to the more advanced phases.

Chapter 7 discusses the most important large-scale statin trials in patients with different stages of CKD. It appears that in patients with CKD stage 1–2, the benefit of statin is similar to that in non-CKD patients. Furthermore, in patients with more advanced stage 3–5 CKD, the recently conducted Study of Heart and Renal Protection (SHARP) trial was able to demonstrate a clear reduction in CV events. In patients on dialysis, current evidence from the 4D and AURORA studies does not suggest that benefit of statins can be generally derived, but decisions should be tailored to the individual patient. Finally, the Assessment of LEscol in Renal Transplantation (ALERT) trial has demonstrated that patients with a kidney transplant may also benefit from statin therapy. In summary, available evidence clearly supports the use of statins in CKD patients not on dialysis and in those with a kidney transplant, in particular in the presence of concomitant CV risk factors or established CV disease.

The conclusions in this chapter to a large extent conform to the conclusions formulated in a more recent meta-analysis and systematic review of statin therapy in CKD patients [1]

This meta-analysis concluded that the quality of the evidence indicating that statins reduce all-cause and cardiovascular mortality and major cardiovascular events in persons not receiving dialysis by about one-fifth to one-quarter during approximately 5 years of treatment ranges between moderate and high. In absolute terms, 1,000 persons with CKD not receiving dialysis would need to receive statin treatment to prevent approximately five deaths each year. By contrast, moderate- to high-quality evidence indicates that statins have little or no effect on all-cause mortality, cardiovascular mortality, and major cardiovascular events in persons receiving dialysis, despite decreases in serum cholesterol levels of 1.0 mmol/L or 40 mg/dL. The systematic review concluded, however, that the evidence for statin treatment in kidney transplant recipients is rather sparse and uncertain [1].

In Chap. 8 the pharmacokinetic and pharmacodynamic properties of lipid-lowering drugs in CKD patients without and with the need of dialysis and in patients following transplantation are described. This chapter also discusses the safety, drug dosing, and drug interactions that are important in this group of patients.

Although it is understandable that in a discussion of the treatment of dyslipidemia most attention is given to statin drugs, Chap. 9 correctly covers the important topic of non-statin therapeutic possibilities. Besides lifestyle changes like weight loss, omega-3 polyunsaturated fatty acid (PUFA) consumption, and physical exercise, these possibilities further include fibrates, nicotinic acid, bile acid sequestrants, omega-3 fatty acids (fish oil), and inhibitors of cholesteryl ester transfer protein (CETPi). The discussion in this chapter on ezetemide, an inhibitor of intestinal cholesterol absorption, likely interacting with the NPC1L1 protein of the intestinal brush border, is particularly relevant to the nephrologist. This drug was in combination with a statin, one of the components in the SHARP trial, well known to every nephrologist.

As discussed in many previous chapters in the book, hemodialysis or peritoneal dialysis (PD) leads to some particular changes in the lipid and lipoprotein profiles, with PD patients having in general a more atherogenic lipid profile compared with their HD counterparts. Chapter 10 discusses in some detail the particularities of the dyslipidemia in these patient populations. Despite the fact that two of the most important prospective RCTs with statins were rather negative, the authors of this chapter believe that besides other measures related to the HD or PD technique, statins mainly constitute the current therapeutic armamentarium against dyslipidemia also in dialysis patients. This opinion is presumably partly based on the recent post hoc analysis of the AURORA trial in diabetic hemodialysis patients [2]. This analysis showed a significant reduction in cardiac events (defined as cardiac death and nonfatal MI) of 32 % (RR: 0.68; 95 % CI: 0.51–0.90). It is imperative to remember that this is a post hoc analysis of a neutral study and as such should be considered hypothesis generating as opposed to directing clinical practice. The authors emphasize, however, that future RCTs should take into account the particular characteristics of dialysis dyslipidemia to obtain evidence-based answers in this currently controversial topic.

Chapter 11 discusses in more detail the mechanisms, consequences, and management of dyslipidemia in kidney transplant patients. Mainly based on the original and extensions of the ALERT trial, this chapter concludes that statin therapy effectively lowers atherogenic lipid levels in kidney transplant patients with few drug interactions and good tolerability compared to placebo. The data from the ALERT trial demonstrate benefit to CV survival after treatment with fluvastatin during the long-term follow-up compared to controls, and are consistent with the effects of statins in the general populations. Statins should thus be administered to all transplant patients with dyslipidemia. As discussed earlier, the recent meta-analysis concluded that the evidence for this therapy in transplant patients was of rather low quality [1]. However, transplant patients, despite their often unusual lipid profiles, will have a range of GFR between that of the general population and advanced CKD, and should thus, on an individual basis, receive lipid-lowering statin therapy.

The excellent Chap. 12 reviews in great detail the characteristics, pathophysiology, and treatment of the dyslipidemia observed in patients with nephrotic syndrome, progression of CKD, and diabetic nephropathy.

Chapter 13 on dyslipidemia in children with kidney diseases starts by reminding the reader that the process of atherosclerosis already begins in childhood, but that the data on this topic in this population are limited. The pattern of dyslipidemia differs amongst the major categories of renal diseases: nephrotic syndrome, chronic renal insufficiency/ESRD, and renal transplantation. Some children with certain diseases encounter several stages progressively, and the exposure to dyslipidemia can thus be more extended than in adult-onset kidney disease. The authors also remind us that in view of the different disease profiles between adults and children, adult data cannot directly be translated in children.

As the incidence of kidney dysfunction increases with aging, understanding and treating abnormalities in lipid metabolism become central in geriatric patients with CKD. Chapter 14 discusses this important topic, but because no large RCT about outcomes of dyslipidemia is available in this particular age group, data from subgroup analysis of several landmark prevention trials teach us that lipid-lowering agents also in the elderly with kidney dysfunction seem to have a benefit. Attention should, of course, be paid to the greater risk of adverse drug effects, and the lowest possible dose of medications should be used.

Although not available in many clinical centers, Chap. 15 deals with a problem that is of great interest to the nephrologist, i.e., the background, physiopathology, techniques, and outcomes of selective LDL-apheresis strategies in the treatment of familial hypercholesterolemia. This disease is a well-known genetic disorder characterized by elevated levels of low-density lipoprotein cholesterol (LDL-C), leading to a rapid evolutive atherosclerotic vascular disease with expected premature onset of coronary heart disease. Several strategies are now available and are discussed in this interesting chapter.

The final Chap. 16 discusses several guidelines available to the physician in the treatment of the CKD patient with CKD dyslipidemias. It is of interest that at the time this Foreword is being written, the KDIGO Clinical Practice Guideline for Lipid Management in Chronic Kidney Disease has been published [3]. It is rewarding for the authors of this book that rapid scanning of all the KDIGO recommendations did not reveal any major inconsistencies.

This is somewhat in contrast to the recent discussion that has taken place between the National Lipid Association (NLA) and the American College of Cardiology and the American Heart Association about the 2013 ACC/AHA Guideline on the Treatment of Blood Cholesterol to Reduce Atherosclerotic Cardiovascular Risk in Adults [4]. In contrast to many other stakeholders, the NLA did not want to endorse these guidelines because it felt that the guidelines did not go far enough to address gaps in clinical care, because the guidelines were limited to reviewing only high-quality RCTs but had excluded other important types of clinical evidence. The NLA also does not find evidence-based support for the guideline's recommendation for removing LDL-C (and non-HDL-C) treatment targets [5].

This book will at least help the nephrologists in the sometimes-difficult decision on when and with what drug the dyslipidemia of their kidney patient should be treated. The recent 2013 ACC/AHA Guideline does not discuss this particular problem.

It is, of course, evident that in a multi-authored book some overlap between the chapters is unavoidable; this is, however, a minor drawback. I believe that the major objective of this book, which is to advise about the management of dyslipidemia and use of lipid-lowering medications in adults and children with known CKD, is certainly achieved. The target audience of this book should not only include nephrologists, but also primary care physicians and non-nephrology specialists (e.g., cardiologists, diabetologists) caring for adults and children with CKD worldwide. They will find useful information in this monograph.

Ghent, Belgium Norbert Lameire, M.D., Ph.D.

References

1. Palmer SC, Craig JC, Navaneethan SD, Tonelli M, Pellegrini F, Strippoli GF. Benefits and harms of statin therapy for persons with chronic kidney disease: a systematic review and meta-analysis. Ann Intern Med. 2012;157(4):263–75.
2. Holdaas H, Holme I, Schmieder RE, Jardine AG, Zannad F, Norby GE, et al. Rosuvastatin in diabetic hemodialysis patients. J Am Soc Nephrol. 2011;22(7):1335–41.
3. Kidney Disease: Improving Global Outcomes (KDIGO) Lipid Work Group. KDIGO Clinical practice guideline for lipid management in chronic kidney disease. Kidney Int. 2013;suppl 3(3):259–305.
4. Stone NJ, Robinson J, Lichtenstein AH, Merz CN, Blum CB, Eckel RH, et al. ACC/AHA guideline on the treatment of blood cholesterol to reduce atherosclerotic cardiovascular risk in adults: a report of the American College of Cardiology/American Heart Association task force on practice guidelines. Circulation 2013; Nov 12 [Epub ahead of print].
5. The NLA position statement on the 2013 ACC/AHA guideline on blood cholesterol. https://www.lipid.org/.

Preface

For more than 100 years, it has been recognized that lipids play an important role in the expansion of cardiovascular disease. Furthermore, therapeutic strategies targeting hyperlipidemia/dyslipidemia have had a profound impact on decreasing cardiovascular mortality and morbidity in various disease populations. In chronic kidney disease, lipids may be involved not only in vascular disease but also in the progression to end-stage renal disease. Our understanding of the pathogenesis and clinical consequences of lipid disorders in CKD patients has increased enormously. Recently, large-scale randomized controlled trials have attempted to attest the importance of controlling lipid metabolisms in CKD patients. It will therefore be suitable for a new book to provide an updated overview of all available clinical and basic scientific data for clinicians and researchers in this area.

This new book summarizes the rapid advances made in the field of lipid disorders, in nephrology. Three chapters address the epidemiology, pathogenesis, and adverse events associated with hyperlipemia. Other chapters review the importance of lipids in different CKD categories: dialysis, transplantation, nephrotic syndrome, pediatric and geriatric populations. Additionally, a world-renowned panel of expert contributors has been challenged to summarize current clinical trials and to make treatment recommendations based on the results of these trials and their own best clinical practice.

This book is very timely, especially in light of recent developments in this area of interest, particularly with the release of recent guidelines. In early November 2013, the Kidney Disease: Improving Global Outcomes (KDIGO) released The Clinical Practice Guideline for Lipid Management in Chronic Kidney Disease, which presented a controversial approach to lipid management. The Work Group found little evidence to justify ongoing assessment of dyslipidemia and recommended that patients be treated with statins or statin/ezetimibe combinations without the need for follow-up testing. Co-chair David Wheeler of the University College London opined that "this 'fire and forget' approach is simple, cost-effective and will improve outcomes for patients".

Later that month, the American College of Cardiology and the American Heart Association released a new clinical practice guideline for the treatment of blood dyslipidemias in people at high risk for cardiovascular diseases caused by atherosclerosis. The new guideline identified four major groups of patients for whom HMG-CoA reductase inhibitors are believed to have the greatest chance of preventing complications such as cerebrovascular accidents and myocardial infractions. In addition, the guideline also emphasized the importance of adopting a certain lifestyle to prevent and control dyslipidemias.

This new guideline represented a significant departure from previous guidelines because it did not focus on specific target levels of low-density lipoprotein cholesterol (LDL), despite there have been no changes in the definition of optimal LDL. Nevertheless, it focused on defining groups for whom decreasing LDL is believed to be most beneficial. Furthermore, this new guideline recommends moderate- or high-intensity statin therapy for these four groups: those who have cardiovascular disease; those with an LDL of 190 mg/dL or higher; those with type 2 diabetes who are between 40 and 75 years of age; and those with an estimated 10-year risk of cardiovascular disease of 7.5 % or higher who are between 40 and 75 years of age.

It is our hope that this book will shed some light on our understanding of the rationale behind these recently developed guidelines and that it will help practitioners in their clinical practice, particularly when dealing with dyslipidemias in patients with chronic kidney disease.

The perfect medicine book should be pleasant to read, easy to understand, evidence-based, and remarkably practical. The present book is a result of these goals. The book is designed to be both easily readable and at the same time to provide an extensively referenced work written by experts in specific fields. Overall, this comprehensive book will continue the tradition of excellent papers of nephrology. It will be of great interest not only to nephrologists, but also to internists, cardiologists, and endocrinologists, as well as all healthcare providers with particular interest in lipid-related disorders.

Certainly, this book would not have been possible were it not for so many people. First of all, we would like to thank all of our contributing authors, who have spent countless hours in producing high-quality, updated information. We spent a significant amount of time communicating via telephone and email as we reviewed the chapters and discussed recommendations, most of which were agreed upon but, on occasion, disputed. We express our sincerest gratitude for their openness to this very collegial collaboration, which has been a truly rewarding experience for all of us. We appreciate the help and support of all the staff of Springer publications, most especially Diane Lamsback, our Developmental Editor; and Gregory Sutorius, our Editor, both of whom have been very patient with our procrastination and stubbornness at times.

We thank all our teachers and mentors, who devoted their own time and effort to educate and train us to become who we are. We thank all the medical students, interns, residents, and fellows who, in one way or another, have inspired us to persevere in this most noble teaching profession. Most of all, we thank all of our patients, who have been truly instrumental in our learning and devotion to this field of medicine. On behalf of all the contributors to this book, we hope that all of our efforts may contribute to relieving your suffering and lead to recovery.

Iasi, Romania — Adrian Covic
Istanbul, Turkey — Mehmet Kanbay
Chicago, IL, USA — Edgar V. Lerma

Contents

Contributors

Baris Afsar, M.D. Department of Nephrology, Konya Numune State Hospital, Konya, Selcuklu, Turkey

Valentina Batini, M.D. Department of Nephrology and Dialysis, Hospital of Livorno, Livorno, Tuscany, Italy

Stefano Bianchi, M.D. Department of Nephrology and Dialysis, Hospital of Livorno, Livorno, Tuscany, Italy

Adrian Covic, M.D., Ph.D., F.R.C.P. (London), F.E.R.A. "C.I. Parhon" University Hospital, Iasi, Romania

Tevfik Ecder, M.D. Department of Internal Medicine, Division of Nephrology, Istanbul Faculty of Medicine, Istanbul, Turkey

Kai-Uwe Eckardt, M.D. Department of Nephrology and Hypertension, University Hospital Erlangen and Community Hospital Nuremberg, Erlangen, Bavaria, Germany

Cumali Gokce Department of Endocrinology, Mustafa Kemal University, School of Medicine, Serinyol, Antakya, Hatay, Turkey

David Goldsmith, M.A., M.B., B.Chir., F.R.C.P. (London), F.R.C.P. (Edin.), F.A.S.N., F.E.R.A. Renal Department, Guy's Hospital London, London, UK

Alan G. Jardine, B.Sc., M.D., F.E.S.C., F.E.B.S. Institute of Cardiovascular and Medical Sciences, University of Glasgow, Glasgow, UK

Mehmet Kanbay, M.D. Division of Nephrology, Department of Medicine, Istanbul Medeniyet University School of Medicine, Istanbul, Turkey

Theodoros Kassimatis, M.D., Ph.D. Nephrology Department, Asklepieion General Hospital, Athens, Greece

Minso Kim, M.D. Department of Pediatrics, NYU Langone Medical Center, New York, NY, USA

Agata Kujawa-Szewieczek, M.D. Department of Nephrology, Endocrinology and Metabolic Diseases, Medical University of Silesia in Katowice, Katowice, Poland

Norbert Lameire, M.D., Ph.D. University Hospital, Ghent, Belgium

Jessica Lassiter, Pharm.D. Department of Pharmacy, University of Michigan Health System, Ann Arbor, MI, USA

Edgar V. Lerma, M.D., F.A.C.P., F.A.S.N., F.A.H.A., F.A.S.H., F.N.L.A., F.N.K.F. Department of Medicine, University of Illinois at Chicago College of Medicine, Chicago, IL, USA

John Moorhead, M.B.Ch.B., F.R.C.P. Centre for Nephrology, University College London Medical School, Royal Free Campus, London, UK

Istvan Mucsi, M.D., Ph.D. Department of Medicine, Division of Nephrology, McGill University Health Centre, Royal Victoria Hospital, Montreal, QC, Canada

Ali Olyaei, Pharm.D. Department of Nephrology and Hypertension, Oregon Health and Sciences University, Portland, OR, USA

Zeynep Birsin Özçakar, M.D. Division of Pediatric Nephrology and Rheumatology, Department of Pediatrics, Ankara University School of Medicine, Ankara Üniversitesi Tıp Fakültesi, Cebeci Kampüsü, Ankara, Turkey

Zeynel Abidin Ozturk, M.D. Division of Geriatrics, Department of Internal Medicine, School of Medicine, Gaziantep University Faculty of Medicine, Gaziantep, Turkey

Rajan Kantilal Patel, M.B.Ch.B., Ph.D. Renal Research Group, Institute of Cardiovascular and Medical Sciences, University of Glasgow, Glasgow, UK

Grzegorz Piecha, M.D. Department of Nephrology, Endocrinology and Metabolic Diseases, Medical University of Silesia in Katowice, Katowice, Poland

Xiong Zhong Ruan, Ph.D., M.D. Centre for Nephrology, University College London Medical School, Royal Free Campus, London, UK

Markus P. Schneider, M.D. Department of Nephrology and Hypertension, University Hospital Erlangen and Community Hospital Nuremberg, Erlangen, Bavaria, Germany

Serdar Sivgin, M.D. Department of Hematology and Stem Cell Transplantation, Hematology Oncology Hospital, Erciyes University, Kayseri, Turkey

Yalcin Solak, M.D. Department of Nephrology, Karaman State Hospital, Karaman Devlet Hastanesi, Karaman, Turkey

Halil Zeki Tonbul, M.D. Department of Nephrology, Meram School of Medicine Necmettin Erbakan Üniversitesi, Meram Tıp Fakültesi, Nefroloji Bölümü, Meram, Konya, Turkey

Howard Trachtman, M.D. Division of Pediatric Nephrology, Department of Pediatrics, NYU Langone Medical Center, New York, NY, USA

Faruk Turgut, M.D. Department of Nephrology, Mustafa Kemal University, School of Medicine, Serinyol, Antakya, Hatay, Turke

Ihsan Ustun Department of Endocrinology, Mustafa Kemal University, School of Medicine, Serinyol, Antakya, Hatay, Turkey

Zekeriya Ulger, M.D. Division of Geriatrics, Department of Internal Medicine, School of Medicine, Gazi University Hospital, Ankara, Turkey

Zac Varghese, Ph.D., F.R.C.P. Centre for Nephrology, University College London Medical School, Royal Free Campus, London, UK

Andrzej Więcek, M.D., F.R.C.P. (Edin.) Department of Nephrology, Endocrinology and Metabolic Diseases, Medical University of Silesia in Katowice, Katowice, Poland

Fatoş Yalçınkaya, M.D. Division of Pediatric Nephrology and Rheumatology, Department of Pediatrics, Ankara University School of Medicine, Ankara Üniversitesi Tıp Fakültesi, Cebeci Kampüsü, Ankara, Turkey

[illegible], M.D., [illegible] Medicine [illegible]

[illegible], M.D., [illegible] New York, NY, USA

[illegible], M.D., Department of [illegible] School of Medicine [illegible], Turkey

[illegible] Department of [illegible] University [illegible] Medicine [illegible]

[illegible], M.D., [illegible] Medicine [illegible]

[illegible]

[illegible]

[illegible]

Chapter 1
Epidemiology/Prevalence of Dyslipidemia in the General Population and in Patients with Chronic Kidney Disease

Tevfik Ecder

Dyslipidemia as a Major Cardiovascular Risk Factor

Epidemiologic studies have established smoking, diabetes, dyslipidemia, and hypertension as independent risk factors for coronary heart disease (CHD) [1–3]. High blood cholesterol is a leading risk factor in the development of atherosclerosis and CHD. The World Health Organization estimates that dyslipidemia is associated with more than half of global cases of ischemic heart disease and more than four million deaths per year [4].

There is a close association between serum cholesterol levels and cardiovascular morbidity and mortality in the general population. In a meta-analysis of individual data from 61 prospective studies, consisting of almost 900,000 adults without previous disease, 1 mmol/L lower total cholesterol was associated with about a half, a third, and a sixth lower ischemic heart disease mortality in both sexes at ages 40–49, 50–69, and 70–89 years, respectively, throughout the main range of cholesterol in most developed countries, with no apparent threshold [5].

The Multiple Risk Factor Intervention Trial (MRFIT) screened 350,977 men aged 35–57 years and followed them for an average of 12 years. A strong, positive, graded relationship was found between serum cholesterol level measured at initial screening and death from CHD [6]. Moreover, this relationship persisted over the 12-year follow-up period. Likewise, in a prospective study, 44,985 men in the United States without a history of cardiovascular disease at baseline were followed-up for 25 years [7]. The four conventional cardiovascular risk factors of smoking, hypertension, hypercholesterolemia, and type 2 diabetes accounted for the majority of risk associated with the development of clinically significant peripheral artery disease.

T. Ecder, M.D. (✉)
Department of Internal Medicine, Division of Nephrology, Istanbul Faculty of Medicine, Capa, Istanbul 34390, Turkey
e-mail: ecder@istanbul.edu.tr

A. Covic et al. (eds.), *Dyslipidemias in Kidney Disease*, DOI 10.1007/978-1-4939-0515-7_1,

In order to estimate the long-term effects of cardiovascular risk factors, Framingham Offspring cohort was investigated [8]. In this study, 4,506 participants of the Framingham Offspring cohort aged 20–59 years free of cardiovascular disease at baseline examination were prospectively followed for the development of hard cardiovascular events (coronary death, myocardial infarction, stroke). The 30-year hard cardiovascular disease event rates adjusted for the competing risk of death were 7.6 % for women and 18.3 % for men. Standard risk factors (male sex, systolic blood pressure, total and high-density lipoprotein [HDL] cholesterol, smoking, and diabetes mellitus), measured at baseline, were significantly related to the incidence of hard cardiovascular disease and remained significant when updated regularly on follow-up for more than 30 years.

In order to compare the relationship between serum total cholesterol and long-term mortality from CHD in different cultures, total cholesterol was measured at baseline and at 5- and 10-year follow-up in 12,467 men aged 40 through 59 years in 16 cohorts in five European countries, the United States, and Japan [3]. For a cholesterol level of around 5.45 mmol/L (210 mg/dL), CHD mortality rates varied from 4 to 5 % in Japan and Mediterranean Southern Europe to about 15 % in Northern Europe. Across these different cultures, cholesterol was linearly related to CHD mortality, and the relative increase in CHD mortality rates with a given cholesterol increase was the same.

Systematic reviews and meta-analysis reported that reduction in total and low-density lipoprotein (LDL) cholesterol by statins was associated with marked reductions in nonfatal and fatal cardiovascular events [9, 10]. A prospective meta-analysis of data from 90,056 individuals in 14 randomized trials of statins showed that statin therapy can safely reduce the 5-year incidence of major coronary events, coronary revascularization, and stroke by about one-fifth per mmol/L reduction in LDL-cholesterol, irrespective of the initial lipid profile or other presenting characteristics. Furthermore, lowering LDL cholesterol with statin therapy even in people at low risk of vascular disease (5-year risk of major vascular events lower than 10 %) was associated with benefit [11].

Dyslipidemia in the General Population

Dyslipidemia is a common cardiovascular risk factor. According to the report of the American Heart Association Statistics Committee and Stroke Statistics Committee in 2011, an estimated 33.6 million adults 20 years or older have total serum cholesterol levels of 240 mg/dL or greater, for a prevalence of 15 % of the American population [12]. Analysis of 30-year national trends in serum lipid levels showed improvements in total cholesterol and LDL cholesterol, which may in part be explained by the increase in the use of lipid-lowering drug therapy [13]. In another epidemiologic study, in order to describe prevalence of major cardiovascular risk factors and cardiovascular diseases among Hispanic/Latino individuals of diverse backgrounds in the United States, the data of 15,079 participants of the Hispanic Community Health Study was analyzed [14]. Hypercholesterolemia prevalence was highest among Central American men (54.9 %) and Puerto Rican women (41 %).

The Multi-Ethnic Study of Atherosclerosis (MESA) which is a population-based study of 6,814 men and women aged 45–84 years, aimed to study the prevalence, treatment, and control of dyslipidemia in different ethnic groups living in the United States [15]. Drug treatment thresholds and goals were defined according to the Third Report of the Adult Treatment Panel (ATP III) [16]. Control to ATP III goal was observed in 75.2 % of participants with treated dyslipidemia and 40.6 % of participants with dyslipidemia. Dyslipidemia was more common in men than in women and was treated and controlled less often in men than in women. Dyslipidemia prevalence differed little across ethnic groups, with the exception of a lower prevalence in Chinese subjects. Drug treatment also differed little across ethnic groups, with the exception of a lower prevalence of treatment reported by Hispanic subjects. Control of dyslipidemia was achieved less commonly in blacks and Hispanics than in non-Hispanic whites. Importantly, control of dyslipidemia was achieved less commonly in high-risk and intermediate-risk than in low-risk individuals.

The awareness of the importance of dyslipidemia as a major cardiovascular risk factor is increasing all over the world. The EUROASPIRE (European Action on Secondary and Primary Prevention by Intervention to Reduce Events) surveys by the European Society of Cardiology were done in selected geographical areas and hospitals in Czech Republic, Finland, France, Germany, Hungary, Italy, the Netherlands, and Slovenia [17–21]. The first EUROASPIRE survey was done in 1995–1996 in nine European countries, the second in 1999–2000 in 15 countries, and the third in 2006–2007 in 22 countries, including eight countries that participated in EUROASPIRE I and II. Although the frequency of obesity increased from 25.0 % in EUROASPIRE I to 32.6 % in II and 38 % in III, the proportion with raised cholesterol (≥4.5 mmol/L) decreased from 94.5 % in EUROASPIRE I to 76.7 % in II and 46.2 % in III [21]. The proportion of patients taking lipid-lowering drugs who achieved the cholesterol target levels of less than 4.5 mmol/L was sevenfold higher in the third survey than in the first. However, in the EUROASPIRE III survey, 42.7 % of patients on treatment had still not reached this target.

In a cross-sectional study on 11,554 individuals representative of the population aged ≥18 years in Spain, 50.5 % had hypercholesterolemia (total cholesterol ≥200 mg/dL or drug treatment) and 44.9 % had high levels of LDL cholesterol (≥130 mg/dL or drug treatment), with no substantial sex-related differences [22]. Of note, cholesterol control was poor, particularly among those with the highest cardiovascular risk, such as diabetics or patients with cardiovascular disease.

A total of 10,872 participants were included in a population-based, national survey in Turkey on populations aged over 18 years [23]. In this study, the prevalence of dyslipidemia, defined as patients having anti-lipid treatment or total cholesterol >240 mg/dL or LDL cholesterol >130 mg/dL or HDL cholesterol <40 mg/dL for men, <46 mg/dL for women or serum triglyceride >150 mg/dL, was 76.3 %.

Dyslipidemia in Patients with Chronic Kidney Disease

The incidence and prevalence of chronic kidney disease (CKD) are increasing worldwide. Chronic renal failure is associated with premature atherosclerosis and increased incidence of cardiovascular morbidity and mortality. Thus, cardiovascular disease is a major cause of morbidity and mortality in patients with CKD. Both traditional risk factors and nontraditional risk factors associated with CKD, including inflammation, oxidant stress, and malnutrition, may further increase cardiovascular risk in these patients [24–26]. In dialysis patients, the relationship between serum cholesterol levels and mortality is complex. Observational studies show that a lower level of total cholesterol predicts higher risk of both all-cause mortality and cardiovascular mortality in dialysis patients [27, 28]. Since hypercholesterolemia is an established cardiovascular risk factor in the general population, this relationship in dialysis patients is called "reverse epidemiology" [29]. However, hypocholesterolemia also correlates closely with low serum albumin and serum C-reactive protein (CRP) levels, which are markers of malnutrition and inflammation [28]. A study by Liu et al. [30] reported that in the absence of malnutrition or inflammation, elevated total cholesterol was associated with increased risk of cardiovascular disease in dialysis patients.

Data from the population-based Atherosclerosis Risk in Communities (ARIC) Study showed that risk factors for CHD in the general population also are associated with an increased risk for CHD among the population with CKD [26]. In this study, with the exception of HDL cholesterol, which showed a weaker association, and anemia, which showed a stronger association, the relationship of CHD risk factors was similar for people with and without CKD. Clinical trials have also reported that dyslipidemia is associated with increased rate of progression of CKD [31]. Moreover, high cholesterol is an independent risk factor associated with a decline in renal function in healthy subjects [32].

Dyslipidemia is common in patients with CKD. CKD is associated with metabolic abnormalities of plasma lipoproteins. Hypertriglyceridemia is a common lipid abnormality in patients with CKD. The concentrations of triglyceride-rich lipoproteins (very-low-density lipoprotein [VLDL], chylomicrons and their remnants) start to increase in early stages of CKD. These parameters are almost always high in patients with nephrotic syndrome and in dialysis patients, especially in peritoneal dialysis (PD) patients [33]. Increases in plasma apoprotein (apo)C-III levels may be responsible for the increased triglyceride levels in patients with CKD. Apoprotein C-III is a potent inhibitor of the enzyme lipoprotein lipase, which degrades triglyceride-rich particles [33].

HDL levels are decreased in patients with CKD [30]. Reductions in plasma concentrations of apoA-I and apoA-II cholesterol are thought to play a role in the low HDL cholesterol levels [32, 34]. Chronic inflammation, by decreasing albumin levels, also contributes to the low levels of HDL cholesterol in these patients. Since albumin acts as a carrier of free cholesterol from peripheral tissues to HDL, its reduction may result in reduced HDL cholesterol levels [35].

Several studies showed that dyslipidemia is common in kidney transplant recipients [36, 37]. Over 80 % of patients with kidney transplantation have total cholesterol levels above 5.2 mmol/L (200 mg/dL) and over 90 % have LDL cholesterol levels above 2.6 mmol/L (100 mg/dL) [36–39].

In the CREDIT (Chronic Renal Disease in Turkey) study, the prevalence rates for hypertension, diabetes, dyslipidemia, obesity, and metabolic syndrome were 32.7 %, 12.7 %, 76.3 %, 20.1 %, and 31.3 %, respectively, in the general population [23]. The prevalence of hypertension was higher in subjects with CKD than in those without CKD (56.3 and 31 %, $P<0.001$). Similarly, the prevalence rates of diabetes (26.6 % vs. 10.1 %), dyslipidemia (83.4 % vs. 75.8 %), obesity (29.2 % vs. 20 %), and metabolic syndrome (46 % vs. 29.8 %) were significantly higher in subjects with CKD compared with subjects without CKD ($P<0.001$ for all analyses). In addition, the CREDIT-C study, which investigated a cohort of 3,622 children aged 5–18 years, the prevalence of hypercholesterolemia was 5.8 % [40]. Importantly, the mean glomerular filtration rate (GFR) was lower in children with hypercholesterolemia (120.53 ± 27.33 vs. 129.29 ± 22.71, $P<0.001$).

Although clinical trials in the general population and in people with established cardiovascular disease have reported a strong association between reducing lipid levels and the risk of cardiovascular morbidity and mortality, data on patients with CKD is conflicting. Meta-analyses of large randomized controlled trials showed that lipid-lowering treatment with statins is effective in reducing the risk for cardiovascular disease in early stages of CKD [41, 42]. However, the benefit of such therapies may be limited in patients with stage 5 CKD [43, 44]. The SHARP (Study of Heart and Renal Protection) trial investigated the effects of lowering LDL cholesterol with simvastatin plus ezetimibe in 9,270 patients with CKD (3,023 on dialysis and 6,247 not) [45]. During a median follow-up of 4.9 years, there was a significant reduction in major atherosclerotic events in patients randomized to simvastatin plus ezetimibe therapy compared to placebo. However, the study did not have sufficient power to assess the effects on major atherosclerotic events separately in dialysis and non-dialysis patients.

References

1. Khot UN, Khot MB, Bajzer CT, Sapp SK, Ohman EM, Brener SJ, et al. Prevalence of conventional risk factors in patients with coronary heart disease. JAMA. 2003;290:898–904.
2. Stamler J, Vaccaro O, Neaton JD, Wentworth D. Diabetes, other risk factors, and 12-yr cardiovascular mortality for men screened in the Multiple Risk Factor Intervention Trial. Diabetes Care. 1993;16(2):434–44.
3. Verschuren WM, Jacobs DR, Bloemberg BP, Kromhout D, Menotti A, Aravanis C, et al. Serum total cholesterol and long-term coronary heart disease mortality in different cultures. Twenty-five-year follow-up of the seven countries study. JAMA. 1995;274:131–6.
4. World Health Organization. Quantifying selected major risks to health. In: The World Health report 2012—reducing risks, promoting healthy life. Chap. 4. Geneva: World Health Organization; 2002. p. 47–97.

5. Lewington S, Whitlock G, Clarke R, Sherliker P, Emberson J, Halsey J, et al. Blood cholesterol and vascular mortality by age, sex, and blood pressure: a meta-analysis of individual data from 61 prospective studies with 55,000 vascular deaths. Lancet. 2007;370:1829–9.
6. Neaton JD, Blackburn H, Jacobs D, Kuller L, Lee DJ, Sherwin R, et al. Serum cholesterol level and mortality findings for men screened in the Multiple Risk Factor Intervention Trial. Multiple Risk Factor Intervention Trial Research Group. Arch Intern Med. 1992;152:1490–500.
7. Joosten MM, Pai JK, Bertoia ML, Rimm EB, Spiegelman D, Mittleman MA, et al. Associations between conventional cardiovascular risk factors and risk of peripheral artery disease in men. JAMA. 2012;308:1660–7.
8. Pencina MJ, D'Agostino RB, Larson MG, Massaro JM, Vasan RS. Predicting the 30-year risk of cardiovascular disease. The Framingham Study. Circulation. 2009;119:3078–84.
9. Cholesterol Treatment Trialists' (CTT) Collaborators. Efficacy and safety of cholesterol-lowering treatment: prospective meta-analysis of data from 90,056 participants in 14 randomised trials of statins. Lancet. 2005;366:1267–78.
10. Cholesterol Treatment Trialists' (CTT) Collaborators. Efficacy and safety of more intensive lowering of LDL cholesterol: a meta-analysis of data from 170,000 participants in 26 randomised trials. Lancet. 2010;376:1670–81.
11. Cholesterol Treatment Trialists' (CTT) Collaborators. The effects of lowering LDL cholesterol with statin therapy in people at low risk of vascular disease: meta-analysis of individual data from 27 randomised trials. Lancet. 2012;380:581–90.
12. Go AS, Mozaffarian D, Roger VL, Benjamin EJ, Berry JD, Borden WB, et al. Heart disease and stroke statistics—2013 update: a report from the American Heart Association. Circulation. 2013;127(1):e6–e245.
13. Cohen JD, Cziraky MJ, Cai Q, Wallace A, Wasser T, Crouse JR, et al. 30-year trends in serum lipids among United States adults: results from the National Health and Nutrition Examination Surveys II, III, and 1999–2006. (Erratum in: Am J Cardiol. 2010;106: 1826). Am J Cardiol. 2010;106:969–75.
14. Daviglus ML, Talavera GA, Avilés-Santa ML, Allison M, Cai J, Criqui MH, et al. Prevalence of major cardiovascular risk factors and cardiovascular diseases among Hispanic/Latino individuals on diverse backgrounds in the United States. JAMA. 2012;308(17):1775–84.
15. Goff DC, Bertoni AG, Kramer H, et al. Dyslipidemia, prevalence, treatment, and control in the Multi-Ethnic Study of Atherosclerosis (MESA): gender, ethnicity, and coronary artery calcium. Circulation. 2006;113:647–56.
16. National Cholesterol Education Program (NCEP) Expert Panel in Detection, Evaluation, and Treatment of High Blood Cholesterol in Adults (Adult Treatment Panel III). Third report of the National Cholesterol Education Program (NCEP) Expert Panel in Detection, Evaluation, and Treatment of High Blood Cholesterol in Adults (Adult Treatment Panel III): final report. Circulation. 2002;106:3143–421.
17. EUROASPIRE Study Group. EUROASPIRE. A European Society of Cardiology survey of secondary prevention of coronary heart disease: principal results. Eur Heart J. 1997;18: 1569–82.
18. EUROASPIRE II Study Group. Lifestyle and risk factor management and use of drug therapies in coronary patients from 15 countries. Principal results from EUROASPIRE II Euro Heart Survey Programme. Eur Heart J. 2001;22:554–72.
19. EUROASPIRE I and II Group. Clinical reality of coronary prevention guidelines: a comparison of EUROASPIRE I and II in nine countries. Lancet. 2001;357:995–1001.
20. Kotseva K, Wood D, De Backer G, De Bacquer D, Pyorala K, Keil U, for the EUROASPIRE Study Group. EUROASPIRE III: a survey on lifestyle, risk factors and use of cardioprotective drug therapies in coronary patients from twenty two European countries. Eur J Cardiovasc Prev Rehabil. 2009;16:121–37.
21. Kotseva K, Wood D, De Backer G, De Bacquer D, Pyorala K, Keil U, for the EUROASPIRE Study Group. Cardiovascular prevention guidelines in daily practice: a comparison of EUROASPIRE I, II, and III surveys in eight European countries. Lancet. 2009;373:929–40.

22. Guallar-Castillon P, Gil-Montero M, Leon-Munos LM, Graciani A, Bayan-Bravo A, Taboada JM, et al. Magnitude and management of hypercholesterolemia in the adult population of Spain, 2008–2010: the ENRICA Study. Rev Esp Cardiol. 2012;65(6):551–8.
23. Süleymanlar G, Utaş C, Arinsoy T, Ateş K, Altun B, Altiparmak MR, et al. A population-based survey of chronic renal disease in Turkey—the CREDIT study. Nephrol Dial Transplant. 2011;26:1862–71.
24. Foley RN, Parfrey PS, Sarnak MJ. Clinical epidemiology of cardiovascular disease in chronic renal disease. Am J Kidney Dis. 1998;32:S112–9.
25. Coresh J, Longenecker JC, Miller III ER, Young HJ, Klag MJ. Epidemiology of cardiovascular risk factors in chronic renal disease. J Am Soc Nephrol. 1998;9:S24–30.
26. Muntner P, He J, Astor BC, Folsom AR, Coresh J. Traditional and nontraditional risk factors predict coronary heart disease in chronic kidney disease: results from the Atherosclerosis Risk in Communities Study. J Am Soc Nephrol. 2005;16:529–38.
27. Lowrie EG, Lew NL. Death risk in hemodialysis patients: the predictive value of commonly measured variables and an evaluation of death rate differences between facilities. Am J Kidney Dis. 1990;15:458–82.
28. Iseki K, Yamazato M, Tozawa M, Takishita S. Hypocholesterolemia is a significant predictor of death in a cohort of chronic dialysis patients. Kidney Int. 2002;61:1887–93.
29. Kalantar-Zadeh K, Block G, Humphreys MH, Kopple JD. Reverse epidemiology of cardiovascular risk factors in maintenance dialysis patients. Kidney Int. 2003;63:793–808.
30. Liu Y, Coresh J, Eustace JA, Longenecker JC, Jaar B, Fink NE, et al. Association between cholesterol level and mortality in dialysis patients: role of inflammation and malnutrition. JAMA. 2004;291:451–9.
31. Manttari M, Tiula E, Alikoski T, Manninen V. Effects of hypertension and dyslipidemia on the decline in renal function. Hypertension. 1995;26:670–5.
32. Schaeffner ES, Kurth T, Curhan GC, Glynn RJ, Rexrode KM, Baigent C, et al. Cholesterol and the risk of renal dysfunction in apparently healthy men. J Am Soc Nephrol. 2003; 14:2084–91.
33. Harper CR, Jacobson TA. Managing dyslipidemia in chronic kidney disease. J Am Coll Cardiol. 2008;51:2375–84.
34. Bagdade J, Casaretto A, Albers J. Effects of chronic uremia, hemodialysis, and renal transplantation on plasma lipids and lipoproteins in man. J Lab Clin Med. 1976;87:38–48.
35. Vaziri ND, Deng G, Liang K. Hepatic HDL receptor, SR-B1 and Apo A-I expression in chronic renal failure. Nephrol Dial Transplant. 1999;14:1462–6.
36. Vaziri ND, Moradi H. Mechanisms of dyslipidemia of chronic renal failure. Hemodial Int. 2006;10:1–7.
37. Aakhus S, Dahl K, Wideroe TE. Hyperlipidemia in renal transplant recipients. J Intern Med. 1996;239:407–15.
38. Moore R, Thomas D, Morgan E, Wheeler D, Griffin P, Salaman J, et al. Abnormal lipid and lipoprotein profiles following renal transplantation. Transplant Proc. 1993;25:1060–1.
39. Gonyea JE, Anderson CF. Weight change and serum lipoproteins in recipients of renal allografts. Mayo Clin Proc. 1992;67:653–7.
40. Soylemezoglu O, Duzova A, Yalcinkaya F, Arinsoy T, Süleymanlar G. Chronic renal disease in children aged 5–18 years: a population-based survey in Turkey, the CREDIT-D study. Nephrol Dial Transplant. 2012;27 Suppl 3:iii146–iii51.
41. Sandhu S, Wiebe N, Fried LF, Tonelli M. Statins for improving renal outcomes: a meta-analysis. J Am Soc Nephrol. 2006;17:2006–16.
42. Strippoli GFM, Navaneethan SD, Johnson DW, Perkovic V, Pellegrini F, Nicolucci A, et al. Effects of statins in patients with chronic kidney disease: meta-analysis and meta-regression of randomized controlled trials. BMJ. 2008;336:645–51.
43. Wanner C, Krane V, Marz W, Olschewski M, Mann JF, Ruf G, et al. Atorvastatin in patients with type 2 diabetes mellitus undergoing hemodialysis. N Engl J Med. 2005;353:238–48.

44. Fellstrom BC, Jardine AG, Schmieder RE, Holdaas H, Bannister K, Beutler J, et al. Rosuvastatin and cardiovascular events in patients undergoing hemodialysis. N Engl J Med. 2009;360:1395–407.
45. Baigent C, Landray MJ, Reith C, Emberson J, Wheeler DC, Tomson C, et al. The effects of lowering LDL cholesterol with simvastatin plus ezetimibe in patients with chronic kidney disease (Study of Heart and Renal Protection): a randomised placebo-controlled trial. Lancet. 2011;377:2181–92.

Chapter 2
Lipid Nephrotoxicity: New Concept for an Old Disease

Xiong Zhong Ruan, Zac Varghese, and John Moorhead

Introduction

In 1982 Moorhead and colleagues published the "Lipid Nephrotoxicity Hypothesis" in Lancet [1], which stimulated lipid studies in the context of kidney diseases. This chapter was the first to introduce the concept that the compensatory hepatic synthesis of lipoproteins in response to urinary loss of albumin could cause progressive kidney disease and that pathogenesis of atherosclerosis and renal injury and glomerulosclerosis could have a common pathway. In this "two-hit" model, the original disease could coexist or be replaced by lipid-mediated damage. Persistent albuminuria stimulates excess lipoprotein synthesis by the liver, thereby maintaining the lipid injury cycle. It also proposed that many of the features of progressive glomerular and tubulo-interstitial diseases share biological mechanisms with those of atherosclerosis, including dyslipidemia, oxidative stress, inflammatory stress, and genetic factors. The term glomerular atherosclerosis was proposed. Lipid-loaded cells derived from macrophages and mesangial cells (MCs), which share many properties of vascular smooth muscle cells (VSMCs) and take up both unaltered and altered LDL cholesterol, should be considered in the context of lipid-mediated vascular and renal injury. Against this background, it is not surprising that cardiovascular disease (CVD) is the most important cause of morbidity and mortality at all stages of progressive kidney disease and that chronic kidney disease (CKD) is now considered as a risk factor for CVD.

Since then, many laboratory and clinical studies [1, 2] have supported the hypothesis that hyperlipidemia resulting from compensatory hepatic synthesis of lipoproteins in response to urinary loss of albumin contributed to the progression of both atherosclerosis and glomerulosclerosis. However, kidney injury does not always

X.Z. Ruan, Ph.D., M.D. (✉) • Z. Varghese, Ph.D., F.R.C.P.
J. Moorhead, M.B.Ch.B., F.R.C.P.
Centre for Nephrology, University College London Medical School,
Royal Free Campus, London, UK
e-mail: x.ruan@ucl.ac.uk; zacvarghese@aol.com; jfmoorhead@gmail.com

A. Covic et al. (eds.), *Dyslipidemias in Kidney Disease*, DOI 10.1007/978-1-4939-0515-7_2

occur in the presence of hyperlipidemia alone; for example, the higher risk of cardiovascular death in dialysis individuals is associated with low plasma cholesterol (reverse epidemiology), suggesting that multiple factors accompanying with CKD may interfere lipid-mediated kidney injury. In this chapter, we will discuss the promises and exceptions to the original hypothesis, updating the lipid nephrotoxicity hypothesis by analyzing dyslipidemia of CKD, the renal pathophysiological changes induced by dyslipidemia, recent developments of and some apparent exceptions to the hypothesis, and how inflammatory stress alters lipid homeostasis.

Original Lipid Nephrotoxicity Hypothesis: Promises and Exceptions

Intensive laboratory studies have demonstrated that dyslipidemia in CKD can be both consequence [3] and cause [1] of the progression of CKD and CVD, a disease spectrum offering a substantial study platform for the original hypothesis. Although many studies support the hypothesis that lipid abnormalities contribute to renal injury, the latter does not occur in the presence of hyperlipidemia alone [4]. For example, the Watanabe heritable hyperlipidemic (WHHL) rabbit model, which is characterized by a deficiency of low-density lipoprotein (LDL) receptors and hypercholesterolemia, develops atherosclerosis but not renal lesions [5]. There is also no evidence of kidney disease in the hypercholesterolemic Nagase analbuminemic rat model [6]. In humans familial hypercholesterolemia is not usually associated with renal failure, and kidney disease rarely occurs in patients with primary hyperlipidemias [7]. In contrast normolipidemic patients with kidney disease often develop both glomerulosclerosis and atherosclerosis [8, 9]. Interestingly, while atherosclerosis regresses with reduction of serum cholesterol, human kidney disease does not. In other words, the plasma level of cholesterol per se does not correlate with glomerulosclerosis.

Since renal injury does not always occur in the presence of hyperlipidemia alone [4], and glomerulosclerosis can occur without lipid deposition, a precursor condition such as intra-renal hypertension, increased glomerular capillary shear stress, hyperfiltration, decreased nephron mass, or inflammatory stress appears to be required for the induction and progression of lipid-induced renal dysfunction.

Atherogenic Dyslipidemia in CKD: Enhanced Disease Progression

The lipid profile of CKD patients is typified by high circulating levels of very low-density lipoprotein (VLDL) triglycerides, intermediate-density lipoprotein (IDL) and chylomicron remnants (CM), and low plasma high-density lipoprotein (HDL) cholesterol. Reduced clearance and increased plasma levels of small dense LDL particles aid easier entrance into arterial walls where faster oxidation causes renal and vascular damage [10]. The LDL cholesterol level is not usually increased and may even be reduced. A higher risk of death from CVD is associated with low plasma cholesterol (reverse epidemiology) [8, 11]. In addition to causing quantitative reductions in HDL cholesterol and apoA-1 concentrations, CKD results in deficiency of HDL-associated enzymes (paraoxonase, glutathione peroxidase, and lecithin:cholesterol acyltransferase (LCAT)) and conversion of HDL from an antioxidant/anti-inflammatory agent to a prooxidant and pro-inflammatory agent [12, 13]. These abnormalities can compound the effects of HDL deficiency in promoting an atherogenic diathesis in this population. Lp(a), and apolipoprotein (apo)A-IV are also increased. This lipid profile is similar to the atherogenic dyslipidemia of diabetics, and may sometimes be observed in early stages of primary kidney disease when measured glomerular filtration rate (GFR) is normal [14].

Renal Injury

It has long been established that cholesterol supplementation of the diets of several animal species leads to focal and segmental glomerulosclerosis (FSGS). French et al. showed that feeding guinea pigs a diet containing 1 % cholesterol caused severe glomerular disease [15, 16]. Peric-Golia et al. have demonstrated that feeding normal male Sprague–Dawley rats with a 3–4 % cholesterol diet resulted in hypercholesterolemia accompanied by aortic damage and renal glomerular abnormalities including lipid droplets, hyalinosis, glomerulosclerosis, and interstitial fibrosis [17, 18]. The severity of glomerular injury is greatly increased if dietary-induced hyperlipidemia is combined with either a loss of functioning nephrons, partial nephrectomy, or hypertension [18, 20]. Rats that had a unilateral nephrectomy at 1 month that were fed a diet consisting of 4 % cholesterol developed significantly higher glomerular scarring than cholesterol-fed rats with two kidneys. Chronic renal failure induced by 5/6 nephrectomy results in accumulation of lipids in the remnant kidney, which is associated with upregulation of receptors involved in the influx of oxidized lipids and lipoproteins, activation of fatty acid biosynthesis, and inhibition of pathways involved in fatty acid oxidation [19]. Studies using the puromycin amino nucleoside (PAN) nephrotic rat model have also shown that cholesterol feeding increases the severity of proteinuria and FSGS [18, 20]. Apo B and apo E were encountered in increased amounts in the mesangium and co-localized with Oil Red O-positive lipid deposits [21]. Animals with endogenous hyperlipidemia [22] also develop progressive glomerular damage. Such models include the hyperlipidemic Sprague–Dawley rat developed by Imai et al. [23], the spontaneously hypertensive rat described by Koletsky [24], and the obese Zucker rat [22]. Glomerular injury is also greater when systemic hypertension is combined with hyperlipidemia [25].

Several clinical studies have documented an association between dyslipidemia and the progression of CKD. Atherosclerosis risk in communities (ARIC) [26] with low HDL cholesterol and increased non-HDL cholesterol was associated with increased risk of developing a reduced GFR (≤55 mL/min/1.73 m^2). In the ARIC study, higher HDL cholesterol levels were associated with a decreased risk of progression of CKD, although one study showed an association between high LDL cholesterol levels and progression of kidney disease [27]. The weight of evidence, therefore, suggests that hypertriglyceridemia, accumulation of LDL cholesterol and low HDL cholesterol are associated with increased risk of progression of CKD. Survival statistics in renal transplant patients have also demonstrated that survival with declining renal function is far superior in patients with normalized lipid profiles [28, 29].

Foam cells and lipid deposits are found in FSGS in human renal biopsies [30]. Patients with hereditary LCAT enzyme deficiency are unable to esterify cholesterol normally, and their abnormally large lipid-laden HDL has a defective maturation pattern. In these individuals, lipid deposition in the glomerulus is associated with progressive renal insufficiency. Some patients with hepatorenal syndrome who have lipoproteins with abnormal compositions have been reported to have progressive glomerular damage. A unique form of the nephrotic syndrome was reported in Japanese patients, where mesangial proliferation, mesangial expansion, glomerular deposition of lipoproteins, and FSGS were associated with high levels of circulating apoE [31]. Lee et al. found that 8.4 % of 631 CKD patients had ultrastructurally detectable extracellular lipid in non-sclerotic glomeruli, which suggests that there may be an early pre-sclerotic stage of lipoprotein-mediated damage [30]. Takemura also demonstrated that predominant deposition of apo B and apo E in the mesangial area in mesangial proliferative types of glomerulonephritis and that the distribution and staining intensity of these apolipoproteins correlated with the grade of mesangial proliferation and proteinuria, but were independent of plasma lipid levels [32].

Vascular Injury

The term glomerular atherosclerosis was proposed, because atherosclerosis shares similar pathogenesis with glomerular sclerosis. CVD risk is increased in chronic inflammatory states, up to 33-fold in patients with renal failure and allografts compared to non-uremic subjects. Patients with an "inflammation profile" including CKD, SLE, rheumatoid arthritis, psoriasis, and diabetes are especially prone to this problem. On the face of it, these data could suggest that a relatively normal cholesterol level in inflammatory conditions argues against a causative connection with cardiovascular mortality, which may explain why the phenomenon is often ignored by the atherosclerosis research community. The explanation for this may lie in the fact that the clinical setting responsible for previously "hidden" mechanisms of lipid-mediated vascular damage and cytotoxicity is more complex in CKD than in the general population; the question one should ask is why cholesterol levels are relatively normal or low under inflammatory stress?

Renal Pathophysiological Changes Driven by Atherogenic Dyslipidemia

Lipid-loaded foam cells in the kidney and atherosclerotic plaques support pathophysiological roles for lipids in the progression of both CKD and CVD.

Oxidative Stress

Though initial events involved in lipid-mediated renal damage are unclear, oxidative stress is thought to be especially important. Hyperlipidemia causes significantly higher rates of monocyte reactive oxygen species (ROS) generation, which is strongly associated with impairment of endothelium-dependent relaxation and elevated plasma levels of Ox-LDL. Arteries from hypercholesterolemic animals produced significantly higher rates of oxygen radical than control arteries.

The mechanisms by which hyperlipidemia contributes to systemic oxidative stress in CKD remain unclear. Plasma HDL-cholesterol with its important antioxidant function is reduced in CKD [33]. Inflammatory mediators, including TNFα and IL-1β, are ROS-activating factors in the kidney and may induce oxygen radical production by MCs. Immune-mediated mesangial injury causes increased oxygen radical and eicosanoid production [34]. An important source of ROS is NAD(P)H-oxidase (NOX). The NOX family comprises seven members, Nox1–Nox7. Nox1 and Nox2 (gp91phox-containing NADPH oxidase), together with Nox4 and Nox5, have been identified in the cardiovascular–renal systems and have been implicated in oxidative stress [35] in kidney disease. In addition, the leukocyte-derived enzymes myeloperoxidase (MPO) and xanthine oxidoreductase (XOR) may contribute to oxidative stress pathways in end-stage renal disease (ESRD) with a role in cardiovascular dysfunction [36, 37].

Inappropriate ROS generation may contribute to tissue dysfunction in three ways: (1) dysregulation of redox-sensitive signalling pathways; (2) oxidative damage to biological structures including DNA, proteins, and lipids; and (3) activation of macrophages [38]. Lipid peroxidation is the first step in the generation of Ox-LDL, which can accumulate in renal mesangial cells [39]. The process of lipid peroxidation itself generates free radicals and ROS.

The cytotoxic effects of Ox-LDL, produced in vitro by incubating LDL with $CuSO_4$ include induction of podocyte [40] and endothelial cells apoptosis, which may influence cellular turnover in vascular and renal injuries. All major cell types in the artery wall and kidney, including endothelial cells, SMCs, monocyte–macrophages, and MCs, have been shown to cause oxidative modification of LDL in vitro [41, 42]. Oxidative stress decreases renal NO production and availability [43] and stimulates angiotensin II synthesis, suggesting that activation of the renin-angiotensin system (RAS) may contribute to lipid-induced renal injury. It has been demonstrated that angiotensin II increases TGF-β and plasminogen activator inhibitor-1 (PAI-1) expression, thereby propagating glomerular fibrosis [44]. Oxidized LDL has also been identified in the lesions of FSGS in vivo [45].

Endoplasmic Reticulum Stress

Metabolic stress within the endoplasmic reticulum (ER) induces a coordinated unfolded protein response (UPR), which helps the ER to cope with the accumulation of misfolded proteins. UPR is initiated by three ER transmembrane proteins (namely, PKR-like ER-regulated kinase (PERK), inositol-requiring enzyme-1 (IRE-1), and activating transcription factor-6 (ATF-6)) [46]. Recent studies report that intracellular accumulation of saturated fatty acids and cholesterol results in ER stress, resulting in apoptosis in macrophages; macrophage scavenger receptor type A is essential in regulating ER stress-induced apoptosis [47]. Palmitate also induces ER stress by increasing IRE1 protein levels and activating the c-Jun NH_2-terminal kinase (JNK) pathway [48]. In both cultured cells and whole animals, ER stress leads to activation of the JNK and IKK/NFkB pathways, promoting an inflammatory response. ER stress, in turn, leads to dysregulation of the endogenous sterol response mechanism and concordantly activates oxidative stress pathways [49].

Inflammatory Stress

The presence of oxidative and ER stress activates the NF-κB pathway, which has been associated with inflammatory events in glomerulonephritis, as well the progression of CKD [50]. In addition, lipids may act as pro-inflammatory mediators. At certain concentrations LDL, VLDL, and IDL enhanced the secretion of inflammatory cytokines by MCs, including IL-6, PDGF, and TGFβ. Since HDL down-regulates VCAM-1 and E-selectin on endothelial surfaces and reduces NFκB, low HDL cholesterol levels may augment inflammatory responses [51]. In apoE KO mice [52], blocking the IL-6 receptor prevented progression of proteinuria and renal lipid deposition, as well as the mesangial cell proliferation associated with severe hyperlipoproteinemia. These results strongly support the role of pro-inflammatory cytokines in the pathogenesis of hyperlipidemia-induced glomerular injury. Inflammation also enhances both medial and intimal calcification, which contribute to vascular, and perhaps also renal injury [53, 54].

Ox-LDL binds preferentially to the glomerulus when injected intra-arterially in the rat and to mesangial cells in vitro [55]. Ox-LDL is a potent proinflammatory chemoattractant for macrophages and T lymphocytes with a role in the recruitment of circulating monocytes either directly or by inducing SMC, MCs, and/or endothelial cells to produce chemotactic and adhesive factors such as MCP-1, monocyte colony-stimulating factor (m-CSF), and IL-1β [56, 57]. Modified LDL may also inhibit the motility of resident monocytes once they have differentiated into macrophages within the site [58]. Both oxidized LDL and minimally oxidized LDL stimulated TNF-α secretion by MCs by activating the NFκB pathway [50].

Mesangial Cell Proliferation and Matrix Expansion

MCs have been shown to bind LDL and Ox-LDL, leading to more cell proliferation via multiple downstream effects. LDL also stimulates the expression of extracellular matrix proteins including fibronectin. Furthermore, glomerular macrophages obtained from hypercholesterolemic animals displayed higher expressions of TGF-β mRNA, which contributes to glomerular matrix expansion [59].

Inflammatory Stress Modifies Lipid Homeostasis

CKD is associated with a low-grade, long-term, and chronic inflammatory stress characterized by elevated plasma CRP levels [60]. Inflammatory stress may modify lipid homeostasis, thereby causing tissue lipid accumulation [61].

Inflammation Changes Lipid Composition

Inflammation alters HDL structure and removes its anti-inflammatory functionality. HDL levels are decreased in inflamed individuals without renal failure, and SAA replaces the apo A-I that normally composes about half of the proteins in HDL [36]. The resulting loss of HDL's protective ability during inflammatory stress renders LDL prone to oxidation from increased activity of MPO, an abundantly expressed enzyme of activated neutrophils that chlorinates a tyrosine residue on apo B100 [62]. Inflammation could be responsible for an increase in triglyceride levels in CKD [63]. Ettinger showed that human recombinant TNF-α, IL-1β, and IL-6 resulted in dose-related reductions in the concentrations of apoA-I, apoB, and LCAT activity in HepG2 cells, which may contribute to the hypocholesterolemia of acute inflammation.

Inflammation Causes Cholesterol Redistribution

Recently, kinetic analysis of TG fractional catabolic rates (FCR) and production rates (PR) demonstrated that CKD is associated with decreased clearance of TG-rich lipoproteins without change in synthesis. However, catabolism of LDL cholesterol is increased significantly [64], suggesting that both cholesterol production and degradation are modified in CKD. LDL is the major carrier of cholesterol in humans and plays a more important role than other lipids in forming foam cells. However, the plasma LDL cholesterol level is not increased in CKD and hemodialysis patients and the relationship between cardiovascular mortality and plasma cholesterol levels is reversed [8]. In this section, we will focus on recently observed connections between inflammatory stress, cholesterol homeostasis, and renal injury.

In a retrospective study of nephrotic patients with progressive kidney disease, heavy proteinuria and hypercholesterolemia accompanied kidney disease progression, but plasma cholesterol gradually fell to normal levels as patients approached ESRD [65]. Recently, Liu et al. evaluated the association between plasma cholesterol levels and mortality in 823 dialysis patients from 79 clinics in the United States. They divided the patients into inflamed and non-inflamed on the basis of inflammation markers (CRP and IL-6). The non-inflamed dialysis patients showed a linear relationship between cholesterol levels and mortality and behaved like the normal population in that higher cholesterol was associated with higher mortality. In contrast the higher mortality in inflamed dialysis patients was inversely associated with lower cholesterol levels (J-shaped curve) [8], suggesting that inflammation may divert plasma cholesterol to the tissue compartments, increasing cardiovascular mortality.

We have demonstrated that inflammatory cytokine IL-1β increases intracellular cholesterol influx into VSMCs, MCs, and macrophages by inducing scavenger receptor expression, disrupting LDL receptor feedback regulation and causing unrestrained LDL receptor-mediated uptake [39, 66, 67]. Pro-inflammatory cytokine IL-1β also inhibits ATP-binding cassette A1 (ABCA1)-mediated cholesterol efflux from mesangial cells [68]. Furthermore, in vitro studies have shown that IL-1β increases intracellular cholesterol synthesis in MCs, HepG2 [69], and VSMCs by increasing HMG-CoA reductase transcription and activity, thereby enhancing inflammation-mediated intracellular cholesterol synthesis and inhibiting HMG-CoA reductase degradation. In vivo, chronic systemic inflammation induced by 10 % subcutaneous casein in apoE KO mice and characterized by increased serum SAA and TNF-α, lowered plasma LDL cholesterol and HDL cholesterol levels, and enhanced lipid accumulation in the liver, vessels, and kidneys, promoting nonalcoholic fatty liver disease (NAFLD), atherosclerosis, and renal injury [70]. However, cholesterol biosynthesis and fatty acid oxidation were reported to be reduced in a remnant rat kidney model [19, 71]. The possible reasons for the differences are that inflammatory stress may differ between nephrectomy rat models (unilateral and 5/6th) and systemic casein-induced inflammatory stress in a mouse model. The nephrectomy rat model is characterized by heavy proteinuria, marked elevation of plasma total cholesterol, LDL cholesterol, triglyceride, and free fatty acid concentrations. While suitable for the investigation of renal pathophysiological changes, this model does not adequately mirror lipid homeostasis in CKD patients whose LDL cholesterol level is not increased; nor is the casein-induced systemic inflammatory stress model affected by uremia-related factors. These points reinforce views that across-species cholesterol homeostasis may be differently regulated according to the type and stage of kidney disease as well as variations in inflammatory stress. HMG-CoA reductase-mediated cholesterol synthesis in kidney may be decreased in the CRF nephrectomy rat model but increased in the presence of serious inflammatory stress or in the early stages of CKD.

Zhao et al., using a unilateral nephrectomy model, showed adipose tissue redistribution to kidney from the peri-renal capsule, omentum, mesentery, and abdominal wall, suggesting that lipid redistribution may also take place between tissues [72, 73]. Furthermore, we and others have shown that inflammatory stress causes cholesterol accumulation in the normally cholesterol-poor ER, indicating that cholesterol redistribution can occur intracellularly between organelles. Cholesterol relocation at this level could potentially trigger lipid-induced apoptosis or ER stress [74].

Hence, inflammatory stress accompanied by CKD modifies cholesterol homeostasis by diverting cholesterol from blood to tissues, which causes cholesterol to accumulate in peripheral tissues such as kidney, vessel wall, and liver, lowering circulating cholesterol levels. Tissue cholesterol redistribution and accumulation in response to inflammation may occur at several levels and sites: from circulation to tissue, tissue to tissue, and organelle to organelle. Therefore, plasma LDL cholesterol in patients with CKD may be a poor marker of the risk of lipid-mediated vascular or renal injury and unhelpful or even misleading in the evaluation of the clinical efficacy of lipid-lowering drugs.

The Impact of Statins on CKD

Statins have revolutionized the treatment of high plasma cholesterol and atherosclerosis, confirming their benefits in vascular disease [75]. They are effective in correcting dyslipidemia and are relatively safe [76]. Statin prescription is now common in patients with CKD, an approach endorsed by the recent Kidney Disease Outcomes Quality Initiative (K/DOQI) guidelines, although its value in preventing the progression of CVD and CKD is not yet clear.

Effect of Statins on Renal Protection: Evidence from CVD Trial

The majority of clinical trials in statins excluded patients with kidney disease as judged by serum creatinine (Cr), which leaves large subgroups of patients with normal Cr but abnormal estimated glomerular filtration rates (eGFR) using the modification of diet in renal disease (MDRD) calculation. A post hoc subgroup analysis of the Cholesterol and Recurrent Events trial (CARE) study [77] demonstrated that pravastatin may slow renal function loss in individuals with moderate to severe kidney disease, especially in those with proteinuria. The GREACE study, performed to evaluate the effect of atorvastatin on renal function [78], demonstrated that statin treatment prevented decline in renal dysfunction based on eGFR and potentially improved renal function, offsetting an additional factor associated with CHD risk. A pooled analysis of data demonstrated that among patients who received long-term rosuvastatin treatment (>96 weeks), eGFR was unchanged or tended to increase rather than to decrease when compared with baseline [79]. Furthermore, a post hoc subgroup analysis of data from three randomized double-blind controlled trials (LIPID, CARE, and WOSCOPS) demonstrated that pravastatin (40 mg/day) reduced the adjusted rate of kidney function loss by 34 % in patients with moderate CKD [80]. These data suggest a protective effect of statins on renal function, though the value may be limited due to the fact that the patients in these studies had preexisting cardiac disease.

Effect of Statins on Renal Protection: Evidence from CKD Trials

The first meta-analysis of 13 controlled prospective studies demonstrated a lower, though small, rate of decline in eGFR with treatment compared with controls [81]. In a second meta-analysis of 27 studies comprising 39,704 participants, 21 studies included data for eGFR and 20 for proteinuria. Overall, the change in the weighted mean differences for eGFR and reduction in proteinuria were significant in statin recipients. Both analyses, together with small prospective controlled studies [82, 83], support emerging trial evidence that treatment with statins reduces proteinuria and possibly the rate of kidney function loss. However, recently the randomized, double-blind, controlled SHARP trial involving patients with advanced CKD demonstrate no benefit on renal protection [84]. The controversy may result from various complicated conditions in CKD patients, such as the stages of the disease or presence or absence of other disorders. The types or doses of statin may also affect the renal outcome.

The Pleiotropic Effects of Statins

In addition to lowering lipids, statins may provide renal protection via pleiotropic effects. Statins act by blocking 3-hydroxy-3-methylglutaryl coenzyme A reductase, thereby inhibiting synthesis of mevalonic acid, a precursor of many nonsteroidal isoprenoid compounds such as farnesyl pyrophosphate and geranylgeranyl-pyrophosphate involved in subcellular localization and intracellular trafficking of several membrane-bound proteins involved in oxidative stress injury (Rho, Ras, Rac, Rab, Ral, and Rap). An important source of ROS is NOX. Statins inhibit the activation of Rac1, which is involved in the activation of NOX by preventing the geranylgeranyl-dependent translocation of Rac1 from the cytosol to the cell membrane thereby reducing ROS generation [85, 86]. By blocking geranylgeranylation of Rho GTPase, statins also decrease the levels of the surface protein endothelin-1, a potent vasoconstrictor and mitogen, which might play a role in retarding glomerulosclerosis [87]. Statins also prolong eNOS mRNA half-life and upregulate eNOS expression, reducing hypertension-induced glomerular injury by inhibiting the expression of Rho [88]. Statins also reduce LDL oxidation via the above mechanisms. Statins suppress receptor CD36 expression on monocytes, which may inhibit the uptake of Ox-LDL and their subsequent conversion to macrophage foam cells [89]. Furthermore, statins have been shown to reduce levels of MCP-1, TNF-α, TGF-β, IL-6, PDGF, and NFκB [89–91], and reduce the proliferation of renal tubular epithelium by impairment of activator protein-1 (Ap-1) [92] as well as by preventing monocytes from maturing into macrophages, inducing apoptosis of these cells [93].

Statin Resistance Under Inflammatory Stress

Some recent experimental evidence showed that statins in therapeutic concentrations failed to prevent cholesterol synthesis in these cells under inflammatory stress, causing statin resistance [69]. The recent TNT study suggests a dose-related effect of atorvastatin on GFR, with 80 mg/day eliciting a greater beneficial effect than 10 mg/day [94]. This raises the possibility that a variable response to statins may be due to statin resistance in some patients, which higher statin doses and anti-inflammatory treatments might overcome. A further point requiring investigation is the presently unknown ability of statins to reduce apo B concentrations in many clinical trials of CKD patients. Peripheral statin resistance might partly explain why statins at ordinary doses did not reduce cardiovascular events or contributed to the residual risk in large randomized trials (4D and AURORA) in dialysis patients [95, 96].

How Long a Low LDL Cholesterol Status Should be Maintained?

It seems that duration for cholesterol lowering is a very important issue. Recently, it has been demonstrated that lifelong history of reduced LDL cholesterol in patients with PCSK9 mutation was associated with a 28 % reduction in mean LDL cholesterol and an 88 % reduction in the risk of CHD [97, 98], compared to only 40 % reduction normally observed in most of the clinical trials completed in 5 years. These data indicate that moderate lifelong reduction in the plasma level of LDL cholesterol is associated with a substantial reduction in the incidence of coronary events, even in populations with a high prevalence of non-lipid-related cardiovascular risk factors. It may imply that long-term use of lipid-lowering treatment may be important, especially for the patients with chronic inflammatory stress, such as CKD or dialysis.

Conclusion

Clinical and experimental evidence suggest that dyslipidemia promotes progression of CKD by activating inflammatory, oxidative, and ER stress. Inflammation also fundamentally modifies lipid homeostasis by diverting cholesterol from plasma to tissue compartments. Thus, the level of circulating cholesterol is not on its own a reliable predictor of cardiovascular and renal risks in patients with inflammatory stress. Therefore, we suggest that in kidney disease emphasis should be placed on the role of inflammatory cytokines on cholesterol redistribution together with plasma cholesterol levels or hypercholesterolemia. Increased understanding of the pathogenesis of lipid-mediated renal and vascular injury will encourage a search for reliable methods of risk assessment in at-risk patients in whom higher doses of statins for longer periods, carefully monitored for side effects on liver, muscle, and myocardium, may be required to prevent lipid-mediated renal and vascular injury.

References

1. Moorhead JF, Chan MK, El-Nahas M, Varghese Z. Lipid nephrotoxicity in chronic progressive glomerular and tubulo-interstitial disease. Lancet. 1982;2:1309–11.
2. Grone HJ, Walli A, Grone E, Niedmann P, Thiery J, Seidel D, Helmchen U. Induction of glomerulosclerosis by dietary lipids. A functional and morphologic study in the rat. Lab Invest. 1989;60:433–46.
3. Chan MK, Varghese Z, Moorhead JF. Lipid abnormalities in uremia, dialysis and transplantation. Kidney Int. 1981;19:625–37.
4. Ruan XZ, Varghese Z, Moorhead JF. Inflammation modifies lipid-mediated renal injury. Nephrol Dial Transplant. 2003;18:27–32.
5. Keane WF, Kasiske BL, O'Donnell MP, Kim Y. The role of altered lipid metabolism in the progression of renal disease: experimental evidence. Am J Kidney Dis. 1991;17:38–42.
6. Zatz R, Prado EBA, Prado MJBA, Santos MM, Fujihara CK. Aging analbuminemic rats fail to develop focal glomerulosclerosis. Kidney Int. 1989;35:442A (Abstr.).
7. McIntyre N. Familial LCAT deficiency and fish-eye disease. J Inherit Metab Dis. 1988;11 Suppl 1:45–56.
8. Liu Y, Coresh J, Eustace JA, Longenecker JC, Jaar B, Fink NE, Tracy RP, et al. Association between cholesterol level and mortality in dialysis patients: role of inflammation and malnutrition. JAMA. 2004;291:451–9.
9. Tracy RE. Blood pressure related separately to parenchymal fibrosis and vasculopathy of the kidney. Am J Kidney Dis. 1992;20:124–31.
10. Berneis KK, Krauss RM. Metabolic origins and clinical significance of LDL heterogeneity. J Lipid Res. 2002;43:1363–79.
11. Lowrie EG, Lew NL. Death risk in hemodialysis patients: the predictive value of commonly measured variables and an evaluation of death rate differences between facilities. Am J Kidney Dis. 1990;15:458–82.
12. Moradi H, Pahl MV, Elahimehr R, Vaziri ND. Impaired antioxidant activity of high-density lipoprotein in chronic kidney disease. Transl Res. 2009;153:77–85.
13. Vaziri ND, Moradi H, Pahl MV, Fogelman AM, Navab M. In vitro stimulation of HDL anti-inflammatory activity and inhibition of LDL pro-inflammatory activity in the plasma of patients with end-stage renal disease by an apoA-1 mimetic peptide. Kidney Int. 2009; 76:437–44.

14. Wanner C, Ritz E. Reducing lipids for CV protection in CKD patients-current evidence. Kidney Int. 2008;74 Suppl 111:S24–8.
15. French SW, Yamanaka W, Ostwald R. Dietary induced glomerulosclerosis in the guinea pig. Arch Pathol. 1967;83:204–10.
16. Brenner BM. Nephron adaptation to renal injury or ablation. Am J Physiol. 1985;249: F324–37.
17. Peric-Golia L, Peric-Golia M. Aortic and renal lesions in hypercholesterolemic adult, male, virgin Sprague–Dawley rats. Atherosclerosis. 1983;46:57–65.
18. Kasiske BL, O'Donnell MP, Schmitz PG, Kim Y, Keane WF. Renal injury of diet-induced hypercholesterolemia in rats. Kidney Int. 1990;37:880–91.
19. Kim HJ, Moradi H, Yuan J, Norris K, Vaziri ND. Renal mass reduction results in accumulation of lipids and dysregulation of lipid regulatory proteins in the remnant kidney. Am J Physiol Renal Physiol. 2009;296:F1297–306.
20. Lee HS, Jeong JY, Kim BC, Kim YS, Zhang YZ, Chung HK. Dietary antioxidant inhibits lipoprotein oxidation and renal injury in experimental focal segmental glomerulosclerosis. Kidney Int. 1997;51:1151–9.
21. van Goor H, van der Horst ML, Atmosoerodjo J, Joles JA, van Tol A, Grond J. Renal apolipoproteins in nephrotic rats. Am J Pathol. 1993;142:1804–12.
22. Kasiske BL, Cleary MP, O'Donnell MP, Keane WF. Effects of genetic obesity on renal structure and function in the Zucker rat. J Lab Clin Med. 1985;106:598–604.
23. Imai Y, Matsumura H, Miyajami H, Oka K. Serum and tissue lipids and glomerulosclerosis in the spontaneously hypercholesterolemic (SHC) rat, with a note on the effects of gonadectomy. Atherosclerosis. 1977;27:165–78.
24. Koletsky S. Pathologic findings and laboratory data in a new strain of obese hypertensive rats. Am J Pathol. 1975;80:129–42.
25. Grone HJ, Walli AK, Grone EF. Arterial hypertension and hyperlipidemia as determinants of glomerulosclerosis. Clin Investig. 1993;71:834–9.
26. Muntner P, Coresh J, Smith JC, Eckfeldt J, Klag MJ. Plasma lipids and risk of developing renal dysfunction: the atherosclerosis risk in communities study. Kidney Int. 2000;58:293–301.
27. Samuelsson O, Attman PO, Knight-Gibson C, Larsson R, Mulec H, Weiss L, Alaupovic P. Complex apolipoprotein B-containing lipoprotein particles are associated with a higher rate of progression of human chronic renal insufficiency. J Am Soc Nephrol. 1998;9:1482–8.
28. Pascual M, Theruvath T, Kawai T, Tolkoff-Rubin N, Cosimi AB. Strategies to improve long-term outcomes after renal transplantation. N Engl J Med. 2002;346:580–90.
29. Kobashigawa JA, Kasiske BL. Hyperlipidemia in solid organ transplantation. Transplantation. 1997;63:331–8.
30. Lee HS, Lee JS, Koh HI, Ko KW. Intraglomerular lipid deposition in routine biopsies. Clin Nephrol. 1991;36:67–75.
31. Koitabashi Y, Ikoma M, Miyahira T, Fujita R, Mio H, Ishida M, Shimizu K, et al. Long-term follow-up of a paediatric case of lipoprotein glomerulopathy. Pediatr Nephrol. 1990;4:122–8.
32. Takemura T, Yoshioka K, Aya N, Murakami K, Matumoto A, Itakura H, Kodama T, et al. Apolipoproteins and lipoprotein receptors in glomeruli in human kidney diseases. Kidney Int. 1993;43:918–27.
33. Vaziri ND. Causal link between oxidative stress, inflammation, and hypertension. Iran J Kidney Dis. 2008;2:1–10.
34. Oberle GP, Niemeyer J, Thaiss F, Schoeppe W, Stahl RA. Increased oxygen radical and eicosanoid formation in immune-mediated mesangial cell injury. Kidney Int. 1992;42:69–74.
35. Sedeek M, Hebert RL, Kennedy CR, Burns KD, Touyz RM. Molecular mechanisms of hypertension: role of Nox family NADPH oxidases. Curr Opin Nephrol Hypertens. 2009; 18:122–7.
36. Kaysen GA, Eiserich JP. The role of oxidative stress-altered lipoprotein structure and function and microinflammation on cardiovascular risk in patients with minor renal dysfunction. J Am Soc Nephrol. 2004;15:538–48.

37. Suzuki I, Yamauchi T, Onuma M, Nozaki S. Allopurinol, an inhibitor of uric acid synthesis—can it be used for the treatment of metabolic syndrome and related disorders? Drugs Today (Barc). 2009;45:363–8.
38. Gavras I, Gavras H. Angiotensin II as a cardiovascular risk factor. J Hum Hypertens. 2002;16 Suppl 2:S2–6.
39. Ruan XZ, Varghese Z, Powis SH, Moorhead JF. Human mesangial cells express inducible macrophage scavenger receptor. Kidney Int. 1999;56:440–51.
40. Bussolati B, Deregibus MC, Fonsato V, Doublier S, Spatola T, Procida S, Di CF, et al. Statins prevent oxidized LDL-induced injury of glomerular podocytes by activating the phosphatidylinositol 3-kinase/AKT-signaling pathway. J Am Soc Nephrol. 2005;16:1936–47.
41. Fernando RL, Varghese Z, Moorhead JF. Oxidation of low-density lipoproteins by rat mesangial cells and the interaction of oxidized low-density lipoproteins with rat mesangial cells in vitro. Nephrol Dial Transplant. 1993;8:512–8.
42. Heinecke JW, Baker L, Rosen H, Chait A. Superoxide-mediated oxidation of low density lipoprotein by arterial smooth muscle cells. J Clin Invest. 1986;77:757–61.
43. Rahman MM, Varghese Z, Fuller BJ, Moorhead JF. Renal vasoconstriction induced by oxidized LDL is inhibited by scavengers of reactive oxygen species and L-arginine. Clin Nephrol. 1999;51:98–107.
44. Chalmers L, Kaskel FJ, Bamgbola O. The role of obesity and its bioclinical correlates in the progression of chronic kidney disease. Adv Chronic Kidney Dis. 2006;13:352–64.
45. Lee HS. Oxidized LDL, glomerular mesangial cells and collagen. Diabetes Res Clin Pract. 1999;45:117–22.
46. Ron D, Walter P. Signal integration in the endoplasmic reticulum unfolded protein response. Nat Rev Mol Cell Biol. 2007;8:519–29.
47. Tabas I. Consequences of cellular cholesterol accumulation: basic concepts and physiological implications. J Clin Invest. 2002;110:905–11.
48. Bachar E, Ariav Y, Ketzinel-Gilad M, Cerasi E, Kaiser N, Leibowitz G. Glucose amplifies fatty acid-induced endoplasmic reticulum stress in pancreatic beta-cells via activation of mTORC1. PLoS One. 2009;4:e4954.
49. Kovacs WJ, Tape KN, Shackelford JE, Wikander TM, Richards MJ, Fliesler SJ, Krisans SK, et al. Peroxisome deficiency causes a complex phenotype because of hepatic SREBP/Insig dysregulation associated with endoplasmic reticulum stress. J Biol Chem. 2009;284:7232–45.
50. Guijarro C, Egido J. Transcription factor-kappa B (NF-kappa B) and renal disease. Kidney Int. 2001;59:415–24.
51. Ashby DT, Rye KA, Clay MA, Vadas MA, Gamble JR, Barter PJ. Factors influencing the ability of HDL to inhibit expression of vascular cell adhesion molecule-1 in endothelial cells. Arterioscler Thromb Vasc Biol. 1998;18:1450–5.
52. Tomiyama-Hanayama M, Rakugi H, Kohara M, Mima T, Adachi Y, Ohishi M, Katsuya T, et al. Effect of interleukin-6 receptor blockage on renal injury in apolipoprotein e-deficient mice. Am J Physiol Renal Physiol. 2009;297(3):F679–84.
53. Moe SM, Chen NX. Inflammation and vascular calcification. Blood Purif. 2005;23:64–71.
54. Al-Aly Z. Vascular calcification in uremia: what is new and where are we going? Adv Chronic Kidney Dis. 2008;15:413–9.
55. Coritsidis G, Rifici V, Gupta S, Rie J, Shan ZH, Neugarten J, Schlondorff D. Preferential binding of oxidized LDL to rat glomeruli in vivo and cultured mesangial cells in vitro. Kidney Int. 1991;39:858–66.
56. Berliner JA, Territo MC, Sevanian A, Ramin S, Kim JA, Bamshad B, Esterson M, et al. Minimally modified low density lipoprotein stimulates monocyte endothelial interactions. J Clin Invest. 1990;85:1260–6.
57. Cases A, Coll E. Dyslipidemia and the progression of renal disease in chronic renal failure patients. Kidney Int Suppl. 2005;99:S87–93.

58. Quinn MT, Parthasarathy S, Fong LG, Steinberg D. Oxidatively modified low density lipoproteins: a potential role in recruitment and retention of monocyte/macrophages during atherogenesis. Proc Natl Acad Sci U S A. 1987;2995:2998.
59. Ding G, van Goor H, Frye J, Diamond JR. Transforming growth factor-beta expression in macrophages during hypercholesterolemic states. Am J Physiol. 1994;267:F937–43.
60. Landray MJ, Wheeler DC, Lip GY, Newman DJ, Blann AD, McGlynn FJ, Ball S, et al. Inflammation, endothelial dysfunction, and platelet activation in patients with chronic kidney disease: the chronic renal impairment in Birmingham (CRIB) study. Am J Kidney Dis. 2004;43:244–53.
61. Mayr M, Kiechl S, Willeit J, Wick G, Xu Q. Infections, immunity, and atherosclerosis: associations of antibodies to Chlamydia pneumoniae, Helicobacter pylori, and cytomegalovirus with immune reactions to heat-shock protein 60 and carotid or femoral atherosclerosis. Circulation. 2002;102:833–9.
62. Cockerill GW, Huehns TY, Weerasinghe A, Stocker C, Lerch PG, Miller NE, Haskard DO. Elevation of plasma high-density lipoprotein concentration reduces interleukin-1-induced expression of E-selectin in an in vivo model of acute inflammation. Circulation. 2001;103:108–12.
63. Ridker PM, Hennekens CH, Buring JE, Rifai N. C-reactive protein and other markers of inflammation in the prediction of cardiovascular disease in women. N Engl J Med. 2000;342:836–43.
64. Batista MC, Welty FK, Diffenderfer MR, Sarnak MJ, Schaefer EJ, Lamon-Fava S, Asztalos BF, et al. Apolipoprotein A-I, B-100, and B-48 metabolism in subjects with chronic kidney disease, obesity, and the metabolic syndrome. Metabolism. 2004;53:1255–61.
65. Moorhead JF, Persaud W, Varghese Z, Sweny P. Serum cholesterol falls spontaneously in nephrotic patients with progressive renal disease. Ren Fail. 1993;15:389–93.
66. Ruan XZ, Varghese Z, Powis SH, Moorhead JF. Dysregulation of LDL receptor under the influence of inflammatory cytokines: a new pathway for foam cell formation. Kidney Int. 2001;60:1716–25.
67. Ruan XZ, Moorhead JF, Tao JL, Ma KL, Wheeler DC, Powis SH, Varghese Z. Mechanisms of dysregulation of low-density lipoprotein receptor expression in vascular smooth muscle cells by inflammatory cytokines. Arterioscler Thromb Vasc Biol. 2006;26:1150–5.
68. Ruan XZ, Moorhead JF, Fernando R, Wheeler DC, Powis SH, Varghese Z. PPAR agonists protect mesangial cells from interleukin 1 beta-induced intracellular lipid accumulation by activating the ABCA1 cholesterol efflux pathway. J Am Soc Nephrol. 2003;14:593–600.
69. Chen Y, Ruan XZ, Li Q, Huang A, Moorhead JF, Powis SH, Varghese Z. Inflammatory cytokines disrupt LDL-receptor feedback regulation and cause statin resistance: a comparative study in human hepatic cells and mesangial cells. Am J Physiol Renal Physiol. 2007;293:F680–7.
70. Ma KL, Ruan XZ, Powis SH, Chen Y, Moorhead JF, Varghese Z. Inflammatory stress exacerbates lipid accumulation in hepatic cells and fatty livers of apolipoprotein E knockout mice. Hepatology. 2008;48:770–81.
71. Moradi H, Yuan J, Ni Z, Norris K, Vaziri ND. Reverse cholesterol transport pathway in experimental chronic renal failure. Am J Nephrol. 2009;30:147–54.
72. Ruan XZ, Moorhead JF, Varghese Z. Lipid redistribution in renal dysfunction. Kidney Int. 2008;74:407–9.
73. Zhao HL, Sui Y, Guan J, He L, Zhu X, Fan RR, Xu G, et al. Fat redistribution and adipocyte transformation in uninephrectomized rats. Kidney Int. 2008;74:467–77.
74. Devries-Seimon T, Li Y, Yao PM, Stone E, Wang Y, Davis RJ, Flavell R, et al. Cholesterol-induced macrophage apoptosis requires ER stress pathways and engagement of the type A scavenger receptor. J Cell Biol. 2005;171(1):61–73.
75. Cheung BM, Lauder IJ, Lau CP, Kumana CR. Meta-analysis of large randomized controlled trials to evaluate the impact of statins on cardiovascular outcomes. Br J Clin Pharmacol. 2004;57:640–51.

76. Kidney Disease Outcomes Quality Initiative (K/DOQI) Group. K/DOQI clinical practice guidelines for managing dyslipidaemias in patients with kidney disease. Am J Kidney Dis. 2003;41(4 Suppl 3):I–IV. S1–S91.
77. Tonelli M, Moye L, Sacks FM, Cole T, Curhan GC. Effect of pravastatin on loss of renal function in people with moderate chronic renal insufficiency and cardiovascular disease. J Am Soc Nephrol. 2003;14:1605–13.
78. Athyros VG, Mikhailidis DP, Papageorgiou AA, Symeonidis AN, Pehlivanidis AN, Bouloukos VI, Elisaf M. The effect of statins versus untreated dyslipidaemia on renal function in patients with coronary heart disease. A subgroup analysis of the Greek atorvastatin and coronary heart disease evaluation (GREACE) study. J Clin Pathol. 2004;57:728–34.
79. Vidt DG, Cressman MD, Harris S, Pears JS, Hutchinson HG. Rosuvastatin-induced arrest in progression of renal disease. Cardiology. 2004;102:52–60.
80. Tonelli M, Keech A, Shepherd J, Sacks F, Tonkin A, Packard C, Pfeffer M, et al. Effect of pravastatin in people with diabetes and chronic kidney disease. J Am Soc Nephrol. 2005;16:3748–54.
81. Fried LF, Orchard TJ, Kasiske BL. Effect of lipid reduction on the progression of renal disease: a meta-analysis. Kidney Int. 2001;59:260–9.
82. Bianchi S, Bigazzi R, Caiazza A, Campese VM. A controlled, prospective study of the effects of atorvastatin on proteinuria and progression of kidney disease. Am J Kidney Dis. 2003;41:565–70.
83. Lee TM, Su SF, Tsai CH. Effect of pravastatin on proteinuria in patients with well-controlled hypertension. Hypertension. 2002;40:67–73.
84. Baigent C, Landray MJ, Reith C, et al. Lancet. 2011;377:2181–92.
85. Dusi S, Donini M, Rossi F. Mechanisms of NADPH oxidase activation in human neutrophils: p67phox is required for the translocation of rac 1 but not of rac 2 from cytosol to the membranes. Biochem J. 1995;308(Pt 3):991–4.
86. Habibi J, Whaley-Connell A, Qazi MA, Hayden MR, Cooper SA, Tramontano A, Thyfault J, et al. Rosuvastatin, a 3-hydroxy-3-methylglutaryl coenzyme a reductase inhibitor, decreases cardiac oxidative stress and remodeling in Ren2 transgenic rats. Endocrinology. 2007;148:2181–8.
87. Campese VM, Shaohua Y, Huiquin Z. Oxidative stress mediates angiotensin II-dependent stimulation of sympathetic nerve activity. Hypertension. 2005;46:533–9.
88. Wolfrum S, Jensen KS, Liao JK. Endothelium-dependent effects of statins. Arterioscler Thromb Vasc Biol. 2003;23:729–36.
89. Chmielewski M, Bryl E, Marzec L, Aleksandrowicz E, Witkowski JM, Rutkowski B. Expression of scavenger receptor CD36 in chronic renal failure patients. Artif Organs. 2005;29:608–14.
90. McFarlane SI, Muniyappa R, Francisco R, Sowers JR. Clinical review 145: pleiotropic effects of statins: lipid reduction and beyond. J Clin Endocrinol Metab. 2002;87:1451–8.
91. Massy ZA, Kim Y, Guijarro C, Kasiske BL, Keane WF, O'Donnell MP. Low-density lipoprotein-induced expression of interleukin-6, a marker of human mesangial cell inflammation: effects of oxidation and modulation by lovastatin. Biochem Biophys Res Commun. 2000;267:536–40.
92. Zelvyte I, Dominaitiene R, Crisby M, Janciauskiene S. Modulation of inflammatory mediators and PPARgamma and NFkappaB expression by pravastatin in response to lipoproteins in human monocytes in vitro. Pharmacol Res. 2002;45:147–54.
93. Vamvakopoulos JE, Green C. HMG-CoA reductase inhibition aborts functional differentiation and triggers apoptosis in cultured primary human monocytes: a potential mechanism of statin-mediated vasculoprotection. BMC Cardiovasc Disord. 2003;3:6.
94. Shepherd J, Kastelein JJ, Bittner V, Deedwania P, Breazna A, Dobson S, Wilson DJ, et al. Effect of intensive lipid lowering with atorvastatin on renal function in patients with coronary heart disease: the Treating to New Targets (TNT) study. Clin J Am Soc Nephrol. 2007;2: 1131–9.

95. Wanner C, Krane V, Marz W, Olschewski M, Mann JF, Ruf G, Ritz E. Atorvastatin in patients with type 2 diabetes mellitus undergoing hemodialysis. N Engl J Med. 2005;353:238–48.
96. Fellstrom BC, Jardine AG, Schmieder RE, Holdaas H, Bannister K, Beutler J, Chae DW, et al. Rosuvastatin and cardiovascular events in patients undergoing hemodialysis. N Engl J Med. 2009;360:1395–407.
97. Cohen JC, Boerwinkle E, Mosley Jr TH, Hobbs HH. Sequence variations in PCSK9, low LDL, and protection against coronary heart disease. N Engl J Med. 2006;354:1264–72.
98. Brown MS, Goldstein JL. Biomedicine. Lowering LDL—not only how low, but how long? Science. 2006;311:1721–3.

Chapter 3
Hyperlipidemia as a Risk Factor for Progression of CKD in Nondiabetics

Agata Kujawa-Szewieczek, Grzegorz Piecha, and Andrzej Więcek

Introduction

Hyperlipidemia is a well-established cardiovascular (CV) risk factor in the general population, as well as in patients with chronic kidney disease (CKD) [1]. Several lines of evidence suggest that mechanisms and factors contributing to the pathogenesis of cardiovascular and kidney injury may be similar [2]. Therefore, it has been hypothesized that progression of CKD may be mediated, among other factors, by abnormalities in lipid metabolism. Besides the baseline predisposition to dyslipidemia in the general population, patients with CKD are additionally exposed to secondary lipid disorders, which are resulting from renal dysfunction. Bearing in mind the additional potential anti-inflammatory and antioxidant effect of statins, it can be expected that this lipid-lowering treatment could have beneficial effects on renal function. In the last two decades, the potential nephroprotective effects of statins have been evaluated in numerous experimental models [3–6]. Moreover, some evidence that CKD patients benefit from lipid-lowering therapy comes from meta-analyses and post-hoc analyses of large cardiovascular statin trails in the general population [7–10]. Nevertheless, it should be noted that most of these studies were created to assess CV but not renal outcomes. At the present time, there is no strong evidence indicating that statins may modulate renal function. Further prospective, randomized, controlled studies designed specifically for CKD populations are needed to investigate the association between the use of statins and CKD, in particular.

A. Kujawa-Szewieczek, M.D. • G. Piecha, M.D. • A. Więcek, M.D., F.R.C.P. (Edin) (✉)
Department of Nephrology, Endocrinology and Metabolic Diseases,
Medical University of Silesia in Katowice, Francuska 20-24, Katowice 40-027, Poland
e-mail: agata.szewieczek@gmail.com; g.piecha@gmx.de; awiecek@spskm.katowice.pl

A. Covic et al. (eds.), *Dyslipidemias in Kidney Disease*, DOI 10.1007/978-1-4939-0515-7_3

Lipid Abnormalities Secondary to CKD

The causes of disorders in lipid metabolism in patients suffering from CKD are complex and depend on the degree of renal failure. In a cross-sectional study of over 16,000 patients from NHANES III population, lower glomerular filtration rate (GFR) was associated with decreased apolipoprotein A-I (apoA-I) and increased apolipoprotein B (apoB) serum concentrations [11].

The atherogenic lipid profile in patients with CKD is characterized by lower serum concentration of high-density lipoproteins (HDL), and higher serum concentrations of triglycerides (TG), apoB, lipoprotein (a) [Lp(a)], remnant intermediate (IDL) and very low-density lipoproteins (VLDL) as well as a greater proportion of oxidized low-density lipoproteins (oxLDL). The degree of disturbances in lipoprotein metabolism is associated with the rate of declining of GFR.

The main dyslipidemic disturbance observed in CKD patients is the elevated concentration of triglycerides and TG-rich VLDL and IDL remnants [12, 13]. Decreased activity of peripheral lipoprotein lipase (LPL) and hepatic lipase (HL) seems to be the main cause of these lipid abnormalities. One potential mechanism responsible for increased TG levels in CKD appears to be the elevated serum concentration of apolipoprotein C-III (apoC-III)—a direct inhibitor of LPL [14]. Moreover, several lines of evidence suggest a role for the hyperparathyroidism in the delayed catabolism of TG [15, 16]. Besides the impaired lipolysis, a down-regulation of lipoprotein receptors may be involved in the development of dyslipoproteinemia in patients with CKD. A correlation between decreased clearance of TG-rich lipoproteins and reduced expression of hepatic LDL receptor-related protein (LRP) and VLDL receptor has been found in experimental models of CKD [17, 18].

Although in patients with CKD total and LDL cholesterol concentrations are usually within the target range or even lower, the serum concentrations of lipid subfractions may not fully reflect the CV risk attributed to lipid abnormalities. Compared to individuals with normal renal function, patients with CKD usually are characterized by a greater proportion of oxidized LDL particles, which are recognized by scavenger receptors and induce formation of foam cells in atherosclerotic plaques [19, 20]. Furthermore, LDL particles in CKD patients tend to be smaller and denser, and, therefore, more atherogenic [21, 22].

Low HDL cholesterol is observed in the majority of patients with kidney disease. It is most probably caused by a decreased activity of lecithin-cholesterol acetyltransferase (LCAT), an enzyme involved in esterification of cholesterol and maturation of HDL from pre-β-HDL to HDL3 and HDL2 [23, 24]. Increased activity of cholesterol ester transfer protein (CETP) and acyl CoA: cholesterol acyltransferase (ACAT) is also related to the lower HDL concentration in CKD [25]. Moreover, patients with kidney disease have been shown to have lower plasma concentration of apoA-I and apoA-II due to reduced expression of these proteins in the liver [26]. The change in HDL concentration may also be affected by the presence of inflammation and decreased albumin concentration in patients with renal failure [12].

Elevated concentrations of total and LDL cholesterol as well as increased serum triglycerides concentrations are the typical lipid abnormalities of patients with nephrotic syndrome [27]. Both proteinuria and hypoalbuminemia stimulate the activity of 3-hydroxy-3-methylglutaryl CoA (HMG-CoA) reductase and ACAT [28], as well as may decrease the expression of the LDL receptor in the liver [29]. Impaired clearance of TG-rich lipoproteins [30] and elevated hepatic synthesis of VLDL [31] seems to be the main cause of hypertriglyceridemia in patients with massive proteinuria.

The results of HDL measurements in patients with nephrotic syndrome are inconsistent. Some authors have reported higher [32] levels of HDL cholesterol, while others have found lower [33] or normal [34] concentration of this lipoprotein in the presence of proteinuria.

Dyslipidemia in hemodialysis patients is characterized by hypertriglyceridemia, low HDL concentration, and usually normal levels of total and LDL cholesterol [35–37], similar to CKD patients not requiring renal replacement therapy. It has been observed, however, that additional factors, like repeated use of heparin [38] or type of membranes used [39], may affect lipid metabolism in these patients.

In the majority of published studies, peritoneal dialysis patients had a more atherogenic lipid profile (higher total and LDL cholesterol, triglycerides and Lp(a) concentration, greater proportion of oxidized and small, dense LDL particles) than those on hemodialysis [21, 22, 40–42]. Two important factors may explain this phenomenon. First, glucose absorption from the dialysate solution and coexisting insulin resistance may promote TG synthesis through elevated availability of free fatty acids [43, 44]. Secondly, the loss of protein, including apolipoproteins, across the peritoneal membrane may lead to lipid abnormalities similar to those in the nephrotic syndrome [45].

Pathogenesis of Kidney Injury due to Dyslipidemia

In 1982 Moorhead et al. hypothesized that progression of CKD may be mediated by abnormalities in lipid metabolism [46]. It has been suggested that hyperlipidemia as well as oxidized Lp(a) and LDL particles may play an important role in kidney injury [5, 47]. Although potential mechanisms of these abnormalities are not completely elucidated, it seems credible that circulating LDL particles, by binding to the glycoaminoglycans in the glomerular basement membrane, may lead to an increased permeability of the membrane. Filtered lipoproteins may stimulate proliferation of mesangial cells and contribute to glomerular damage. Even though some of the filtered lipoproteins are reabsorbed in proximal tubules, the rest will be altered passing down the nephron and, if intraluminal pH is close to the isoelectric point of the apolipoprotein, it will precipitate causing tubulointerstitial damage [46, 48].

Over the past three decades there have been numerous studies performed in order to better understand the role of hyperlipidemia in the pathogenesis and progression of kidney disease. More rapid progression of CKD in patients with lipid disorders is a consequence of both renal microvasculature and renal parenchymal dysfunction. It is supposed that macrophages located in different parts of the renal parenchyma may uptake the oxidized LDL particles through scavenger receptors, a process that would transform the macrophages into foam cells [2]. After some intracellular modification, these cells start to generate oxidized low-density lipoproteins, further activating multiple proinflammatory and profibrogenic factors. At the same time the atherosclerotic process, in the form of endothelial damage, foam cell accumulation, and smooth muscle cell proliferation, can be observed in the renal microvasculature.

Increased oxidative stress appears to play an important role in the pathogenesis of any CKD [49]. The expression of the NADPH oxidase, the main enzyme involved in the production of reactive oxygen species (ROS), has been shown in glomerular mesangial cells [50]. Factors that might stimulate the activity of mesangial cell NADPH oxidase include interleukin-1 (IL-1) [50], angiotensin II, and platelet-derived growth factor (PDGF) [51]. The local synthesis of ROS leads to modification of lipoproteins and generation of oxidized LDL remnants. These reactive lipoproteins can be re-used in the formation of ROS, which further enhance the oxidative stress forming a "vicious circle" [52].

No receptors for lipoproteins have been detected on mesangial cells. It is suspected, however, that oxidized lipoproteins can interact directly with various membrane proteins without the specificity of an agonist-receptor binding. There is some evidence from experimental studies that oxLDL can stimulate the production of angiotensin II and transforming growth factor-β1 (TGF-β1) [53]. Subsequently, these factors either directly, through specific receptors, or indirectly, by activation of the NADPH oxidase and generation of ROS may lead to extracellular signal-regulated kinase 1/2 (ERK 1/2) and Smad activation, which in turn results in overproduction of collagen-rich mesangial matrix [52].

Lee and Kim [54], in the study of over 900 renal biopsy specimens, have suggested that the distribution of oxLDL in some parts of glomeruli may be involved in the pathogenesis of glomerulosclerosis. It is suspected that LDL particles and oxidized lipids may stimulate the production of proinflammatory and profibrogenic agents through the activation of multiple signaling cascades. These lipoproteins could increase the expression of PDGF [55, 56], monocyte chemotactic protein-1 (MCP-1) [57, 58], macrophage colony-stimulating factor (M-CSF) [56], inteleukin-6 (IL-6) [55, 59], tumor necrosis factor-α (TNF-α) [55], and finally lead to accelerated proliferation of mesangial matrix and inflow of inflammatory cells into the glomerulus. The increased activation of TGF-β and fibronectin, in both cultured mesangial and glomerular epithelial cells, appears to play an important role in the lipid-mediated glomerulosclerosis and interstitial fibrosis [60–64]. The stimulation of Smad3 [65], ERK [64] and the increase in production of connective tissue growth factor (CTGF) [66], collagen (type I, III, IV) [65] and plasminogen activator inhibitor-1 (PAI-1) [64] may have an impact on fibrogenesis.

In experimental studies, oxidized Lp(a) and LDL particles cause apoptotic cell death in cultured human umbilical vein endothelial cells (HUVEC) and in the smooth muscle cells isolated from the aorta [67–69]. Other authors have noted that oxLDL can induce apoptosis in glomerular mesangial cells through stimulation of the ROS formation [5, 69]. Moreover, it has been reported that oxidized LDL, but not native LDL, may induce the loss of nephrin (a principal component of the slit diaphragm) and apoptosis in cultured human podocytes, which may lead to proteinuria [5].

Agarwal et al. [70] proposed that there could be a predisposition to renal tubular epithelial cells injury upon exposure to reactive lipoproteins among patients with proteinuria. The authors have demonstrated that oxidized LDL, but not native LDL, may initiate tubulointerstitial disease in vitro and the use of antioxidants might prevent cytotoxicity of the lipoproteins.

Oxidized LDL may decrease the generation of nitric oxide (NO), thus affecting the endothelial function and impairing endothelium-dependent vasodilation [71–73]. Moreover, it has also become evident that these highly reactive LDL particles lead to enhanced production of endothelin-1 [74] and thromboxane [75]. Galle et al. [76] have documented that the oxLDL remnants can directly stimulate renin release in cultured juxtaglomerular cells, further contributing to angiotensin II-dependent kidney damage.

Samuelsson et al. [77] have noted that there is a significant association between higher serum concentrations of triglycerides and apoE-containing lipoproteins and more rapid progression of renal function decline in patients with glomerulonephritis. It has been reported that VLDL remnants may increase the expression of MCP-1 in mesangial cells and stimulate the infiltration of monocytes into the glomeruli. After phagocytosis of lipoproteins and conversion into foam cells, monocytes can contribute to the pathogenesis of glomerulosclerosis [78]. Moreover, Joles et al. have documented that both hypercholesterolemia and hypertriglyceridemia can lead to podocyte injury and proteinuria in uninephrectomized rats [79].

Lipid Abnormalities and Progression of CKD

Several lines of evidence suggest that hyperlipidemia may contribute to progression of CKD. The potential nephroprotective effects of statins have been evaluated in numerous experimental models as well as in clinical studies.

Hattori et al. [80] have reported that a high-cholesterol diet in rats (containing 3 % cholesterol, 0.6 % sodium cholate, and 15 % olive oil) led to hypercholesterolemia as well as macrophage infiltration into the glomeruli, and was associated with proteinuria and focal glomerular injury at 6 weeks of observation. Joles et al. [79] studied the effects of lipid disorders on kidney function in uninephrectomized male rats with dietary hypercholesterolemia. They have noted that hypercholesterolemia leads to podocyte injury and proteinuria in animals after uninephrectomy as well as in animals with intact kidneys. Other authors demonstrated that there is a correlation between high dietary fat intake and kidney volume, cyst growth, and decline in renal function in the animal model of polycystic kidney disease [81].

The potential nephroprotective effect of statins, with particular regard to anti-inflammatory and anti-fibrotic effect, was investigated in numerous in vivo and in vitro studies. A protective role of rosuvastatin against puromycin and adriamycin-induced p21-dependent apoptosis in mouse podocytes has been reported by Cormack-Aboud et al. [3], suggesting that statins may decrease proteinuria and delay the progression of CKD. Moreover, statins may exert anti-proteinuric effects through the stimulation of Akt activity and inhibition of the oxLDL-induced apoptosis and loss of nephrin in cultured human podocytes [5]. Fluvastatin significantly decreased urinary albumin excretion and glomerular sclerosis, as well as increased nephrin expression in podocytes in a murine model of HIV-associated nephropathy [4]. In a group of salt-loaded, spontaneously hypertensive stroke-prone rats, treatment with rosuvastatin significantly decreased the severity of kidney disease, regardless of changes in blood pressure and lipid levels. The authors have demonstrated that rosuvastatin can exert a protective action through the preservation of renal morphology, particularly podocyte integrity, and by reducing the inflammation and preventing the impairment of matrix metalloproteinase system. None of the evaluated parameters have been improved by treatment with simvastatin, which indicates there are differences in potential renoprotective effects between statins independent of their cholesterol-lowering effects [6].

Takemura et al. [80], analyzing the results of the renal biopsies from patients with glomerular kidney disease, have showed the presence of apoB and apoE lipoproteins in the glomerular epithelial and mesangial cells and mesangial matrix. The authors have indicated the correlation between lipids accumulation, proteinuria, and the progression of mesangial proliferation. Attman et al. [40] described a relationship between accumulation of triglyceride-rich apoB-containing lipoproteins and a more rapid loss of renal function among patients with nondiabetic kidney disease. The same authors in a prospective study in 73 patients with primary CKD of a nondiabetic etiology have found that elevated total cholesterol, LDL cholesterol and apoB plasma concentrations, but not reduced concentrations of HDL cholesterol, were significantly associated with more rapid progression of kidney disease [77]. Similarly, other investigators have noted that the increase of apoB lipoprotein concentration from 0.77 to 1.77 g/L was associated with over two times higher risk of CKD progression in the group of 169 patients followed-up for about 4 years [83].

Schaeffner et al. [84] assessed the role of dyslipidemia in the early stages of kidney disease development; it involved the analysis of 4,483 healthy men, with serum creatinine concentration <1.5 mg/dL at baseline, participating in the Physicians' Health Study (PHS). After 14 years of follow-up, 134 patients (3.0 %) had elevated serum creatinine concentration (defined as ≥1.5 mg/dL) and 244 (5.4 %) had reduced estimated creatinine clearance (defined as ≤55 mL/min). In the multivariate analysis the total serum cholesterol concentration ≥240 mg/dL and HDL concentration <40 mg/dL were factors independently associated with the increased risk for creatinine elevation (RR 1.77 and 2.34, respectively). Similar, although less significant correlation was found between serum concentration of cholesterol fractions and reduced estimated GFR.

Two thousand seven hundred and two participants of the Helsinki Heart Study (HHS), middle-aged men with dyslipidemia (defined as non–HDL-C of 5.2 mmol/L) and baseline serum creatinine concentration ≤136 μmol/L, were tested for a potential association between lipid disorders and kidney disease progression. The decline in renal function was estimated from the linear regression slopes of the reciprocal serum creatinine concentration vs. time over the 5-year follow-up. During the study period, there was a 3 % increase in mean measured serum creatinine levels. It has been observed that the progression of CKD was 20 % faster in subjects with LDL/HDL cholesterol ratio >4.4 compared to those with a ratio <3.2 [85].

The influence of statins on kidney outcomes remains controversial. In contrast to some studies reporting positive association between lipid-lowering treatment and CKD progression [7–10, 86], several large-scale prospective and retrospective studies did not confirm these findings [87–93]. Nevertheless, it should be noted that most of these studies were created to assess CV but not renal outcomes. The main renal outcomes evaluated in these studies were eGFR (or creatinine clearance) (Table 3.1) and proteinuria (or albuminuria) (Table 3.2).

In the post-hoc analysis of the Greek Atorvastatin and Coronary Heart Disease Evaluation (GRACE) study, the effect of atorvastatin on kidney function was compared with the "usual care," defined as lifestyle modification and lipid-lowering therapy (including statins) in 1,600 patients with coronary heart disease and dyslipidemia. An increase in creatinine clearance by approximately 12 % ($p<0.0001$) and 4.9 % ($p=0.003$) was observed in groups treated with 10–80 mg of atorvastatin or "usual care," respectively. Whereas in subjects who had discontinued therapy or never received statins, a decline in renal function by 5.2 % ($p<0.0001$) was observed [7]. This nephroprotective effect of atorvastatin appeared to be dose-related and was more pronounced in participants at early stages of CKD.

This observation has been confirmed in the subanalysis of the Treating to New Targets (TNT) study, in which a significant difference in mean change from baseline eGFR at the end of the 5-year follow-up was noted between patients with CHD treated with atorvastatin in dose 10 mg ($n=4{,}829$; increase of 3.5 ± 0.14 mL/min/1.73 m^2) and 80 mg daily ($n=4{,}827$; increase of 5.2 ± 0.14 mL/min/1.73 m^2) [8].

Tonelli et al. [9] have reported that, compared to placebo, pravastatin reduced the rate of renal function decline by approximately 34 % in the group of 3,402 patients with moderate CKD (defined as an eGFR of 30–59.9 mL/min/1.73 m^2) but did not reduce the risk of a ≥25 % decrease of eGFR.

The subanalysis of the LIVES (LIVALO Effectiveness and Safety) study revealed a significant improvement in eGFR (increase of 5.4 mL/min/1.73 m^2, $p<0.001$) among 958 patients with hypercholesterolemia and eGFR of <60 mL/min/1.73 m^2 at baseline, treated with pitavastatin for 104 weeks [86].

In a subsequent meta-analysis of 27 randomized, controlled trials, therapy with statin was associated with reduced rate of decline in eGFR (1.22 mL/min/year slower) compared to placebo [10]. However, this effect was significant only in the cardiovascular disease (CVD) subpopulation but not in participants with glomerulonephritis, diabetes mellitus, or arterial hypertension.

In contrast to previous studies, other authors failed to confirm the impact of statins on renal function. In a recently performed secondary analysis of the JUPITER (Justification for the Use of Statins in Prevention-an Intervention Trial Evaluating Rosuvastatin) trial, treatment with rosuvastatin (20 mg daily) was associated with 44 % reduction in all-cause mortality in participants with moderate CKD. After 12 months of observation, the decrease of GFR between rosuvastatin and placebo group was comparable, from 73.3 to 66.8 and from 73.6 to 66.6, respectively [88].

Table 3.1 The effects of lipid-lowering therapy on renal outcomes—the influence on eGFR or creatinine clearance

Study	Population	Duration	Treatment	The impact on eGFR or creatinine clearance
Post-hoc analysis				
GREACE [7]	1,600 patients	3 years	Atorvastatin 10–80 mg/day vs. usual care	*Atorvastatin group*: Mean CrCl (mL/min) 76 (at baseline) vs. 84 (at 48 months); $p<0.0001$ Increase in CrCl of 12 % *Usual care, patients not treated with statins*: Mean CrCl (mL/min) 77 (at baseline) vs. 72 (at 48 months); $p<0.0001$ Decrease in CrCl of 5.3 %
TNT [8]	9,656 patients	5 years	Atorvastatin 10 vs. 80 mg/day	*Atorvastatin 10 mg group*: Increase of 3.5 ± 0.14 mL/min/1.73 m^2 in mean change from baseline eGFR Increase of 5.6 % *Atorvastatin 80 mg group*: Increase of 5.2 ± 0.14 mL/min/1.73 m^2 in mean change from baseline eGFR Increase of 8.3 % $p<0.0001$ for treatment difference
PPP [9]	18,659 patients	5 years	Pravastatin 40 mg/day vs. placebo	*Pravastatin group*: Reduced the rate of decline in eGFR by 8 % (0.08 mL/min/1.73 m^2/year, 95 % CI 0.01–0.15) Reducing the risk of acute renal failure (RR 0.60, 95 % CI 0.41–0.86) No significant reduction in the frequency of a ≥25 % decline in kidney function by eGFR (RR 0.94, 95 % CI 0.88–1.01) Among patients with moderate CKD at baseline, the rate of renal function decline by approximately 34 % (0.22 mL/min/1.73 m^2/year, 95 % CI 0.07–0.37)
LIVES [86]	3,119 patients	104 weeks	Pitavastatin 1–4 mg/day	*Among patients with eGFR <60 mL/min at baseline*: Increase of 2.4 ± 1.6 mL/min/1.73 m^2 in mean change from baseline eGFR after 12 weeks treatment Increase of 5.6 ± 14.0 mL/min/1.73 m^2 in mean change from baseline eGFR after 104 weeks treatment $p<0.001$

JUPITER [88]	17,795 patients	1 year	Rosuvastatin 20 mg/day vs. placebo	*Rosuvastatin group*: The decrease of GFR from 73.3 to 66.8 mL/min/1.73 m^2 after 12 months *Placebo group*: The decrease of GFR from 73.6 to 66.6 mL/min/1.73 m^2 after 12 months
ALLHAT [89]	10,060 patients	4.8 years	Pravastatin 40 mg/day vs. usual care	*Pravastatin vs. usual care*: Occurrence of ESRD similar (1.36/100 patient years vs. 1.45/100, $p=0.9$) No significant difference in the 6-year event rates for the composite endpoint of ESRD or a 25 % decline in eGFR (RR 0.95, 95 % CI 0.86–1.04; p=0.3)
Randomized clinical trials				
SHARP [87]	6,247 patients	4.9 years	Simvastatin 20 mg/day plus ezetimibe 10 mg/day vs. placebo	*Main renal outcome*: ESRD (the need of dialysis or transplantation) RR 0.97, 95 % CI 0.89–1.05; $p=$NS *Tertiary renal outcomes*: ESRD or death RR 0.97, 95 % CI 0.90–1.04; $p=$NS ESRD or doubling of baseline creatinine RR 0.93, 95 % CI 0.86–1.01; $p=0.09$
PLANET II [94]	237 patients	52 weeks	Rosuvastatin in dose 10 mg and 40 mg/day and atorvastatin 80 mg/day	*The changes from baseline in eGFR at 52 weeks*: *Rosuvastatin 10 mg* -2.71 ± 13.08 mL/min/1.73 m^2 *Rosuvastatin 40 mg* -3.30 ± 12.32 mL/min/1.73 m^2 *Atorvastatin 80 mg* -1.74 ± 13.96 mL/min/1.73 m^2

CKD chronic kidney disease, *eGFR* estimated glomerular filtration rate, *CrCl* creatinine clearance, *ESRD* end-stage renal disease

Table 3.2 The effects of lipid-lowering therapy on renal outcomes: the impact on proteinuria or albuminuria

Study	Population	Duration	Treatment	The impact on proteinuria or albuminuria
Abe et al. [95]	91 patients	24 weeks	Rosuvastatin	Parameters at baseline and after 24 weeks of treatment: *Urinary albumin/creatinine ratio* (mg/g Cr) 308 ± 38 (at baseline) vs. 195 ± 25 (after 24 weeks of treatment); $p < 0.0001$
Bianchi et al. [96]	56 patients	1 year	Atorvastatin	Parameters at baseline and after 1 year of treatment: *Urine protein excretion* (g/day) 2.2 ± 0.1 (at baseline) vs. 1.2 ± 1.0 (after 1 year of treatment); $p < 0.01$
Ozsoy et al. [97]	31 patients	6 weeks	Atorvastatin	Parameters at baseline and after 6 weeks of treatment: 22 % reduction of *urinary protein excretion* from 1.80 g/24 h to 1.42 g/24 h; $p = 0.005$
PLANET II [94]	237 patients	52 weeks	Rosuvastatin in dose 10 and 40 mg/day and atorvastatin 80 mg/day	*Urine protein/creatinine ratio over baseline urine protein/creatinine ratio at week 52*: Rosuvastatin 10 mg 0.94, 95 % CI 0.72–1.21 Rosuvastatin 40 mg 1.08, 95 % CI 0.93–1.26 Atorvastatin 80 mg 0.76, 95 % CI 0.64–0.91

Rahman et al. [89] performed a post-hoc analysis of the ALLHAT (Antihypertensive and Lipid-Lowering Treatment to Prevent Heart Attack Trial) study data to evaluate the association between pravastatin in dose 40 mg/day or usual care and the progression of CKD. One hundred and fourteen patients from the group of 10,060 participants have reached end-stage renal disease (ESRD), and the occurrence of ESRD during the 6 years' observation was similar between patients treated with pravastatin (1.36/100 patient years) and those receiving usual care (1.45/100, $p = 0.9$). There was also no difference in the event rates for the composite endpoint of ESRD, a 25 % or a ≥50 % decline in eGFR during a 6 years' follow-up.

The PREVEND IT (Prevention of Renal and Vascular End Stage Disease Intervention Trial) is the only published randomized, double-blind, placebo-controlled trial performed to assess the role of statins in patients with microalbuminuria and mild CKD (eGFR <60 mL/min/1.73 m^2). Contrary to previous findings, subjects treated with pravastatin had no significant change in GFR after 4 years [90].

The Assessment of LEscol in Renal Transplantation (ALERT) trial [91] compared fluvastatin ($n=1{,}050$) with placebo ($n=1{,}052$) in patients after renal transplantation. After a mean follow-up of 5 years, fluvastatin failed to influence the composite primary endpoint, defined as cardiac death, nonfatal myocardial infarction, or coronary intervention procedure ($p=0.139$). During a 2-year extension of the ALERT trial, 1,652 renal transplant recipients who received fluvastatin demonstrated a lower risk of major cardiac events, cardiac death, or nonfatal myocardial infarction [92]. However, there was no association between statin treatment and renal outcomes, defined as the incidence of renal graft loss, doubling of serum creatinine or less deterioration in the GFR over time. A possible impact of statins on patient and graft survival was evaluated among 2,041 first-time renal allograft recipients also by Wiesbauer et al. [93]. The authors observed that use of statin was associated with reduced all-cause mortality (adjusted HR 0.64, 95 % CI 0.48–0.86; $p=0.003$) and prolonged patient survival, while no significant effect on graft survival was noted.

Finally, the SHARP (Study of Heart and Renal Protection) trial [87] was created to assess the beneficial effect of the combination of simvastatin plus ezetimibe in patients with CKD and no history of myocardial infarction or coronary revascularization. Of the total 9,438 participants, 6,382 were not on dialysis at the beginning of the study. They were initially randomized to receive simvastatin (20 mg) plus ezetimibe (10 mg), simvastatin (20 mg) or placebo. There was no difference in the incidence of adverse events between simvastatin alone and simvastatin plus ezetimibe group, and after the first year of observation patients who initially received simvastatin were re-randomized to simvastatin plus ezetimibe and placebo groups. The median follow-up was 4.9 years and the main outcome was the first major atherosclerotic event. During the follow-up there was no evidence that this combination therapy increased the risk of cancer, myopathy or hepatitis in CKD patients. On average there was a difference in LDL cholesterol of 0.85 mmol/L and a significant 17 % reduction in major atherosclerotic events as well as in major vascular events in patients treated with simvastatin plus ezetimibe. Nevertheless, the SHARP trial showed no protection from reaching ESRD (defined as the need of dialysis or transplantation) in 6,247 participants not on dialysis at the beginning of the study (RR 0.97, 95 % CI 0.89–1.05; $p=\text{NS}$). There was also no difference in the occurrence of tertiary renal outcomes, defined as ESRD or death (RR 0.97, 95 % CI 0.90–1.04; $p=\text{NS}$) and ESRD or doubling of baseline creatinine (RR 0.93, 95 % CI 0.86–1.01; $p=0.09$). Moreover, secondary analysis, after subdivided disease stage at the beginning of the study, also revealed lack of effect on progression to ESRD.

Recently a new randomized, double-blind, multicentre PLANET II (Prospective Evaluation of Proteinuria and Renal Function in Nondiabetic Patients with Progressive Renal Disease) study was created to assess the role of statins in the decline of kidney function. The aim of this study was to evaluate effects of rosuvastatin 10 mg, rosuvastatin 40 mg and atorvastatin 80 mg on urinary protein excretion in hypercholesterolemic (fasting LDL cholesterol level ≥90 mg/dL at baseline) nondiabetic patients with moderate proteinuria (urinary protein/creatinine ratios of 500–5,000 mg/g at baseline). Two hundred and thirty-seven patients were enrolled into the study and all of them were receiving treatment with angiotensin-converting enzyme (ACE) inhibitors and/or angiotensin receptor blockers (ARBs) for at least 3 months before beginning of the trial. The changes from baseline in eGFR at 52 weeks of follow-up for rosuvastatin 10 mg, 40 mg and atorvastatin group were −2.71 ± 13.08, −3.30 ± 12.32 and −1.74 ± 13.96 mL/min, respectively. Therefore, it can be assumed that the incidence of renal adverse effects may be higher among patients treated with rosuvastatin, and this effect may be dose-related [94].

There are few studies, with a small number of patients, short follow-up and without a control group, which reported positive association between statin treatment and reduction of proteinuria (see Table 3.2). Abe et al. performed a prospective, open-label study of 91 patients with CKD (stages 1–3) treated with ACE inhibitors to assess the effect of rosuvastatin (in dose 2.5–10 mg/day) on kidney function. After 24 weeks of observation, they noted a significant decrease in urinary albumin/creatinine ratio (308 ± 38 mg/g Cr at baseline vs. 195 ± 25 mg/g Cr after 24 weeks of treatment; $p < 0.0001$) and serum cystatin C concentration (1.08 ± 0.04 mg/L at baseline vs. 1.03 ± 0.04 mg/L after 24 weeks of treatment; $p < 0.0001$) [95]. Similarly, 1-year treatment with atorvastatin resulted in decline of the urine protein excretion (from 2.2 ± 0.1 g/24 h to 1.2 ± 1.0 g/24 h; $p < 0.01$) in a group of 56 patients who were treated at the same time with ACE inhibitors or ARBs [96]. Other authors have reported 22 % reduction of urinary protein excretion (from 1.80 g/24 h to 1.42 g/24 h; $p = 0.005$) after 6 weeks of atorvastatin use in 20 patients with glomerulonephritis and proteinuria >0.3 g/24 h [97].

Contrary to previous reports, there was no association between the treatment with pravastatin 40 mg/day and urinary albumin excretion in both PREVENT intervention trial and in the PREVENT cohort study [90]. Moreover, other authors even suggested that some statins at high doses may increase proteinuria [98]. In the ECLIPSE study, 1,036 patients with hypercholesterolemia and high risk of CVD were randomized to treatment with rosuvastatin (10–40 mg/day) or atorvastatin (10–80 mg/day). During 24-week follow-up, there was a dose-related increase in the incidents of proteinuria (from 0.2 to 1.8 %) and hematuria (from 2.9 to 4.0 %) among participants treated with rosuvastatin [99]. However, Shepherd et al. analyzed data from 16,876 patients who received rosuvastatin in doses of 5–40 mg/day and showed that the development of proteinuria did not result in acute or progressive renal disease [100]. Alpha-1 microglobulin was found to be the main excreted protein in those patients, which led to the hypothesis that the cause of proteinuria might be the inhibition of HMG-CoA reductase in renal tubular cells [101].

In view of the inconsistent results of published studies, some investigators conducted a meta-analysis of available data. Fried et al.'s analysis of results of 12 small trials ($n = 362$) indicated the association between lipid-lowering treatment and reduction of proteinuria [102]. Similarly, Douglas et al. performed a meta-analysis of 15 studies ($n = 1{,}384$) and found that statins decreased albuminuria and/or proteinuria in 13 of 15 trials. This effect was more pronounced among participants with higher proteinuria at baseline [103]. Finally, Navaneethan et al. [104] in a Cochrane database review of 50 trials including approximately 30,144 patients with kidney disease did not confirm the beneficial effects of statins on eGFR but found statins reduced urinary protein excretion in six studies (MD −0.73 g/24 h, 95 % CI −0.95 to −0.52).

Again, referring to the recently presented PLANET II study, there was an antiproteinuric effect of statins in the group of 237 patients receiving treatment with ACE inhibitors and/or ARB. After 26 and 52 weeks of follow-up, atorvastatin has led to more than 20 % reduction of proteinuria, while no antiproteinuric effects of rosuvastatin (in doses 10 and 40 mg) could be demonstrated [94].

Conclusion

In regard to hyperlipidemia as a risk factor of CVD, there is evidence suggesting that patients with CKD may benefit similarly or even more from statin therapy than those with normal renal function. Despite this clear information, the use of statins in patients with kidney disease is significantly less frequent. After recent publication of the data from the SHARP trial, given the safety and potential efficacy of statins, this lipid-lowering treatment should be administered more frequently to individuals with CKD stage 1–4, as well as to those undergoing dialysis. Meta-analyses and post-hoc analyses of large cardiovascular statin trails in the general population also suggested a potential nephroprotective effect of HMG-Co-A reductase inhibitors. In the last two decades the role of statins in progression of CKD has been evaluated in numerous experimental models and in clinical studies, which led to inconsistent results. At the present time, there is no strong evidence indicating that statins may modulate renal function. Moreover, rosuvastatin use, particularly in high doses, would not be recommended routinely in this group of patients. Further prospective, randomized, controlled studies designed specifically for CKD population are needed to investigate the association between the use of statins and CKD, in particular.

References

1. Kujawa-Szewieczek A, Więcek A, Piecha G. The lipid story in chronic kidney disease: a long story with a happy end? Int Urol Nephrol. 2013;45(5):1273–87.
2. Magil AB. Interstitial foam cells and oxidized lipoprotein in human glomerular disease. Mod Pathol. 1999;12:33–40.
3. Cormack-Aboud FC, Brinkkoetter PT, Pippin JW, Shankland SJ, Durvasula RV. Rosuvastatin protects against podocyte apoptosis in vitro. Nephrol Dial Transplant. 2009;24:404–12.
4. Sakurai N, Kuroiwa T, Ikeuchi H, Hiramatsu N, Takeuchi S, Tomioka M, et al. Fluvastatin prevents podocyte injury in a murine model of HIV-associated nephropathy. Nephrol Dial Transplant. 2009;24:2378–83.
5. Bussolati B, Deregibus MC, Fonsato V, Doublier S, Spatola T, Procida S, et al. Statins prevent oxidized LDL-induced injury of glomerular podocytes by activating the phosphatidylinositol 3-kinase/AKT-signaling pathway. J Am Soc Nephrol. 2005;16:1936–47.
6. Gianella A, Nobili E, Abbate M, Zoja C, Gelosa P, Mussoni L, et al. Rosuvastatin treatment prevents progressive kidney inflammation and fibrosis in stroke-prone rats. Am J Pathol. 2007;170:1165–77.

7. Athyros VG, Mikhailidis DP, Papageorgiou AA, Symeonidis AN, Pehlivanidis AN, Bouloukos VI, et al. The effect of statins versus untreated dyslipidaemia on renal function in patients with coronary heart disease. A subgroup analysis of the Greek atorvastatin and coronary heart disease evaluation (GREACE) study. J Clin Pathol. 2004;57:728–34.
8. Shepherd J, Kastelein JJ, Bittner V, Deedwania P, Breazna A, Dobson S, et al. Effect of intensive lipid lowering with atorvastatin on renal function in patients with coronary heart disease: the Treating to New Targets (TNT) study. Clin J Am Soc Nephrol. 2007;2:1131–9.
9. Tonelli M, Isles C, Craven T, Tonkin A, Pfeffer MA, Shepherd J, et al. Effect of pravastatin on rate of kidney function loss in people with or at risk for coronary disease. Circulation. 2005;112:171–8.
10. Sandhu S, Wiebe N, Fried LF, Tonelli M. Statins for improving renal outcomes: a meta-analysis. J Am Soc Nephrol. 2006;17:2006–16.
11. Muntner P, Hamm LL, Kusek JW, Chen J, Whelton PK, He J. The prevalence of nontraditional risk factors for coronary heart disease in patients with chronic kidney disease. Ann Intern Med. 2004;140:9–17.
12. Chmielewski M, Carrero JJ, Nordfors L, Lindholm B, Stenvinkel P. Lipid disorders in chronic kidney disease: reverse epidemiology and therapeutic approach. J Nephrol. 2008;21: 635–44.
13. Attman PO, Knight-Gibson C, Tavella M, Samuelsson O, Alaupovic P. The compositional abnormalities of lipoproteins in diabetic renal failure. Nephrol Dial Transplant. 1998;13:2833–41.
14. Hirano T, Sakaue T, Misaki A, Murayama S, Takahashi T, Okada K, et al. Very low-density lipoprotein-apoprotein CI is increased in diabetic nephropathy: comparison with apoprotein CIII. Kidney Int. 2003;63:2171–7.
15. Nishizawa Y, Shoji T, Kawagishi T, Morii H. Atherosclerosis in uremia: possible roles of hyperparathyroidism and intermediate density lipoprotein accumulation. Kidney Int Suppl. 1997;62:90–2.
16. Arnadottir M, Nilsson-Ehle P. Has parathyroid hormone any influence on lipid metabolism in chronic renal failure? Nephrol Dial Transplant. 1995;10:2381–2.
17. Vaziri ND, Liang K. Down-regulation of VLDL receptor expression in chronic experimental renal failure. Kidney Int. 1997;51:913–9.
18. Kim C, Vaziri ND. Down-regulation of hepatic LDL receptor-related protein (LRP) in chronic renal failure. Kidney Int. 2005;67:1028–32.
19. Heeringa P, Tervaert JW. Role of oxidized low-density lipoprotein in renal disease. Curr Opin Nephrol Hypertens. 2002;11:287–93.
20. Kasahara J, Kobayashi K, Maeshima Y, Yamasaki Y, Yasuda T, Matsuura E, et al. Clinical significance of serum oxidized low-density lipoprotein/beta2-glycoprotein I complexes in patients with chronic renal diseases. Nephron Clin Pract. 2004;98:15–24.
21. Deighan CJ, Caslake MJ, McConnell M, Boulton-Jones JM, Packard CJ. Atherogenic lipoprotein phenotype in end-stage renal failure: origin and extent of small dense low-density lipoprotein formation. Am J Kidney Dis. 2000;35:852–62.
22. O'Neal D, Lee P, Murphy B, Best J. Low-density lipoprotein particle size distribution in end-stage renal disease treated with hemodialysis or peritoneal dialysis. Am J Kidney Dis. 1996;27:84–91.
23. Guarnieri GF, Moracchiello M, Campanacci L, Ursini F, Ferri L, Valente M, et al. Lecithin-cholesterol acyltransferase (LCAT) activity in chronic uremia. Kidney Int Suppl. 1978; 13:26–30.
24. McLeod R, Reeve CE, Frohlich J. Plasma lipoproteins and lecithin: cholesterol acyltransferase distribution in patients on dialysis. Kidney Int. 1984;25:683–8.
25. Vaziri ND. Dyslipidemia of chronic renal failure: the nature, mechanisms, and potential consequences. Am J Physiol Renal Physiol. 2006;290:262–72.
26. Vaziri ND, Deng G, Liang K. Hepatic HDL receptor, SR-B1 and Apo A-I expression in chronic renal failure. Nephrol Dial Transplant. 1999;14:1462–6.

27. Joven J, Villabona C, Vilella E, Masana L, Albertí R, Vallés M. Abnormalities of lipoprotein metabolism in patients with the nephrotic syndrome. N Engl J Med. 1990;323:579–84.
28. Vaziri ND, Sato T, Liang K. Molecular mechanisms of altered cholesterol metabolism in rats with spontaneous focal glomerulosclerosis. Kidney Int. 2003;63:1756–63.
29. Vaziri ND. Molecular mechanisms of lipid disorders in nephrotic syndrome. Kidney Int. 2003;63:1964–76.
30. Kashyap ML, Srivastava LS, Hynd BA, Brady D, Perisutti G, Glueck CJ, et al. Apolipoprotein CII and lipoprotein lipase in human nephrotic syndrome. Atherosclerosis. 1980;35:29–40.
31. Vaziri ND, Kim CH, Phan D, Kim S, Liang K. Up-regulation of hepatic acyl CoA: diacylglycerol acyltransferase-1 (DGAT-1) expression in nephrotic syndrome. Kidney Int. 2004; 66:262–7.
32. Ohta T, Matsuda I. Lipid and apolipoprotein levels in patients with nephrotic syndrome. Clin Chim Acta. 1981;117:133–43.
33. Alexander JH, Schapel GJ, Edwards KD. Increased incidence of coronary heart disease associated with combined elevation of serum triglyceride and cholesterol concentrations in the nephrotic syndrome in man. Med J Aust. 1974;2:119–22.
34. Joven J, Rubiés-Prat J, Espinel E, Ras MR, Piera L. High-density lipoproteins in untreated idiopathic nephrotic syndrome without renal failure. Nephrol Dial Transplant. 1987;2:149–53.
35. Cheung AK, Wu LL, Kablitz C, Leypoldt JK. Atherogenic lipids and lipoproteins in hemodialysis patients. Am J Kidney Dis. 1993;22:271–6.
36. Rapoport J, Aviram M, Chaimovitz C, Brook JG. Defective high-density lipoprotein composition in patients on chronic hemodialysis. A possible mechanism for accelerated atherosclerosis. N Engl J Med. 1978;299:1326–9.
37. Attman PO, Alaupovic P. Lipid and apolipoprotein profiles of uremic dyslipoproteinemia-relation to renal function and dialysis. Nephron. 1991;57:401–10.
38. Nässtrõm B, Stegmayr B, Olivecrona G, Olivecrona T. Lipoprotein lipase in hemodialysis patients: indications that low molecular weight heparin depletes functional stores, despite low plasma levels of the enzyme. BMC Nephrol. 2004;5:17.
39. Blankestijn PJ, Vos PF, Rabelink TJ, van Rijn HJ, Jansen H, Koomans HA. High-flux dialysis membranes improve lipid profile in chronic hemodialysis patients. J Am Soc Nephrol. 1995;5:1703–8.
40. Attman PO, Samuelsson OG, Moberly J, Johansson AC, Ljungman S, Weiss LG, et al. Apolipoprotein B-containing lipoproteins in renal failure: the relation to mode of dialysis. Kidney Int. 1999;55:1536–42.
41. Kronenberg F, Lingenhel A, Neyer U, Lhotta K, König P, Auinger M, et al. Prevalence of dyslipidemic risk factors in hemodialysis and CAPD patients. Kidney Int Suppl. 2003;84:113–6.
42. Kronenberg F, König P, Neyer U, Auinger M, Pribasnig A, Lang U, et al. Multicenter study of lipoprotein(a) and apolipoprotein(a) phenotypes in patients with end-stage renal disease treated by hemodialysis or continuous ambulatory peritoneal dialysis. J Am Soc Nephrol. 1995;6:110–20.
43. Johansson AC, Samuelsson O, Attman PO, Haraldsson B, Moberly J, Knight-Gibson C, et al. Dyslipidemia in peritoneal dialysis—relation to dialytic variables. Perit Dial Int. 2000;20:306–14.
44. Prinsen BH, Rabelink TJ, Romijn JA, Bisschop PH, de Barse MM, de Boer J, et al. A broad-based metabolic approach to study VLDL apoB100 metabolism in patients with ESRD and patients treated with peritoneal dialysis. Kidney Int. 2004;65:1064–75.
45. Steele J, Billington T, Janus E, Moran J. Lipids, lipoproteins and apolipoproteins A-I and B and apolipoprotein losses in continuous ambulatory peritoneal dialysis. Atherosclerosis. 1989;79:47–50.
46. Moorhead JF, Chan MK, El-Nahas M, Varghese Z. Lipid nephrotoxicity in chronic progressive glomerular and tubulo-interstitial disease. Lancet. 1982;2:1309–11.
47. Galle J, Heermeier K, Wanner C. Atherogenic lipoproteins, oxidative stress, and cell death. Kidney Int Suppl. 1999;71:62–5.

48. Gyebi L, Soltani Z, Reisin E. Lipid nephrotoxicity: new concept for an old disease. Curr Hypertens Rep. 2012;14:177–81.
49. Vaziri ND. Roles of oxidative stress and antioxidant therapy in chronic kidney disease and hypertension. Curr Opin Nephrol Hypertens. 2004;13:93–9.
50. Jones SA, Hancock JT, Jones OT, Neubauer A, Topley N. The expression of NADPH oxidase components in human glomerular mesangial cells: detection of protein and mRNA for p47phox, and p22phox. J Am Soc Nephrol. 1995;5:1483–91.
51. Galle J, Heermeier K. Angiotensin II and oxidized LDL: an unholy alliance creating oxidative stress. Nephrol Dial Transplant. 1999;14:2585–9.
52. Lee HS, Song CY. Oxidized low-density lipoprotein and oxidative stress in the development of glomerulosclerosis. Am J Nephrol. 2009;29:62–70.
53. Park SY, Song CY, Kim BC, Hong HK, Lee HS. Angiotensin II mediates LDL-induced superoxide generation in mesangial cells. Am J Physiol Renal Physiol. 2003;285:909–15.
54. Lee HS, Kim YS. Identification of oxidized low density lipoprotein in human renal biopsies. Kidney Int. 1998;54:848–56.
55. Lee HS, Kim BC, Kim YS, Choi KH, Chung HK. Involvement of oxidation in LDL-induced collagen gene regulation in mesangial cells. Kidney Int. 1996;50:1582–90.
56. Nishida Y, Yorioka N, Oda H, Yamakido M. Effect of lipoproteins on cultured human mesangial cells. Am J Kidney Dis. 1997;29:919–30.
57. Kamanna VS, Pai R, Roh DD, Kirschenbaum MA. Oxidative modification of low-density lipoprotein enhances the murine mesangial cell cytokines associated with monocyte migration, differentiation, and proliferation. Lab Invest. 1996;74:1067–79.
58. Rovin BH, Tan LC. LDL stimulates mesangial fibronectin production and chemoattractant expression. Kidney Int. 1993;43:218–25.
59. Massy ZA, Kim Y, Guijarro C, Kasiske BL, Keane WF, O'Donnell MP. Low-density lipoprotein-induced expression of interleukin-6, a marker of human mesangial cell inflammation: effects of oxidation and modulation by lovastatin. Biochem Biophys Res Commun. 2000;267:536–40.
60. Ding G, Pesek-Diamond I, Diamond JR. Cholesterol, macrophages, and gene expression of TGF- 1 and fibronectin during nephrosis. Am J Physiol. 1993;33:577–84.
61. Eddy AA. Interstitial inflammation and fibrosis in rats with diet-induced hypercholesterolemia. Kidney Int. 1996;50:1139–49.
62. Lee HS, Kim BC, Hong HK, Kim YS. LDL stimulates collagen mRNA synthesis in mesangial cells through induction of PKC and TGF expression. Am J Physiol. 1999;277:369–76.
63. Song CY, Kim BC, Hong HK, Lee HS. Oxidized LDL activates PAI-1 transcription through autocrine activation of TGF signalling in mesangial cells. Kidney Int. 2005;67:1743–52.
64. Ding G, van Goor H, Ricardo SD, Orlowski JM, Diamond JR. Oxidized LDL stimulates the expression of TGF and fibronectin inhuman glomerular epithelial cells. Kidney Int. 1997;51:147–54.
65. Hong HK, Song CY, Kim BC, Lee HS. ERK contributes to the effects of Smad signalling on oxidized LDL-induced PAI-1 expression in human mesangial cells. Transl Res. 2006;148: 171–9.
66. Sohn M, Tan Y, Klein RL, Jaffa AA. Evidence for low-density lipoprotein-induced expression of connective tissue growth factor in mesangial cells. Kidney Int. 2005;67:1286–96.
67. Harada-Shiba M, Kinoshita M, Kamido H, Shimokado KJ. Oxidized low density lipoprotein induces apoptosis in cultured human umbilical vein endothelial cells by common and unique mechanisms. Biol Chem. 1998;273:9681–7.
68. Galle J, Schneider R, Heinloth A, Wanner C, Galle PR, Conzelmann E, et al. Lp(a) and LDL induce apoptosis in human endothelial cells and in rabbit aorta: role of oxidative stress. Kidney Int. 1999;55:1450–61.
69. Sharma P, Reddy K, Franki N, Sanwal V, Sankaran R, Ahuja TS, et al. Native and oxidized low density lipoproteins modulate mesangial cell apoptosis. Kidney Int. 1996;50:1604–11.
70. Agarwal A, Balla J, Balla G, Croatt AJ, Vercellotti GM, Nath KA. Renal tubular epithelial cells mimic endothelial cells upon exposure to oxidized LDL. Am J Physiol. 1996;271:814–23.

71. Keil A, Blom IE, Goldschmeding R, Rupprecht HD. Nitric oxide down-regulates connective tissue growth factor in rat mesangial cells. Kidney Int. 2002;62:401–11.
72. Wu ZL, Liang MY, Qiu LQ. Oxidized low-density lipoprotein decreases the induced nitric oxide synthesis in rat mesangial cells. Cell Biochem Funct. 1998;16:153–8.
73. Hein TW, Kuo L. LDLs impair vasomotor function of the coronary microcirculation: role of superoxide anions. Circ Res. 1998;83:404–14.
74. Tan MS, Lee YJ, Shin SJ, Tsai JH. Oxidized low-density lipoprotein stimulates endothelin-1 release and mRNA expression from rat mesangial cells. J Lab Clin Med. 1997;129:224–30.
75. Oda H, Keane WF. Recent advances in statins and the kidney. Kidney Int Suppl. 1999;71:2–5.
76. Galle J, Heinloth A, Schwedler S, Wanner C. Effect of HDL and atherogenic lipoproteins on formation of O2– and renin release in juxtaglomerular cells. Kidney Int. 1997;51:253–60.
77. Samuelsson O, Mulec H, Knight-Gibson C, Attman PO, Kron B, Larsson R, et al. Lipoprotein abnormalities are associated with increased rate of progression of human chronic renal insufficiency. Nephrol Dial Transplant. 1997;12:1908–15.
78. Lynn EG, Siow YL, O K. Very low-density lipoprotein stimulates the expression of monocyte chemoattractant protein-1 in mesangial cells. Kidney Int. 2000;57:1472–83.
79. Joles JA, Kunter U, Janssen U, Kriz W, Rabelink TJ, Koomans HA, et al. Early mechanisms of renal injury in hypercholesterolemic or hypertriglyceridemic rats. J Am Soc Nephrol. 2000;11:669–83.
80. Hattori M, Nikolic-Paterson DJ, Miyazaki K, Isbel NM, Lan HY, Atkins RC, et al. Mechanisms of glomerular macrophage infiltration in lipid-induced renal injury. Kidney Int Suppl. 1999;71:47–50.
81. Jayapalan S, Saboorian MH, Edmunds JW, Aukema HM. High dietary fat intake increases renal cyst disease progression in Han:SPRD-cy rats. J Nutr. 2000;130:2356–60.
82. Takemura T, Yoshioka K, Aya N, Murakami K, Matumoto A, Itakura H, et al. Apolipoproteins and lipoprotein receptors in glomeruli in human kidney diseases. Kidney Int. 1993;43:918–27.
83. Ozsoy RC, van der Steeg WA, Kastelein JJ, Arisz L, Koopman MG. Dyslipidaemia as predictor of progressive renal failure and the impact of treatment with atorvastatin. Nephrol Dial Transplant. 2007;22:1578–86.
84. Schaeffner ES, Kurth T, Curhan GC, Glynn RJ, Rexrode KM, Baigent C, et al. Cholesterol and the risk of renal dysfunction in apparently healthy men. J Am Soc Nephrol. 2003;14: 2084–91.
85. Mänttäri M, Tiula E, Alikoski T, Manninen V. Effects of hypertension and dyslipidemia on the decline in renal function. Hypertension. 1995;26:670–5.
86. Kimura K, Shimano H, Yokote K, Urashima M, Teramoto T. Effects of pitavastatin (LIVALO tablet) on the estimated glomerular filtration rate (eGFR) in hypercholesterolemic patients with chronic kidney disease. Sub-analysis of the LIVALO Effectiveness and Safety (LIVES) study. J Atheroscler Thromb. 2010;17:601–9.
87. Baigent C, Landray MJ, Reith C, Emberson J, Wheeler DC, Tomson C, et al. The effects of lowering LDL cholesterol with simvastatin plus ezetimibe in patients with chronic kidney disease (Study of Heart and Renal Protection): a randomised placebo-controlled trial. Lancet. 2011;377:2181–92.
88. Ridker PM, MacFadyen J, Cressman M, Glynn RJ. Efficacy of rosuvastatin among men and women with moderate chronic kidney disease and elevated high-sensitivity C-reactive protein: a secondary analysis from the JUPITER (Justification for the Use of Statins in Prevention-an Intervention Trial Evaluating Rosuvastatin) trial. J Am Coll Cardiol. 2010;55:1266–73.
89. Rahman M, Baimbridge C, Davis BR, Barzilay J, Basile JN, Henriquez MA, et al. Progression of kidney disease in moderately hypercholesterolemic, hypertensive patients randomized to pravastatin versus usual care: a report from the Antihypertensive and Lipid-Lowering Treatment to Prevent Heart Attack Trial (ALLHAT). Am J Kidney Dis. 2008;52:412–24.
90. Atthobari J, Brantsma AH, Gansevoort RT, Visser ST, Asselbergs FW, van Gilst WH, et al. The effect of statins on urinary albumin excretion and glomerular filtration rate: results from

both a randomized clinical trial and an observational cohort study. Nephrol Dial Transplant. 2006;21:3106–14.

91. Holdaas H, Fellström B, Jardine AG, Holme I, Nyberg G, Fauchald P, et al. Effect of fluvastatin on cardiac outcomes in renal transplant recipients: a multicentre, randomised, placebo-controlled trial. Lancet. 2003;361:2024–31.
92. Holdaas H, Fellström B, Cole E, Nyberg G, Olsson AG, Pedersen TR, et al. Long-term cardiac outcomes in renal transplant recipients receiving fluvastatin: the ALERT extension study. Am J Transplant. 2005;5:2929–36.
93. Wiesbauer F, Heinze G, Mitterbauer C, Harnoncourt F, Hörl WH, Oberbauer R. Statin use is associated with prolonged survival of renal transplant recipients. J Am Soc Nephrol. 2008;19:2211–8.
94. de Zeeuw. Prospective evaluation of proteinuria and renal function in nondiabetic patients with progressive renal disease: XLVII European Renal Association-European Dialysis and Transplant Association (ERA-EDTA) congress 2010, June 25–28, Munich, Germany
95. Abe M, Maruyama N, Yoshida Y, Ito M, Okada K, Soma M. Efficacy analysis of the lipid-lowering and renoprotective effects of rosuvastatin in patients with chronic kidney disease. Endocr J. 2011;58:663–74.
96. Bianchi S, Bigazzi R, Caiazza A, Campese VM. A controlled, prospective study of the effects of atorvastatin on proteinuria and progression of kidney disease. Am J Kidney Dis. 2004;41:565–70.
97. Ozsoy RC, Koopman MG, Kastelein JJ, Arisz L. The acute effect of atorvastatin on proteinuria in patients with chronic glomerulonephritis. Clin Nephrol. 2005;63:245–9.
98. Deslypere JP, Delanghe J, Vermeulen A. Proteinuria as complication of simvastatin treatment. Lancet. 1990;336:1453.
99. Faergeman O, Hill L, Windler E, Wiklund O, Asmar R, Duffield E, et al. Efficacy and tolerability of rosuvastatin and atorvastatin when force-titrated in patients with primary hypercholesterolemia: results from the ECLIPSE study. Cardiology. 2008;111:219–28.
100. Shepherd J, Vidt DG, Miller E, Harris S, Blasetto J. Safety of rosuvastatin: update on 16,876 rosuvastatin-treated patients in a multinational clinical trial program. Cardiology. 2007;107:433–43.
101. Kostapanos MS, Milionis HJ, Gazi I, Kostara C, Bairaktari ET, Elisaf M. Rosuvastatin increases alpha-1 microglobulin urinary excretion in patients with primary dyslipidemia. J Clin Pharmacol. 2006;46:1337–43.
102. Fried LF, Orchard TJ, Kasiske BL. Effect of lipid reduction on the progression of renal disease: a meta-analysis. Kidney Int. 2001;59:260–9.
103. Douglas K, O'Malley PG, Jackson JL. Meta-analysis: the effect of statins on albuminuria. Ann Intern Med. 2006;145:117–24.
104. Navaneethan SD, Pansini F, Perkovic V, Manno C, Pellegrini F, Johnson DW, et al. HMG CoA reductase inhibitors (statins) for people with chronic kidney disease not requiring dialysis. Cochrane Database Syst Rev. 2009;2:CD007784.

Chapter 4
How Lipid-Lowering Agents Work: The Good, the Bad, and the Ugly

Faruk Turgut, Ihsan Ustun, and Cumali Gokce

Introduction

Decline in kidney function results in profound lipid disorders [1]. Among the traditional risk factors, altered serum lipid and lipoprotein profile (dyslipidemia) are noted in both early chronic kidney disease (CKD) and patients with end-stage renal disease (ESRD), regardless of the etiology of renal disease [2]. It is expected that dyslipidemia contributes to the increased cardiovascular morbidity and mortality in CKD patients [3]. However, studies investigating the association between dyslipidemia and mortality in this population are conflicting; some show the expected relation between higher serum cholesterol levels and mortality risk, especially among patients without signs of malnutrition and inflammation [4, 5], but others found no association [6, 7], and some have found that low serum cholesterol values are associated with increased mortality [5, 8].

The long-recognized relationship between CKD and increased cardiovascular mortality has been the impetus for evaluating cardiovascular disease-directed pharmacotherapy in patients throughout the CKD spectrum from mild CKD to kidney transplantation. Therefore, it was assumed that the greatest benefit could be obtained by treating dyslipidemia. The first step of treatment for dyslipidemia is usually therapeutic lifestyle changes. But for some patients, diet changes alone are not enough to lower blood cholesterol levels. These patients need drugs in addition to making lifestyle changes, to bring their cholesterol down to a safe level. Several different classes of drugs are used to treat hyperlipidemia. Table 4.1 shows the most common cholesterol-lowering drugs.

F. Turgut, M.D. (✉)
Department of Nephrology, Mustafa Kemal University, School of Medicine,
Serinyol, Antakya, Hatay 31034, Turkey
e-mail: turgutfaruk@yahoo.com

I. Ustun, M.D. • C. Gokce, M.D.
Department of Endocrinology, Mustafa Kemal University, School of Medicine,
Serinyol, Antakya, Hatay 31034, Turkey

A. Covic et al. (eds.), *Dyslipidemias in Kidney Disease*, DOI 10.1007/978-1-4939-0515-7_4,

Table 4.1 Cholesterol-lowering drugs

Hydroxymethylglutaryl CoA reductase inhibitors (statins)
Fibric acid derivatives (fibrates)
Cholesterol absorption inhibitors
Nicotinic acid (niacin)
Bile acid sequestrants

Cholesterol-lowering drugs differ not only in their mechanism of action but also in the type of lipid reduction and the magnitude of the reduction. Therefore, the indications for a particular drug are influenced by the underlying lipid abnormality. Statins are the most powerful drugs available for lowering LDL cholesterol, and, in general, statins are the most commonly prescribed cholesterol-lowering medications. In the same line, statins are the nephrologists' drug of first choice, after the lifestyle changes fail adequately to lower LDL-cholesterol levels in the setting of normal or moderately elevated triglycerides.

Statins

Currently, several statins in different doses are available in the market (Table 4.2). Pitavastatin is a new statin available in Japan in pharmaceutical form. The absorption of statins varies from 20 to 98 %, and the presence of food increases oral absorption. All statins are rapidly absorbed after oral administration and achieve the peak concentrations level within 4 h. Statins are primarily metabolized by the liver via the through P-450 III A4 and P-450 2C8, while the amount of renal elimination varies among the statins. Lovastatin and simvastatin are prodrugs that are converted into their active forms in the liver, whereas the other statins are active in their parent forms.

Mechanism of Action

In humans, cholesterol is synthesized from acetyl-CoA via multiple reactions (Fig. 4.1). 3-hydroxy-3-methylglutaryl coenzyme A (HMG-CoA) reductase is the key rate-limiting enzyme of this biosynthetic pathway. The statins inhibit HMG-CoA reductase and, thereby, statins reduce the hepatocyte cholesterol content and lead to increased expression of LDL receptors. The final result is a pronounced reduction in serum LDL cholesterol. Although the statins share a similar mechanism of action, they differ with respect to potency, availability of various strengths, and dosage forms.

Effects of Statins

The statins are the most powerful drugs for lowering LDL cholesterol, with reductions in the range of 30–63 %. Rosuvastatin, atorvastatin, and simvastatin cause the

Table 4.2 Available statins and fixed-dose combination products containing a statin in the market

Statin	Available doses	Dose range
Lovastatin	20, 40, 60, 80 mg	20–80 mg one daily or divided bid
Simvastatin	5, 10, 20, 40, 80 mg	5–80 mg once daily
Pravastatin	10, 20, 40, 80 mg	10–80 mg once daily
Fluvastatin	20 mg, 40 mg XL, 80 mg	20–80 mg once daily or divided bid, XL once daily
Atorvastatin	10, 20, 40, 80 mg	10–80 mg once daily
Rosuvastatin	5, 10, 20, 40 mg	5–40 mg once daily
Pitavastatin	1, 2, 4 mg	1–4 mg once daily
Fixed-dose combination products		
Lovastatin/Niacin ER	20/500, 20/750, 20/1,000, 40/1,000 mg	20/500 to 80/2,000 mg once daily
Simvastatin/Niacin ER	20/500, 20/750, 20/1,000 mg	10/500 to 40/2,000 mg
Simvastatin/Ezetimibe	10/10, 10/20, 10/40, 10/80 mg	10/10 to 10/80 mg

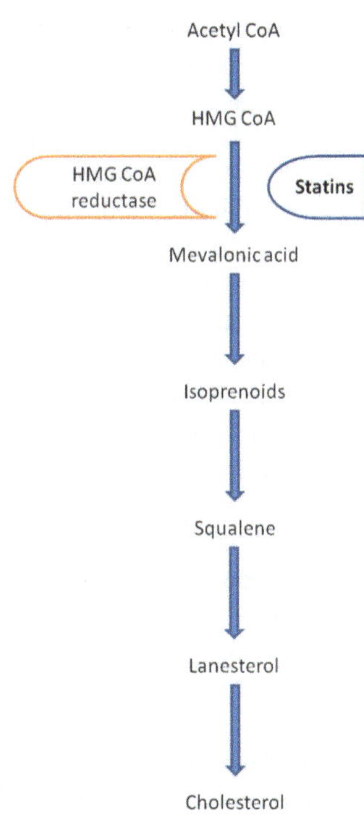

Fig. 4.1 Cholesterol is synthesized from acetyl-CoA via multiple reactions and statins inhibit 3-hydroxy-3-methylglutaryl coenzyme A reductase enzyme, which is the key rate-limiting enzyme of this biosynthetic pathway

greatest reduction in LDL cholesterol, and they are preferred in patients who require a potent statin because of high cardiovascular risk. Statins also decreases triglyceride 6–33 %, and their effects on HDL cholesterol are less pronounced (increase up to 10 %) [9, 10]. The magnitude of triglyceride lowering with statins may be larger in patients with hypertriglyceridemia. The effects of atorvastatin and rosuvastatin on serum triglyceride levels are dose-dependent [10]. In vitro data also support the activity of statins at the receptor level through up-regulation of LDL-cholesterol receptors. The net effects after administration of these drugs are a decrease in total cholesterol, and a slight increase in triglyceride levels and HDL-cholesterol levels. In addition, statins also shift the LDL-cholesterol profile away from a more atherogenic form [11]. These effects are thought to be primary characteristics associated with the attenuation of progression of atherosclerosis and the reduction in cardiovascular events.

All statins show similar function by binding to the active site of HMG-CoA reductase and in this way inhibit the enzyme. However, structural differences in statins are responsible for differences in potency of enzyme inhibition. There are minor differences among the statins. The most difference with atorvastatin and rosuvastatin compared with other statins is a longer half-life [12]. Atorvastatin and rosuvastatin are significantly more potent than other statins, and both these agents can lower LDL cholesterol more than 50 % at maximal prescribed doses [10]. High-dose simvastatin can lower LDL cholesterol by more than 40 %. However, simvastatin dosages of 80 mg are no longer recommended [9]. At doses of up to 40 mg/day, fluvastatin is the least potent statin. However, at doses of 80 mg/day, fluvastatin is as effective on lowering LDL cholesterol as most other statins [13].

Statins have been shown to produce beneficial effects at the endothelial level, displayed by stabilization or regression in atherosclerotic plaque, and at the clinical level, exhibited by reduction in cardiovascular events [11, 14–16]. These beneficial effects of statins are usually assumed to be due to their cholesterol-lowering properties, and that their benefit will follow the reduction in cholesterol pari passu. However, statins, independent of their hipolipidemic effects, may also show additional *pleiotropic* effects such as reduction in oxidative stress, inflammation, and thrombogenesis, and improvement in endothelial dysfunction [17, 18] (Table 4.3). As patients with CKD are at particularly high risk of vascular disease, it may be expected that statins have also substantial beneficial effects in CKD patients due to the pleiotropic effects of statins.

Statins have been extensively studied in a large variety of patient populations and have proven efficacy in the treatment of dyslipidemia, reducing cardiovascular mortality, with regression of coronary calcification especially due to a reduction of LDL-cholesterol level [14, 15, 19]. However, CKD and ESRD patients were excluded from most of the interventional studies, so the effect of statins on mortality and vascular events is still being debated. Currently, most evidence for these patients comes from secondary retrospective analyses of patient subgroups with CKD recruited into clinical trials with cardiovascular endpoints.

The NKF K/DOQI clinical practice guidelines for managing dyslipidemia in CKD patients and the K/DOQI clinical practice guidelines for cardiovascular disease in dialysis patients, both focused entirely on CKD patients advising statin treatment in all adults with stage 5 CKD and LDL-cholesterol levels ≥100 mg/dL with the goal to reduce LDL-cholesterol concentration to values <100 mg/dL [20, 21].

Table 4.3 Pleiotropic effects of statins

Anti-inflammatory	↓ CRP
	↓ Proinflammatory cytokines
Immunomodulatory	↓ Monocyte activation
	↓ T cell proliferation
	↓ TNF-α, IL-6, IL-8
Anti-atherogenic	↓ LDL-cholesterol oxidation
	↓ Superoxide formation
	↓ NAD(P)H oxidase
	↑ Free radical scavenging
Antithrombotic	↓ Tissue factor activation
	↓ Platelet activation
	↑ Fibrinolysis activity
Endothelial function improvement	↓ Endothelin-1 expression
	↓ Complement-mediated injury
	↑ eNOS expression
Plaque stability	↓ Inflammatory cell infiltrate
	↑ Collagen synthesis

In general, dose adjustment in CKD patients is usually not needed for atorvastatin and fluvastatin, which are the statins of choice in patients with CKD. Dose adjustment is warranted with other statins as CKD becomes more advanced (glomerular filtration rate [GFR] < 30 mL/min/1.73 m^2) [21]. A number of studies have evaluated the effect of statin therapy on renal outcomes in CKD patients, namely protein excretion and CKD progression [16, 22–27].

Statins in Predialysis CKD Patients

The evidence for statin use in mild-to-moderate CKD includes many post hoc analyses of trials powered for cardiovascular outcomes. Post hoc analyses from large-scale randomized controlled trials suggest a benefit of statin therapy with respect to cardiovascular and renal endpoints in patients with early CKD comparable to the effect in people without renal disease [16, 23, 28, 29]. A recent meta-analysis from the Cochrane Database summarized several of the trials investigating the effects of statins in patients with CKD not requiring dialysis and found that statin therapy led to a significant reduction of all-cause mortality (relative risk 0.81), cardiovascular mortality (relative risk 0.80), and nonlethal cardiovascular events (relative risk 0.75), as compared with placebo [30]. Finally, the Study of Heart and Renal Protection (SHARP) trial is the only large randomized controlled study assessing the role of statins on cardiovascular outcomes in predialysis patient population [24]. In this study, patients receiving simvastatin/ezetimibe (20/10 mg) combination had a 17 % reduction in major cardiovascular events compared with the placebo group.

CKD Progression

Growing evidence indicates that impaired lipid metabolism in CKD patients may contribute to the progression of kidney disease [31–33]. In the same line, a possible role of high LDL-cholesterol levels is defined in the progression of CKD, particularly in subjects with already reduced kidney function [34].

The effect of statins on CKD progression in mild-to-moderate renal failure is unclear, lying somewhere between minor benefit and equivalence to placebo. Most data on the effects of statins on renal function emerged from secondary/post hoc analyses of major statin trials. Some analyses suggested that statins had a beneficial effect on the rate of CKD progression [22, 35–37]. However, others failed to detect such a beneficial effect of statins on GFR [23, 38, 39].

Recent studies specifically designed in CKD patients revealed that rosuvastatin was associated with a statistically significant decrease in eGFR over 52 weeks of use. However, patients allocated to atorvastatin showed no significant change in eGFR in both studies [40]. Furthermore, the only randomized controlled study directly assessing renal outcomes in CKD patients is the recently published SHARP study. Treatment with simvastatin plus ezetimibe did not significantly reduce CKD progression in this study [24].

Proteinuria

Proteinuria is an indicator of kidney disease and is associated with faster loss of GFR. A number of studies have evaluated the effect of statin therapy on proteinuria. Initial analyses suggested that proteinuria can occur with statins, especially with rosuvastatin [41, 42]. However, later trials that specifically evaluated the effect of statin therapy on protein excretion yielded conflicting results, some studies demonstrating proteinuria reduction [26, 43], others showing no effect [38, 44]. Of note, some of these studies enrolled relatively small number of patients with a short study duration and some of them had no control arm. Similarly, a randomized controlled trial showed statins have no effect on renal outcomes in patients treated with adequate angiotensin blockade and blood pressure control [25]. In PLANET I and II studies, patients treated with atorvastatin showed a significant decrease in proteinuria, whereas patients treated with rosuvastatin did not show such an effect [40].

Overall, most of the available data investigating the effects of statins on cardiovascular and renal outcomes are derived from subgroup or post hoc analyses from studies primarily designed to assess cardiovascular outcomes. Therefore, these findings derived from post hoc analyses might be misleading. Different statins, used at different doses, in different renal or non-renal populations make things more complex. Treatment of dyslipidemia in patients with early stage CKD clearly reduces cardiovascular risk; however, available data do not support a strong nephroprotective role for statins in CKD population.

Statins in Dialysis Patients

The benefits of LDL-cholesterol reduction by using statin might not be translated from the general population to all patients undergoing dialysis. Therefore, studies evaluating the effect of statin therapy in dialysis patients on cardiovascular outcomes were designed. Observational studies in hemodialysis patients reported that statins reduce total mortality [45, 46]. However, the 4D trial (Die Deutsche Diabetes Dialyse Study) is one of the largest randomized trials about statins and mortality in diabetic hemodialysis patients comparing atorvastatin 20 mg/daily to placebo [47]. After 4 years of follow-up, there was no difference between atorvastatin 20 mg and placebo on the primary endpoint or all-cause mortality despite an effective LDL reduction within 4 weeks at 125 to 75 mg/dL. There was also an increase in fatal strokes in the atorvastatin group, although this was likely to be a chance finding, and no effect on any individual component of the primary endpoint. Moreover, the largest trial on statins and cardiovascular events in patients on dialysis is the AURORA trial, in which rosuvastatin significantly lowered LDL-cholesterol concentrations and achieved the targeted levels; however, no significant changes were observed in major cardiovascular events and mortality in the active treatment arm compared with the placebo group [48]. Recently, SHARP was the first randomized controlled trial specifically evaluating the effect of statins on cardiovascular events, defined as the combination of myocardial infarction, coronary death, ischemic stroke, or any revascularization procedure, in predialysis CKD and dialysis patients [24]. The results were presented only for the entire study population, combining dialysis and non-dialysis patients. Mean LDL-cholesterol reductions were equivalent in predialysis and dialysis patients. In apparent contrast to previous studies, simvastatin/ezetimibe combination was associated with a trend towards benefit in lowering the incidence of the atherosclerotic cardiovascular events in the patients on dialysis at the start of the study.

In contrast to the predialysis patient population, statins do not seem to have substantial improvement in cardiovascular outcomes in dialysis patients. SHARP is the key RCT in this field to date and clearly demonstrates a role for statins in preventing cardiovascular events in all stages of CKD patients, however, its findings of a beneficial effect of statins in dialysis patients cannot currently be fully accepted.

Satins in Renal Transplant Patients

Dyslipidemia is frequently encountered after renal transplantation even with normal or near normal renal function [49]. The NKF-K/DOQI clinical practice guidelines recommend treating renal transplant recipients with LDL-cholesterol levels that are greater than 100 mg/dL to a goal LDL cholesterol of less than 100 mg/dL [50].

The Assessment of LEscol in Renal Transplantation (ALERT) is the only randomized controlled trial on the effect of statin therapy on cardiovascular outcomes after renal transplantation [51]. After a mean follow-up of 5.1 years, LDL cholesterol reduced 32 % in the statin group compared with placebo group. Fluvastatin was superior to placebo in reducing cardiac deaths or nonfatal myocardial infarction, but there was no effect on the renal endpoints of graft loss, doubling of serum creatinine, or decline in GFR in the ALERT trial. Furthermore, significant long-term benefits in the primary composite outcome with statin therapy were observed in an extension of the ALERT study [52].

A Cochrane meta-analysis of 16 studies including 3,229 kidney transplant recipients compared statins with placebo [53]. There were nonsignificant trends towards a benefit of statins in terms of cardiovascular mortality and nonfatal cardiovascular events in this meta-analysis. A recent meta-analysis showed an uncertain impact of statin use versus placebo or no treatment on overall mortality but a possible reduction in cardiovascular mortality [54].

In summary, the available data shows a benefit of statin therapy on cardiovascular events in kidney transplant patients.

Tolerability and Safety of Statins

In general, statins are well tolerated, with minor adverse reactions such as gastrointestinal upset and headache. However, statins carry with them rare, but well-known, side effects, including liver and muscle toxicity. There are no clear data that the side effects profile differs significantly among statins. Pravastatin and fluvastatin appear less likely to cause muscle toxicity than other statins.

Statins are also well tolerated in predialysis CKD, dialysis, and post-renal transplant patients in clinical trials. However, the incidence of side effects in clinical practice likely exceeds that reported in clinical trials where patients are carefully selected and have a lower chance of potentially experiencing side effects. Statin adverse events are often dose related, and statins that are more dependent on renal excretion are more likely to need dose adjustments in CKD patients. Atorvastatin has less than 2 % renal excretion and does not require a dose adjustment in advanced CKD patients.

Muscle toxicity associated with statins spans a spectrum of complaints ranging from myalgias to myositis to overt rhabdomyolysis [55]. Muscle toxicity is uncommon with statin therapy alone, with a frequency of 2–11 % for myalgias, 0.5 % for myositis, and less than 0.1 % for rhabdomyolysis [56]. The risk of myopathy/rhabdomyolysis may increase with co-administration of some drugs and in some clinical situations (Table 4.4). Patients should be alerted to report the new onset of myalgias or weakness. Patients may have myalgias without an elevation in serum creatine kinase concentrations. Pravastatin and fluvastatin appear to have less muscle toxicity. Thus, if a patient using a statin other than pravastatin and fluvastatin experiences muscle toxicity (other than rhabdomyolysis), once symptoms have resolved off statin therapy, it is recommended to consider a trial of pravastatin or fluvastatin with careful monitoring.

Table 4.4 Factors that may increase the risk of myopathy/rhabdomyolysis with statins

Higher doses
Combination with other myotoxic drugs (niacin or fibrates)
Increased age
Hypothyroidism
Surgery or trauma
Heavy exercise
Excessive alcohol intake
Renal or liver impairment

Liver toxicity is another serious adverse reaction of statins. Asymptomatic hepatic transaminase elevation (less than three times the upper limit of normal) may occur in 0.5–3 % of patients receiving statins. This is dose dependent and occurs primarily during the first 3 months of therapy. All statins appear to have similar liver toxicity [57]. In most patients, elevation of transaminase is resolved spontaneously with continued therapy. Rare episodes of more severe liver injury have also been reported [58].

All of the statins should be used with caution in CKD patients. Starting with a low-dose statin may decrease the risk of muscle toxicity. The risk of clinically significant myopathy is relatively high in renal transplant patients receiving cyclosporine. Attention should be paid to muscle pain and weakness, which can be sign of rhabdomyolysis. Routine monitoring of serum creatine kinase levels is not recommended in patients on statins. However, it is important to obtain a baseline creatine kinase level and then repeat the test for any complaint of muscle pain and weakness. In the absence of clinical symptoms, a creatine kinase level more than ten times the upper limit of normal that is felt to be due to a statin is an indication for discontinuing the medication.

At the start of treatment, baseline liver tests also should be drawn, and it is not recommended to monitor transaminase levels routinely. Discontinuation or lowering the statin dose is generally recommended if transaminase levels are higher than three times the upper level of normal that is confirmed on a second occasion [57]. Transaminase levels typically return to normal after 2–3 months after discontinuation.

Fibric Acid Derivatives

Fibric acid derivatives, also known as fibrates, are another group of antihyperlipidemic agents, widely used in the treatment of different forms of hyperlipidemia. Fibrates are 2-phenoxy-2-methyl propanoic acid derivatives. This group includes bezafibrate, ciprofibrate, clofibrate, clofibric acid, fenofibrate, and gemfibrozil. Currently, gemfibrozil and fenofibrate, due to their milder adverse effect, are being used as lipid-lowering drugs in humans.

Mechanism of Action

Fibrates do not block cholesterol synthesis but are most noted for their ability to lower triglycerides. In fact, these drugs stimulate beta-oxidation of fatty acids mostly in peroxisomes and partially in mitochondria. Fibrates also activate peroxisome proliferator-activated receptors (PPARs). Although these drugs activate PPARs, there is no direct binding with PPARs. In addition to stimulating fatty acid oxidation-associated molecules, fibrates also increase lipolysis.

Fibrates are metabolized in the kidney and predominantly eliminated via the renal route [59]. Fenofibrate excretion is reduced in patients with moderate CKD (GFR < 50 mL/min/1.73 m^2) and accumulation of the drug with persistent usage is likely in CKD patients [59]. Therefore, fibrates should be used cautiously in CKD patients. Among the group of fibrates, blood levels of gemfibrozil appear to be not altered with kidney function deterioration, unlike other fibrates. Therefore, gemfibrozil should be the preferred agent in CKD patients without dose adjustment [21]. Gemfibrozil may increase serum statin concentrations by inhibiting the P-450 enzyme system. Thus, if a combination therapy with gemfibrozil is likely, then fluvastatin may be the safest choice of statin.

Effects of Fibrates

Hypertriglyceridemia is one of the most common quantitative lipid abnormalities in CKD patients [60]. Although triglyceride level in CKD patients may not be high enough to enhance cardiovascular disease alone, the combination of other alteration in lipid metabolism may facilitate atherosclerosis. Mixed dyslipidemia associated with CKD is characterized by hypertriglyceridemia and low serum HDL cholesterol, which make this population of patients good candidates for fibrates therapy.

Studies assessing the effects of fibrates on cardiovascular events in non-renal population have reported overall benefit [61, 62]. Animal studies showed that fibrates may attenuate lipotoxicity-induced glomerular and tubulointerstitial injuries, with enhancement of renal lipolysis [63, 64]. However, no adequately powered outcome study of fibrate therapy has been reported to date, particularly in CKD patients.

In the VA-HIT (Veterans' Affairs High-Density Lipoprotein Intervention Trial) study, a subgroup of 1,000 men with a creatinine clearance <75 mL/min was identified. In post hoc analysis, these patients with mild to moderate CKD were found to have risk reduction in fatal and nonfatal myocardial infarction with gemfibrozil therapy [65]. Moreover, in post hoc analysis of the same study, gemfibrozil did not exert a clinically relevant effect on rates of kidney function loss in CKD patients [66].

A recent study evaluating the effects of long-term therapy with fenofibrate in type 2 diabetic patients with eGFR ≥ 30 mL/min/1.73 m^2 reported that fenofibrate reduces total cardiovascular events compared with placebo without excess drug-related safety concerns [67].

Small studies showed that reduced-dose fibrates is effective in reducing serum triglycerides and cholesterol in dialysis patients [69]. In the US Renal Data System Dialysis Morbidity and Mortality Study, the hemodialysis patients using statin had a 32 % risk reduction in total mortality, but the patients using fibrate had no reduction cardiovascular or total mortality [45]. A recent meta-analysis of studies assessing the efficacy and safety of fibrates therapy in CKD patients has reported that these drugs improve lipid profile and prevent cardiovascular events in patients with CKD at least as much as the effects in subjects with normal kidney function [69]. In the same analysis, fibrates were found to reduce albuminuria and reversibly increase serum creatinine level.

Available data suggest that fibrates may have a place in reducing cardiovascular risk in patients with mild to moderate CKD. K/DOQI guidelines recommend that a triglyceride-lowering agent should be considered for adult patients with stage 5 CKD and markedly increased fasting triglyceride levels (serum triglycerides ≥500 mg/dL) that cannot be corrected by removing an underlying cause, treatment with lifestyle changes without causing malnutrition [21]. Gemfibrozil may be the fibrate of choice for the treatment of high triglycerides in patients with CKD.

Tolerability and Safety of Fibrates

Fibrates are well tolerated with very few side effects in the general population. The most common side effects are gastrointestinal disturbances, such as nausea and diarrhea. The most prominent side effect is myositis, which particularly occurs when combined with a statin, due to pharmacokinetic interaction [70]. Myopathy usually occurs within 2 months of the start of therapy. All fibrates may cause myositis, and gemfibrozil is the most frequent agent associated with rhabdomyolysis [71].

Fibrates are also associated with increases in serum creatinine concentrations (up to 20 %). Gemfibrozil appears to have the least risk of creatinine elevation [72]. Although the mechanism underlying the rapid elevation is not well understood, the increased creatinine concentration returns to baseline within 2 months after discontinuation of therapy [73]. In addition, long-term use of fenofibrate may increase the risk of gallstone disease in hemodialysis patient [74].

Although fibrates can be used to treat mixed dyslipidemia, they need to be used carefully in patients with CKD. In clinical trials, fibrates are well tolerated in patients with renal impairment [67, 68]. Fibrates are usually not recommended for general use in patients with CKD since CKD alone is a risk factor for rhabdomyolysis, especially when administered concomitantly with statins. There is still controversy concerning the safety of fenofibrate in these patients, and fenofibrate is non-dialyzable [59]. Thus, patients on hemodialysis may be particularly susceptible to toxic effects of fibrates.

Cholesterol Absorption Inhibitors

Cholesterol absorption inhibitor functions by decreasing the absorption of cholesterol in the small intestine. Ezetimibe is currently the only drug in this class. After oral administration, ezetimibe moves quickly from the intestinal lumen, through the intestinal wall (where it is glucuronidated rapidly), into the portal plasma and undergoes enterohepatic recirculation. The glucuronide of ezetimibe is much more effective than the parent drug, mainly because of its localization at the brush border of the intestines. Ezetimibe and its metabolite are excreted 90 % in the feces.

Mechanism of Action

Ezetimibe selectively decreases the absorption of biliary and dietary cholesterol from the intestinal lumen into enterocytes by inhibiting the action of Neimann-Pick C1 like 1 protein [75]. Ezetimibe (10 mg/day) inhibits cholesterol absorption by an average of 54 % in hypercholesterolemic individuals. It primarily decreases LDL cholesterol by 15–25 % from baseline, and this effect can be seen after 12–24 weeks of treatment [76].

Effects of Ezetimibe

Typically, ezetimibe is coupled with a statin to ensure a powerful effect when lowering LDL levels. An additional decrease in absolute LDL-cholesterol levels occurs with statin and ezetimibe combination. If statin therapy alone is insufficient to achieve target levels or if the patient does not tolerate statins, ezetimibe can serve as an alternative, either alone or as combination.

Ezetimibe now represents another option that seems to be safe and effective in CKD patients. The Second United Kingdom Heart and Renal Protection (UK-HARP-II) study showed that the addition of ezetimibe to simvastatin was safe and effective in treating dyslipidemia with CKD [77]. Again, the SHARP study demonstrated benefit of ezetimibe combination with simvastatin in reducing cardiovascular events for patients across a spectrum of CKD stages [24]. It has also been reported that addition of ezetimibe to statin therapy enhances proteinuria-lowering effects of statin in non-diabetic CKD patients [78].

Ezetimibe has also been used in posttransplant patients whose hypercholesterolemia has been difficult to control on statin therapy. Several of these studies have shown that ezetimibe is useful in decreasing LDL-cholesterol and triglyceride levels as monotherapy or in combination therapy with statins [79–82]. There have been as yet no studies of cardiovascular outcomes in patients on ezetimibe alone versus placebo.

Tolerability and Safety of Ezetimibe

The adverse effects of ezetimibe are few and mild [76]. In most studies, ezetimibe does not increase myopathy or rhabdomyolysis, whether used alone or in combination with statins, although cases of myopathy have been reported with this agent [83]. Furthermore, there is no evidence that ezetimibe increases the frequency of statin myopathy when used in combination. The combination of ezetimibe and a statin is relatively safe and well tolerated in patients with CKD [77]. Studies in renal transplanted patients reported that renal function, creatine kinase, liver enzymes, and calcineurin inhibitor levels remained stable with ezetimibe use [79, 81].

Although SHARP study has shown that the combination of simvastatin and ezetimibe is effective and safe in reducing cardiovascular events, it is not recommended to use ezetimibe as a first-line lipid-lowering therapy in patients with CKD on the basis of currently available data. Ezetimibe should be reserved for patients who are intolerant of, or unresponsive, to statins.

Nicotinic Acid

Nicotinic acid, also known as niacin, is a naturally occurring water-soluble vitamin of the B complex (vitamin B_3). Niacin is currently available in three different formulations, including immediate release (IR), sustained release (SR), and a new extended release (ER). Niacin is another option for the treatment of mixed dyslipidemia.

Mechanism of Action

Many of the effects of niacin are considered to result from its action on adipose tissue. Niacin inhibits adipocyte lipolysis, and reduces the production of free fatty acids. Consequently, it reduces substrate supply for synthesis of triglyceride and VLDL cholesterol by the liver [84]. The mechanism of nicotinic acid-induced increase in HDL-cholesterol levels is less clear.

Effects of Niacin

Niacin has profound and unique effects on lipid metabolism. Niacin decreases triglyceride and LDL-cholesterol levels while raising the HDL-cholesterol level. It is particularly useful in treating those patients who, despite statin therapy, still have low levels of HDL cholesterol. The ER niacin formulation has a dose-dependent effect on lipid parameters and decreases LDL cholesterol by 5–25 % and triglyceride by 27–38 %; however, it increases HDL cholesterol by 23–29 % [85, 86].

There are limited data on the efficacy and safety of niacin in CKD patients. In animal studies, niacin administration improves renal tissue lipid metabolism, renal function, and proteinuria in rats with CKD [87, 88]. Observational studies showed that nicotinic acid is efficient and well tolerated in dialysis patients [89].

Tolerability and Safety of Niacin

Administration of pharmacological doses of nicotinic acid is accompanied by unwanted effects including gastrointestinal effects. The most frequent side effect of niacin is flushing, which considerably restricts the use of niacin [84]. General recommendations to decrease the intensity of flushing include pretreatment with inhibitors of cyclooxygenase, the gradual increase of the daily dose, and use of ER formulation. Occasionally, oral administration of niacin may cause hepatotoxicity, hyperuricemia, and hyperglycemia [84]. Although niacin is associated with a high incidence of side effects including flushing, there are scant data on whether side effects are more common among patients with CKD [90].

Pharmacokinetic studies indicate that 34 % of niacin is excreted renally and the dose should be lowered up to 50 % in dialysis patients. According to the K/DOQI guidelines, for those with GFR < 15 mL/min/1.73 m^2, niacin dose should be reduced by 50 %; otherwise, no dosing changes are recommended in patients with CKD [21].

Overall, it is possible to suggest that niacin may have the potential to be an effective drug in treating dyslipidemia associated with CKD. Moreover, niacin usage in the transplant population is not well evaluated but seems to be safe.

Bile Acid Sequestrants

Since bile acids synthesized from cholesterol, their removal via sequestration in the intestine decreases plasma LDL-cholesterol levels. Thus, bile acid sequestrants have been used as a strategy to treat hyperlipidemia. Three bile acid sequestrants are available on the market: cholestyramine, colestipol (first generation), and colesevelam hydrochloride (second generation).

Mechanism of Action

Bile acid sequestrants are large polymers that bind negatively charged bile salts in the small intestine. Binding of bile salts interrupts their enterohepatic circulation and increases their fecal excretion. Consequently, bile acid synthesis is increased from LDL cholesterol. The cholesterol-lowering effect of bile acid sequestrants appears to be mainly mediated through increased bile acid excretion. Colesevelam has a substantially higher affinity to bile acids than cholestyramine and colestipol.

Effect of Bile Acid Sequestrants

Bile acid sequestrants, either as monotherapy or in combination with other cholesterol-lowering drugs, have proven their efficacy in reducing cardiovascular events [91]. As monotherapy, these drugs reduce LDL-cholesterol levels by 9–28 %, and slightly increase HDL cholesterol (0–9 %) in a dose-dependent manner. They can also be used in combination with other lipid-lowering drugs in order to achieve more LDL-cholesterol decrease [92]. In a small study, colesevelam reduced by 20 % non-HDL cholesterol in hemodialysis patients. A substudy of the Lipid Research Clinics Coronary Primary Prevention Trial examined the effect of cholesterol reduction with cholestyramine on kidney function [93]. After a follow-up period of 8 years, there was a significant decrease in total and LDL cholesterol in the treatment group, and no difference in the control group. However, cholesterol reduction with cholestyramine treatment did not meaningfully affect renal function compared with placebo in this study.

Tolerability and Safety of Bile Acid Sequestrants

Bile acid sequestrants are considered safe, although they are associated with gastrointestinal complaints (i.e., constipation, nausea,). Bile acid sequestrants can also decrease the absorption of fat-soluble vitamins, which should be considered during long-term treatment. Bile acid sequestrants often increase triglyceride level; thus, they are not an option in mixed dyslipidemia [21].

Bile acid sequestrants appear to be safe in patients with CKD, because they are not systemically absorbed; however, they can increase triglyceride levels and are contraindicated in patients with elevated triglycerides [94]. Although the data on drug interactions are limited, bile acid sequestrants may interfere with the absorption of drugs such as warfarin and immunosuppressive medications. Thus, they should be used carefully in renal transplant patients.

Limited available data suggest that bile acid sequestrants may be used in patients with CKD. Unfortunately, there are no randomized controlled intervention trials in CKD patients showing that the treatment of dyslipidemia with bile acid sequestrants reduces the incidence of cardiovascular morbidity and mortality.

Conclusion

Patients with CKD have a markedly increased risk of cardiovascular events and death. Although many factors other than hypercholesterolemia may contribute to this high cardiovascular risk, it is likely that mixed dyslipidemia common in these patients plays a major role. Statins are the cornerstone of lipid-lowering therapy in this setting of CKD, except those with triglyceride >500 mg/dL, in which case fibrates, particularly gemfibrozil, are the therapy of choice. Lipid-lowering therapy is generally safe when properly monitored in these patients. However, in some subpopulations of CKD patients, lipid-lowering drugs may not be as safe or as effective in reducing the incidence of cardiovascular disease as they are in the general population. The studies in patients with early stages of CKD provide evidence that cardiovascular and renal outcomes are favorably affected by lipid-lowering drugs. Once patients reach ESRD and started to receive dialysis, the underlying pathogenesis of increased cardiovascular mortality may be less related to atherosclerosis and vascular occlusion and, therefore, less amenable to modification by lipid-lowering therapy.

References

1. Attman PO, Samuelsson O, Alaupovic P. The effect of decreasing renal function on lipoprotein profiles. Nephrol Dial Transplant. 2011;26(8):2572–5.
2. Kasiske BL. Hyperlipidemia in patients with chronic renal disease. Am J Kidney Dis. 1998;32(5 Suppl 3):S142–56.
3. National Cholesterol Education Program (NCEP) Expert Panel on Detection Evaluation, and Treatment of High Blood Cholesterol in Adults (Adult Treatment Panel III). Third report of the National Cholesterol Education Program (NCEP) expert panel on detection, evaluation, and treatment of high blood cholesterol in adults (Adult Treatment Panel III) final report. Circulation. 2002;106(25):3143–421.
4. Contreras G, Hu B, Astor BC, Greene T, Erlinger T, Kusek JW, et al. Malnutrition-inflammation modifies the relationship of cholesterol with cardiovascular disease. J Am Soc Nephrol. 2010;21(12):2131–42.
5. Kilpatrick RD, McAllister CJ, Kovesdy CP, Derose SF, Kopple JD, Kalantar-Zadeh K. Association between serum lipids and survival in hemodialysis patients and impact of race. J Am Soc Nephrol. 2007;18(1):293–303.
6. Chawla V, Greene T, Beck GJ, Kusek JW, Collins AJ, Sarnak MJ, et al. Hyperlipidemia and long-term outcomes in nondiabetic chronic kidney disease. Clin J Am Soc Nephrol. 2010;5(9):1582–7.
7. Kovesdy CP, Anderson JE, Kalantar-Zadeh K. Inverse association between lipid levels and mortality in men with chronic kidney disease who are not yet on dialysis: effects of case mix and the malnutrition-inflammation-cachexia syndrome. J Am Soc Nephrol. 2007;18(1): 304–11.
8. Liu Y, Coresh J, Eustace JA, Longenecker JC, Jaar B, Fink NE, et al. Association between cholesterol level and mortality in dialysis patients: role of inflammation and malnutrition. JAMA. 2004;291(4):451–9.
9. Jellinger PS, Smith DA, Mehta AE, Ganda O, Handelsman Y, Rodbard HW, et al. American Association of Clinical Endocrinologists' guidelines for management of dyslipidemia and prevention of atherosclerosis. Endocr Pract. 2012;18 Suppl 1:1–78.

10. Jones PH, Davidson MH, Stein EA, Bays HE, McKenney JM, Miller E, et al. Comparison of the efficacy and safety of rosuvastatin versus atorvastatin, simvastatin, and pravastatin across doses (STELLAR* Trial). Am J Cardiol. 2003;92(2):152–60.
11. Vaughan CJ, Gotto AM, Basson CT. The evolving role of statins in the management of atherosclerosis. J Am Coll Cardiol. 2000;35(1):1–10.
12. Neuvonen PJ, Backman JT, Niemi M. Pharmacokinetic comparison of the potential over-the-counter statins simvastatin, lovastatin, fluvastatin and pravastatin. Clin Pharmacokinet. 2008;47(7):463–74.
13. Eidelman RS, Lamas GA, Hennekens CH. The new National Cholesterol Education Program guidelines: clinical challenges for more widespread therapy of lipids to treat and prevent coronary heart disease. Arch Intern Med. 2002;162(18):2033–6.
14. Callister TQ, Raggi P, Cooil B, Lippolis NJ, Russo DJ. Effect of HMG-CoA reductase inhibitors on coronary artery disease as assessed by electron-beam computed tomography. N Engl J Med. 1998;339(27):1972–8.
15. Brugts JJ, Yetgin T, Hoeks SE, Gotto AM, Shepherd J, Westendorp RG, et al. The benefits of statins in people without established cardiovascular disease but with cardiovascular risk factors: meta-analysis of randomised controlled trials. BMJ. 2009;338:b2376.
16. Tonelli M, Isles C, Curhan GC, Tonkin A, Pfeffer MA, Shepherd J, et al. Effect of pravastatin on cardiovascular events in people with chronic kidney disease. Circulation. 2004;110(12):1557–63.
17. Muhlestein JB, Anderson JL, Horne BD, Carlquist JF, Bair TL, Bunch TJ, et al. Early effects of statins in patients with coronary artery disease and high C-reactive protein. Am J Cardiol. 2004;94(9):1107–12.
18. Kanat M, Yildiz M, Tunckale A, Ceyhan BO, Karagoz Y, Altuntaş Y, et al. Intensive lipid reduction and proinflammatory markers in the MODEST study. Turk Jem. 2010;14:31–4.
19. Scandinavian Simvastatin Survival Study Group. Randomised trial of cholesterol lowering in 4444 patients with coronary heart disease: the Scandinavian Simvastatin Survival Study (4S). Lancet. 1994;344(8934):1383–9.
20. K/DOQI Workgroup. K/DOQI clinical practice guidelines for cardiovascular disease in dialysis patients. Am J Kidney Dis. 2005;45(4 Suppl 3):S1–153.
21. KDOQIKD Group. K/DOQI clinical practice guidelines for management of dyslipidemias in patients with kidney disease. Am J Kidney Dis. 2003;41(4 Suppl 3):I–IV, S1–91.
22. Kimura K, Shimano H, Yokote K, Urashima M, Teramoto T. Effects of pitavastatin (LIVALO tablet) on the estimated glomerular filtration rate (eGFR) in hypercholesterolemic patients with chronic kidney disease. Sub-analysis of the LIVALO Effectiveness and Safety (LIVES) study. J Atheroscler Thromb. 2010;17(6):601–9.
23. Ridker PM, MacFadyen J, Cressman M, Glynn RJ. Efficacy of rosuvastatin among men and women with moderate chronic kidney disease and elevated high-sensitivity C-reactive protein: a secondary analysis from the JUPITER (Justification for the Use of Statins in Prevention-an Intervention Trial Evaluating Rosuvastatin) trial. J Am Coll Cardiol. 2010;55(12):1266–73.
24. Baigent C, Landray MJ, Reith C, Emberson J, Wheeler DC, Tomson C, et al. The effects of lowering LDL cholesterol with simvastatin plus ezetimibe in patients with chronic kidney disease (Study of Heart and Renal Protection): a randomised placebo-controlled trial. Lancet. 2011;377(9784):2181–92.
25. Ruggenenti P, Perna A, Tonelli M, Loriga G, Motterlini N, Rubis N, et al. Effects of add-on fluvastatin therapy in patients with chronic proteinuric nephropathy on dual renin-angiotensin system blockade: the ESPLANADE trial. Clin J Am Soc Nephrol. 2010;5(11):1928–38.
26. Douglas K, O'Malley PG, Jackson JL. Meta-analysis: the effect of statins on albuminuria. Ann Intern Med. 2006;145(2):117–24.
27. Athyros VG, Mikhailidis DP, Papageorgiou AA, Symeonidis AN, Pehlivanidis AN, Bouloukos VI, et al. The effect of statins versus untreated dyslipidaemia on renal function in patients with coronary heart disease. A subgroup analysis of the Greek atorvastatin and coronary heart disease evaluation (GREACE) study. J Clin Pathol. 2004;57(7):728–34.

28. Heart Protection Study Collaborative Group. MRC/BHF Heart Protection Study of cholesterol lowering with simvastatin in 20,536 high-risk individuals: a randomised placebo-controlled trial. Lancet. 2002;360(9326):7–22.
29. Shepherd J, Kastelein JJ, Bittner V, Deedwania P, Breazna A, Dobson S, et al. Intensive lipid lowering with atorvastatin in patients with coronary heart disease and chronic kidney disease: the TNT (Treating to New Targets) study. J Am Coll Cardiol. 2008;51(15):1448–54.
30. Navaneethan SD, Pansini F, Perkovic V, Manno C, Pellegrini F, Johnson DW, et al. HMG CoA reductase inhibitors (statins) for people with chronic kidney disease not requiring dialysis. Cochrane Database Syst Rev. 2009(2):CD007784.
31. Muntner P, Coresh J, Smith JC, Eckfeldt J, Klag MJ. Plasma lipids and risk of developing renal dysfunction: the atherosclerosis risk in communities study. Kidney Int. 2000;58(1):293–301.
32. Chen J, Muntner P, Hamm LL, Jones DW, Batuman V, Fonseca V, et al. The metabolic syndrome and chronic kidney disease in U.S. adults. Ann Intern Med. 2004;140(3):167–74.
33. de Boer IH, Astor BC, Kramer H, Palmas W, Seliger SL, Shlipak MG, et al. Lipoprotein abnormalities associated with mild impairment of kidney function in the multi-ethnic study of atherosclerosis. Clin J Am Soc Nephrol. 2008;3(1):125–32.
34. Samuelsson O, Mulec H, Knight-Gibson C, Attman PO, Kron B, Larsson R, et al. Lipoprotein abnormalities are associated with increased rate of progression of human chronic renal insufficiency. Nephrol Dial Transplant. 1997;12(9):1908–15.
35. Collins R, Armitage J, Parish S, Sleigh P, Peto R, Heart Protection Study Collaborative Group. MRC/BHF Heart Protection Study of cholesterol-lowering with simvastatin in 5963 people with diabetes: a randomised placebo-controlled trial. Lancet. 2003;361(9374):2005–16.
36. Athyros VG, Papageorgiou AA, Mercouris BR, Athyrou VV, Symeonidis AN, Basayannis EO, et al. Treatment with atorvastatin to the National Cholesterol Educational Program goal versus 'usual' care in secondary coronary heart disease prevention. The GREek Atorvastatin and Coronary-heart-disease Evaluation (GREACE) study. Curr Med Res Opin. 2002;18(4): 220–8.
37. Shepherd J, Kastelein JJ, Bittner V, Deedwania P, Breazna A, Dobson S, et al. Effect of intensive lipid lowering with atorvastatin on renal function in patients with coronary heart disease: the Treating to New Targets (TNT) study. Clin J Am Soc Nephrol. 2007;2(6):1131–9.
38. Atthobari J, Brantsma AH, Gansevoort RT, Visser ST, Asselbergs FW, van Gilst WH, et al. The effect of statins on urinary albumin excretion and glomerular filtration rate: results from both a randomized clinical trial and an observational cohort study. Nephrol Dial Transplant. 2006;21(11):3106–14.
39. Rahman M, Baimbridge C, Davis BR, Barzilay J, Basile JN, Henriquez MA, et al. Progression of kidney disease in moderately hypercholesterolemic, hypertensive patients randomized to pravastatin versus usual care: a report from the Antihypertensive and Lipid-Lowering Treatment to Prevent Heart Attack Trial (ALLHAT). Am J Kidney Dis. 2008;52(3):412–24.
40. Keller DM. PLANET I and II: atorvastatin beats rosuvastatin for protecting kidneys in diabetic and nondiabetic patients. 2010. http://www.theheart.org/article/1095269.do.
41. Alsheikh-Ali AA, Ambrose MS, Kuvin JT, Karas RH. The safety of rosuvastatin as used in common clinical practice: a postmarketing analysis. Circulation. 2005;111(23):3051–7.
42. Deslypere JP, Delanghe J, Vermeulen A. Proteinuria as complication of simvastatin treatment. Lancet. 1990;336(8728):1453.
43. Ozsoy RC, Koopman MG, Kastelein JJ, Arisz L. The acute effect of atorvastatin on proteinuria in patients with chronic glomerulonephritis. Clin Nephrol. 2005;63(4):245–9.
44. Remuzzi G, Macia M, Ruggenenti P. Prevention and treatment of diabetic renal disease in type 2 diabetes: the BENEDICT study. J Am Soc Nephrol. 2006;17(4 Suppl 2):S90–7.
45. Seliger SL, Weiss NS, Gillen DL, Kestenbaum B, Ball A, Sherrard DJ, et al. HMG-CoA reductase inhibitors are associated with reduced mortality in ESRD patients. Kidney Int. 2002;61(1):297–304.
46. Andreucci VE, Fissell RB, Bragg-Gresham JL, Ethier J, Greenwood R, Pauly M, et al. Dialysis Outcomes and Practice Patterns Study (DOPPS) data on medications in hemodialysis patients. Am J Kidney Dis. 2004;44(5 Suppl 2):61–7.

47. Wanner C, Krane V, März W, Olschewski M, Mann JF, Ruf G, et al. Atorvastatin in patients with type 2 diabetes mellitus undergoing hemodialysis. N Engl J Med. 2005;353(3):238–48.
48. Fellström BC, Jardine AG, Schmieder RE, Holdaas H, Bannister K, Beutler J, et al. Rosuvastatin and cardiovascular events in patients undergoing hemodialysis. N Engl J Med. 2009;360(14):1395–407.
49. Moore R, Thomas D, Morgan E, Wheeler D, Griffin P, Salaman J, et al. Abnormal lipid and lipoprotein profiles following renal transplantation. Transplant Proc. 1993;25(1 Pt 2):1060–1.
50. Kasiske B, Cosio FG, Beto J, Bolton K, Chavers BM, Grimm R, et al. Clinical practice guidelines for managing dyslipidemias in kidney transplant patients: a report from the Managing Dyslipidemias in Chronic Kidney Disease Work Group of the National Kidney Foundation Kidney Disease Outcomes Quality Initiative. Am J Transplant. 2004;4 Suppl 7:13–53.
51. Holdaas H, Fellström B, Jardine AG, Holme I, Nyberg G, Fauchald P, et al. Effect of fluvastatin on cardiac outcomes in renal transplant recipients: a multicentre, randomised, placebo-controlled trial. Lancet. 2003;361(9374):2024–31.
52. Holdaas H, Fellström B, Cole E, Nyberg G, Olsson AG, Pedersen TR, et al. Long-term cardiac outcomes in renal transplant recipients receiving fluvastatin: the ALERT extension study. Am J Transplant. 2005;5(12):2929–36.
53. Navaneethan SD, Perkovic V, Johnson DW, Nigwekar SU, Craig JC, Strippoli GF. HMG CoA reductase inhibitors (statins) for kidney transplant recipients. Cochrane Database Syst Rev. 2009(2):CD005019.
54. Palmer SC, Craig JC, Navaneethan SD, Tonelli M, Pellegrini F, Strippoli GF. Benefits and harms of statin therapy for persons with chronic kidney disease: a systematic review and meta-analysis. Ann Intern Med. 2012;157(4):263–75.
55. Rosenson RS. Current overview of statin-induced myopathy. Am J Med. 2004;116(6):408–16.
56. Thompson PD, Clarkson PM, Rosenson RS, Panel NLASSTFMSE. An assessment of statin safety by muscle experts. Am J Cardiol. 2006;97(8A):69C–76.
57. Davidson MH. Safety profiles for the HMG-CoA reductase inhibitors: treatment and trust. Drugs. 2001;61(2):197–206.
58. Cohen DE, Anania FA, Chalasani N, Panel NLASSTFLE. An assessment of statin safety by hepatologists. Am J Cardiol. 2006;97(8A):77C–81.
59. Chapman MJ. Pharmacology of fenofibrate. Am J Med. 1987;83(5B):21–5.
60. Attman PO, Samuelsson O. Dyslipidemia of kidney disease. Curr Opin Lipidol. 2009;20(4):293–9.
61. Jun M, Foote C, Lv J, Neal B, Patel A, Nicholls SJ, et al. Effects of fibrates on cardiovascular outcomes: a systematic review and meta-analysis. Lancet. 2010;375(9729):1875–84.
62. Keech A, Simes RJ, Barter P, Best J, Scott R, Taskinen MR, et al. Effects of long-term fenofibrate therapy on cardiovascular events in 9795 people with type 2 diabetes mellitus (the FIELD study): randomised controlled trial. Lancet. 2005;366(9500):1849–61.
63. Tanaka Y, Kume S, Araki S, Isshiki K, Chin-Kanasaki M, Sakaguchi M, et al. Fenofibrate, a PPARα agonist, has renoprotective effects in mice by enhancing renal lipolysis. Kidney Int. 2011;79(8):871–82.
64. Shin SJ, Lim JH, Chung S, Youn DY, Chung HW, Kim HW, et al. Peroxisome proliferator-activated receptor-alpha activator fenofibrate prevents high-fat diet-induced renal lipotoxicity in spontaneously hypertensive rats. Hypertens Res. 2009;32(10):835–45.
65. Tonelli M, Collins D, Robins S, Bloomfield H, Curhan GC, Veterans' Affairs High-Density Lipoprotein Intervention Trial (VA-HIT) Investigators. Gemfibrozil for secondary prevention of cardiovascular events in mild to moderate chronic renal insufficiency. Kidney Int. 2004;66(3):1123–30.
66. Tonelli M, Collins D, Robins S, Bloomfield H, Curhan GC. Effect of gemfibrozil on change in renal function in men with moderate chronic renal insufficiency and coronary disease. Am J Kidney Dis. 2004;44(5):832–9.

67. Ting RD, Keech AC, Drury PL, Donoghoe MW, Hedley J, Jenkins AJ, et al. Benefits and safety of long-term fenofibrate therapy in people with type 2 diabetes and renal impairment: the FIELD study. Diabetes Care. 2012;35(2):218–25.
68. Makówka A, Dryja P, Chwatko G, Bald E, Nowicki M. Treatment of chronic hemodialysis patients with low-dose fenofibrate effectively reduces plasma lipids and affects plasma redox status. Lipids Health Dis. 2012;11:47.
69. Jun M, Zhu B, Tonelli M, Jardine MJ, Patel A, Neal B, et al. Effects of fibrates in kidney disease: a systematic review and meta-analysis. J Am Coll Cardiol. 2012;60(20):2061–71.
70. Davidson MH, Armani A, McKenney JM, Jacobson TA. Safety considerations with fibrate therapy. Am J Cardiol. 2007;99(6A):3C–18.
71. Wu J, Song Y, Li H, Chen J. Rhabdomyolysis associated with fibrate therapy: review of 76 published cases and a new case report. Eur J Clin Pharmacol. 2009;65(12):1169–74.
72. Broeders N, Knoop C, Antoine M, Tielemans C, Abramowicz D. Fibrate-induced increase in blood urea and creatinine: is gemfibrozil the only innocuous agent? Nephrol Dial Transplant. 2000;15(12):1993–9.
73. Mychaleckyj JC, Craven T, Nayak U, Buse J, Crouse JR, Elam M, et al. Reversibility of fenofibrate therapy-induced renal function impairment in ACCORD type 2 diabetic participants. Diabetes Care. 2012;35(5):1008–14.
74. Liang CC, Wang IK, Kuo HL, Yeh HC, Lin HH, Liu YL, et al. Long-term use of fenofibrate is associated with increased prevalence of gallstone disease among patients undergoing maintenance hemodialysis. Ren Fail. 2011;33(5):489–93.
75. Altmann SW, Davis HR, Zhu LJ, Yao X, Hoos LM, Tetzloff G, et al. Niemann-Pick C1 Like 1 protein is critical for intestinal cholesterol absorption. Science. 2004;303(5661):1201–4.
76. Dujovne CA, Ettinger MP, McNeer JF, Lipka LJ, LeBeaut AP, Suresh R, et al. Efficacy and safety of a potent new selective cholesterol absorption inhibitor, ezetimibe, in patients with primary hypercholesterolemia. Am J Cardiol. 2002;90(10):1092–7.
77. Landray M, Baigent C, Leaper C, Adu D, Altmann P, Armitage J, et al. The second United Kingdom Heart and Renal Protection (UK-HARP-II) study: a randomized controlled study of the biochemical safety and efficacy of adding ezetimibe to simvastatin as initial therapy among patients with CKD. Am J Kidney Dis. 2006;47(3):385–95.
78. Nakamura T, Sato E, Fujiwara N, Kawagoe Y, Ueda Y, Suzuki T, et al. Co-administration of ezetimibe enhances proteinuria-lowering effects of pitavastatin in chronic kidney disease patients partly via a cholesterol-independent manner. Pharmacol Res. 2010;61(1):58–61.
79. Buchanan C, Smith L, Corbett J, Nelson E, Shihab F. A retrospective analysis of ezetimibe treatment in renal transplant recipients. Am J Transplant. 2006;6(4):770–4.
80. Rodríguez-Ferrero ML, Anaya F. Ezetimibe in the treatment of uncontrolled hyperlipidemia in kidney transplant patients. Transplant Proc. 2008;40(10):3492–5.
81. Kohnle M, Pietruck F, Kribben A, Philipp T, Heemann U, Witzke O. Ezetimibe for the treatment of uncontrolled hypercholesterolemia in patients with high-dose statin therapy after renal transplantation. Am J Transplant. 2006;6(1):205–8.
82. Türk TR, Voropaeva E, Kohnle M, Nürnberger J, Philipp T, Kribben A, et al. Ezetimibe treatment in hypercholesterolemic kidney transplant patients is safe and effective and reduces the decline of renal allograft function: a pilot study. Nephrol Dial Transplant. 2008;23(1):369–73.
83. Slim H, Thompson PD. Ezetimibe-related myopathy: a systematic review. J Clin Lipidol. 2008;2(5):328–34.
84. Gille A, Bodor ET, Ahmed K, Offermanns S. Nicotinic acid: pharmacological effects and mechanisms of action. Annu Rev Pharmacol Toxicol. 2008;48:79–106.
85. Capuzzi DM, Guyton JR, Morgan JM, Goldberg AC, Kreisberg RA, Brusco OA, et al. Efficacy and safety of an extended-release niacin (Niaspan): a long-term study. Am J Cardiol. 1998;82(12A):74U–81U; discussion 5U–6U.
86. Insull W, McGovern ME, Schrott H, Thompson P, Crouse JR, Zieve F, et al. Efficacy of extended-release niacin with lovastatin for hypercholesterolemia: assessing all reasonable doses with innovative surface graph analysis. Arch Intern Med. 2004;164(10):1121–7.

87. Cho KH, Kim HJ, Kamanna VS, Vaziri ND. Niacin improves renal lipid metabolism and slows progression in chronic kidney disease. Biochim Biophys Acta. 2010;1800(1):6–15.
88. Cho KH, Kim HJ, Rodriguez-Iturbe B, Vaziri ND. Niacin ameliorates oxidative stress, inflammation, proteinuria, and hypertension in rats with chronic renal failure. Am J Physiol Renal Physiol. 2009;297(1):F106–13.
89. Restrepo Valencia CA, Cruz J. [Safety and effectiveness of nicotinic acid in the management of patients with chronic renal disease and hyperlipidemia associated to hyperphosphatemia]. Nefrologia. 2008;28(1):61–6.
90. Gibbons LW, Gonzalez V, Gordon N, Grundy S. The prevalence of side effects with regular and sustained-release nicotinic acid. Am J Med. 1995;99(4):378–85.
91. Out C, Groen AK, Brufau G. Bile acid sequestrants: more than simple resins. Curr Opin Lipidol. 2012;23(1):43–55.
92. Hou R, Goldberg AC. Lowering low-density lipoprotein cholesterol: statins, ezetimibe, bile acid sequestrants, and combinations: comparative efficacy and safety. Endocrinol Metab Clin North Am. 2009;38(1):79–97.
93. Kshirsagar AV, Shoham DA, Bang H, Hogan SL, Simpson RJ, Colindres RE. The effect of cholesterol reduction with cholestyramine on renal function. Am J Kidney Dis. 2005;46(5):812–9.
94. Jacobson TA, Armani A, McKenney JM, Guyton JR. Safety considerations with gastrointestinally active lipid-lowering drugs. Am J Cardiol. 2007;99(6A):47C–55.

Chapter 5
CVD in CKD: Focus on the Dyslipidemia Problem

Theodoros Kassimatis and David Goldsmith

Introduction

Recent data indicate that the burden of chronic kidney disease (CKD) is steadily increasing in the United States [1]. Cardiovascular (CV) disease (CVD) is the leading cause of morbidity and mortality in patients with CKD [2]. Both decreased glomerular filtration rate (GFR) and increased proteinuria are independent CV risk factors in community-based populations as well as in patients at high CV risk [3–5]. Notably, CVD-associated mortality rates increase progressively with increasing CKD stages and are extremely high in end-stage renal disease (ESRD) patients receiving dialysis (10–30 times higher than age-adjusted CV mortality in the general population) [5–7]. It has been reported that 39 % of incident dialysis patients have ischemic heart disease [8], whereas the annual rate of myocardial infarction and/or angina is approximately 10 % [9]. It is well established that dyslipidemias play a pivotal role in the pathogenesis of CVD in the general population [10]. However, the association of dyslipidemia and CVD in CKD patients is confounded by the presence of the so-called non-traditional CV risk factors (inflammation, vascular calcification, anemia, increased oxidative stress, and endothelial dysfunction), rendering the answer to the question of whether and which CKD patients might benefit from lipid-lowering treatments of major importance [11].

T. Kassimatis, M.D., Ph.D. (✉)
Nephrology Department, Asklepieion General Hospital, Vasileos Pavlou 1, Athens 16673, Greece
e-mail: tkassimatis@yahoo.gr

D. Goldsmith, M.A., M.B., B.Chir. F.R.C.P. (Lond.), F.R.C.P. (Edin.), F.A.S.N., F.E.R.A.
Renal Department, Guy's Hospital London, 6th Floor Borough Wing, London SE1 9RT, UK

A. Covic et al. (eds.), *Dyslipidemias in Kidney Disease*, DOI 10.1007/978-1-4939-0515-7_5,

Table 5.1 The five stages of CKD as defined by the National Kidney Foundation

Stage	Description	GFR (mL/min/1.73 m^2)
1	Kidney damage with normal or ↑GFR	≥90
2	Kidney damage with mildly ↓GFR	60–89
3	Moderately ↓GFR	30–59
4	Severely ↓GFR	15–29
5	Kidney failure	<15 or dialysis

Reprinted from the American Journal of Kidney Diseases, 39/2 (Suppl 1), K/DOQI clinical practice guidelines for chronic kidney disease: evaluation, classification, and stratification, S1–266, Copyright 2002, with permission from Elsevier

Definition and Classification of CKD

CKD is defined based on the presence of either kidney damage (structural or functional abnormalities other than decreased GFR) or decreased kidney function (GFR <60 mL/min/1.73 m^2) for 3 or more months, irrespective of cause. Kidney damage refers to pathologic abnormalities detected by a renal biopsy or imaging studies, urinary albumin excretion >30 mg/day, urinary sediment abnormalities, or renal transplant status. Decreased kidney function refers to a decreased GFR, which is usually estimated (eGFR) using serum creatinine and one of several available equations such as the Modification of Diet in Renal Disease (MDRD) and, more recently, the CKD-Epi formula [12]. The definition and classification of CKD were introduced by the National Kidney Foundation (NKF) Kidney Disease Outcomes Initiative (KDOQI) in 2002 [13] and adopted with minor changes by the international guideline group Kidney Disease Improving Global Outcomes (KDIGO) in 2004 [14]. Until recently, staging of CKD was based on eGFR and a five-stage classification was used (Table 5.1). This classification has been recently modified to an 18-stage classification by adding albuminuria stage, subdivision of stage 3, and the cause of CKD (Table 5.2) [5, 15]. By using this modified 18-stage classification, an improved stratification of CKD progression and its major complications has been achieved, thus providing a better guidance for the monitoring and management of CKD patients. However, as most studies have been based on the original classification, we will refer to this one in this chapter.

Association Between CKD and CVD-Epidemiological Data

It is well established that CV mortality rates increase dramatically with advanced CKD stages. In fact, individuals with CKD are more likely to die of CVD than to develop ESRD [6, 16]. Intriguingly, younger ESRD patients (25–34 years old) exhibit 500-fold greater CV mortality rates than age-matched controls with normal renal function [6]. Accumulating evidence suggests that the link between CKD and increased CV morbidity and mortality holds across populations with various degrees of baseline renal function or CV status.

Table 5.2 Revised chronic kidney disease staging

GFR categories		GFR (mL/min/1.73 m^2)		Terms
G1		>90		Normal or high
G2		60–89		Mildly decreased
G3a		45–59		Mildly to moderately decreased
G3b		30–44		Moderately to severely decreased
G4		15–29		Severely decreased
G5		<15		Kidney failure
		ACR (approximate equivalent)		
Albuminuria categories	AER (mg/24 h)	(mg/mmol)	(mg/g)	Terms
A1	<30	<3	<30	Normal to mildly increased
A2	30–300	3–30	30–300	Moderately increased
A3	>300	>30	>300	Severely increased (including nephrotic syndrome)

Adapted from [15]. KDIGO revised classification also includes CKD cause
GFR glomerular filtration rate, *AER* albumin excretion rate, *ACR* albumin-to-creatinine ratio

In the General Population

There are plenty of observations that demonstrate an independent association between diminished GFR or proteinuria and major adverse CV events (MACE) in the general population [17–21].

In a high-quality meta-analysis of general population cohorts including 105,872 participants with urine albumin-to-creatinine ratio (ACR) measurements and 1,128,310 participants with urine protein dipstick measurements, followed for 7.9 years, Matsushita et al. concluded that eGFR less than 60 mL/min/1.73 m^2 and ACR 1.1 mg/mmol (10 mg/g) or more independently predict all cause and CV mortality risk in the general population. In studies with dipstick measurement of proteinuria, a trace urine-positive dipstick was also associated with increased all-cause and CV mortality independently of the level of kidney function [19].

Go et al. evaluated 1,120,295 subjects for the risk of death, CV events, and hospitalization relative to various levels of GFR over 2.84 years [22]. The adjusted hazard ratio for death was 1.2 with an eGFR of 45–59 mL/min/1.73 m^2 (95 % CI, 1.1–1.2), 1.8 with an eGFR of 30–44 mL/min/1.73 m^2 (95 % CI, 1.7–1.9), 3.2 with an eGFR of 15–29 mL/min/1.73 m^2 (95 % CI, 3.1–3.4), and 5.9 with an estimated GFR of less than 15 mL/min/1.73 m^2 (95 % CI, 5.4–6.5). The adjusted hazard ratio for CV events also increased inversely with the estimated GFR: 1.4 (95 % CI, 1.4–1.5), 2.0 (95 % CI, 1.9–2.1), 2.8 (95 % CI, 2.6–2.9), and 3.4 (95 % CI, 3.1–3.8), respectively. This large study demonstrated effectively the inverse association between GFR and rates of CV morbidity and mortality in patients without a prior history of CVD.

Weiner at al. pooled data from community-based trials including the Atherosclerosis Risk in Communities Study, CV Health Study, Framingham Heart

Study, and Framingham Offspring Study; 22,634 subjects were followed for 10 years. CKD was defined by a GFR between 15 and 60 mL/min/1.73 m^2. A composite of myocardial infarction, fatal coronary heart disease (CHD), stroke, and death was the primary study outcome. In adjusted analyses, CKD was an independent risk factor for the composite study outcome (hazard ratio, 1.19; 95 % CI, 1.07–1.32) [21].

In Patients with CV Risk Factors or Preexistent CVD

A growing number of studies have shown an association between the decrease in GFR and CV events among patients with known risk factors for CVD or preexistent CVD [2, 4, 23–28]. Van der Velde et al. performed a collaborative meta-analysis of ten cohorts with 266,975 patients with a history of hypertension, diabetes, or CV disease. Hazard ratios for CV mortality at eGFRs of 60, 45, and 15 mL/min/1.73 m^2 were 1.11, 1.73, and 3.08, respectively, compared to an eGFR of 95 mL/min/1.73 m^2, whereas similar findings were noted for all-cause mortality. There was also an association between albuminuria and risk for overall and CV mortality. The authors concluded that decreased eGFR and higher albuminuria are risk factors for all-cause and CV mortality in high-risk populations, independent of each other and of CV risk factors.

Mann et al. performed a post hoc analysis of the Heart Outcomes and Prevention Evaluation (HOPE) study [29]. The HOPE study included individuals with an objective evidence of vascular disease or diabetes combined with another CV risk factor and was designed to test the benefit of add-on ramipril vs. placebo. Nine hundred and eighty subjects with mild renal insufficiency (serum creatinine $\geq$ 1.4 mg/dL) and 8,307 subjects with normal renal function (serum creatinine < 1.4 mg/dL) were followed for $\approx$5 years. The cumulative incidence of the primary outcome (composite of CV death, myocardial infarction, or stroke) was significantly higher in individuals with mild renal insufficiency compared to those with normal renal function ($P<0.001$).

Perkovic et al. in the Perindopril Protection against Recurrent Stroke Study (PROGRESS) randomly allocated 6,105 participants with cerebrovascular disease to perindopril-based blood pressure-lowering therapy or placebo. Individuals with CKD were at approximately 1.5-fold greater risk of major vascular events, stroke, and CHD, and were more than twice as likely to die (all $P\leq 0.002$).

With respect to the relationship between albuminuria and CKD in patients with CV risk factors or preexistent CKD, Anavekar et al. [30] in a post hoc analysis of the Irbesartan Diabetic Nephropathy Trial (IDNT) showed that the proportion of patients who exhibited the CV composite endpoint (CV death, nonfatal MI, hospitalization for heart failure, stroke, amputation, and coronary and peripheral revascularization) increased progressively with increasing quartiles of baseline urine ACR. This result was confirmed by a multivariate analysis in which albuminuria was an independent risk factor for CV events with a 1.3-fold increased relative risk for each natural log increase of 1 U in urine ACR. In the IDNT study 1,715 subjects with type-2 diabetes, hypertension, and macroalbuminuria were randomized to irbesartan, amlodipine, or placebo for a mean period of 2.6 years. The patients had mean urine ACR of 1,416.2 mg/g. Moreover, the HOPE study investigators evaluated the risk of CV events associated with baseline microalbuminuria (defined as ACR > 2.0 mg/mmol (equivalent to 17.7 mg/g)). In the overall population, microalbuminuria at baseline approximately doubled the relative risk of the primary composite outcome (myocardial infarction, stroke, or CV death), and this effect was significant in both diabetics (relative risk, 1.97) and nondiabetics (relative risk, 1.61) [31]. Moreover, albuminuria was a continuous risk factor for CV events even below the level of microalbuminuria.

Future CV risk in the general population can be modeled in various ways, one typical approach being the Framingham score (though QRISK and other algorithms may be much superior especially for diverse populations). It has been shown that the Framingham score demonstrates poor overall accuracy in predicting cardiac events in individuals with CKD [32], and this might be due to the increased CV and overall mortality rates in these patients. Modification of the Framingham equations might improve their predictive accuracy, yet new models evaluating CV risk in this population should be developed.

Cardiovascular Risk Factors in CKD: The Role of Dyslipidemia

Evidence that reduced GFR and increased albuminuria independently and continuously predict higher CV event rates in CKD patients with or without preexistent CVD, prompts for the early detection and abrogation of the responsible factors that predispose these patients to the development of CVD. Apart from the traditional CV risk factors that are defined by epidemiological studies such as the Framingham study and are present in the general population, CKD patients also exhibit a variety of non-traditional risk factors that accelerate and aggravate the development of CVD in this population.

Traditional risk factors include smoking, diabetes, hypertension, left ventricular hypertrophy (LVH), older age, and hyperlipidemia. These factors are highly prevalent in the CKD setting [33], and they tend to increase the risk of CVD in early CKD stages [34]. Moreover, metabolic syndrome, a condition characterized by insulin resistance, elevated serum glucose, hypertension, abdominal obesity, and dyslipidemia, might also play a role in the development of CVD. This syndrome is also frequently detected in patients with CKD [35].

Although hypercholesterolemia is one of the most widely recognized CV risk factors in the general population as well as in patients with preexistent CVD [10, 36–39], this association in CKD has been difficult to establish. In fact, some studies have shown that low cholesterol levels associate with increased mortality in dialysis patients [11, 40, 41], whereas another study failed to detect any association between hyperlipidemia and mortality in nondiabetic stage 3–4 CKD patients [42]. However, this reverse epidemiology of lower cholesterol predicting a higher mortality is likely due to cholesterol-lowering effect of malnutrition and systemic inflammation, both present in CKD patients [11, 43]. Furthermore, the presence of numerous non-traditional risk factors in the CKD setting further confounds the association of CKD and CVD, thus increasing the prevalence of CVD even in patients with mild to moderate CKD [44]. These factors include increased oxidative stress, amplified inflammatory status, anemia, abnormalities in mineral-bone metabolism, endothelial dysfunction, and reduced nitric oxide (NO) activity [45–48].

The role of oxidative stress and inflammation in the development of CVD in CKD has recently been increasingly supported. In patients with CKD the balance between the production of reactive oxygen species (ROS)/free radicals (FR) and antioxidant defenses is shifted towards amplified oxidative stress. The increase in ROS/FR is caused by numerous factors such as uremic toxins, diabetes mellitus, chronic inflammation, and the dialysis treatments per se [49, 50]. Oxidative stress in uremia can be increased through activation of various ROS-producing enzymatic systems such as the reduced nicotinamide adenine dinucleotide (NAD(P)H) oxidase, xanthine oxidase, uncoupled endothelial NO synthase, and myeloperoxidase (MPO) [51, 52]. Among them, NAD(P)H oxidase seems to be the most important source of oxidative stress in vessels [53], whereas MPO, an enzymatic constituent of neutrophils and macrophages, is also highly expressed in atheromatic lesions [54]. MPO might also play a role in accelerated atherosclerosis in dialysis patients as it has been reported to be released from white blood cells during hemodialysis. Oxidative modification of macromolecules such as lipids, proteins, and nucleic acids results in structural and functional changes and accelerates atherosclerosis. In this regard, elevated plasma levels of oxidized low-density lipoprotein (LDL) have been shown to correlate with CHD [55]. Patients with CKD have increased levels of oxidized LDL [56].

Increased oxidative stress also induces the expression of inflammatory biomarkers. In this regard, both CKD and ESRD are characterized by elevated levels of inflammatory markers such as C-reactive protein (CRP), an acute phase protein reactant, TNF-α, IL-6, fibrinogen, factors VIIc and VIIIc, and the adhesion molecules VCAM-1 and ICAM-1 [57–59]. In the MDRD study elevated levels of CRP [60] were associated with an increased risk of all-cause and CV mortality in stage 3 and 4 CKD patients. Moreover, in dialysis patients increased levels of CRP and IL-6 have been associated with a significant increased risk of sudden cardiac death independently of traditional CVD risk factors [47, 61].

Endothelial dysfunction, which is present in CKD, is an important early event in the pathogenesis of atherosclerosis, contributing to plaque initiation and progression [62]. Microalbuminuria might be a manifestation of impaired endothelial function [63], thus explaining the link between microalbuminuria and increased CV morbidity and mortality reported in many epidemiology studies (see section on "Association Between CKD and CVD-Epidemiological Data"). Reduced NO production seems to be the main culprit for the endothelial dysfunction observed in CKD [64, 65]. In hemodialysis patients, increased levels of asymmetrical dimethylarginine (ADMA), an endogenous inhibitor of NO synthase, have been reported and independently predict overall mortality and CV outcomes [66].

Moreover, in patients with mild to advanced CKD, ADMA level is inversely related to GFR and represents an independent risk factor for progression to ESRD and mortality [67]. ADMA, now considered one of the strongest markers of atherosclerosis [68], is increased under inflammatory conditions and might serve as a link between inflammation and endothelial dysfunction [69]. Finally, the term protein-energy wasting (PEW) has been recently introduced to describe the role of malnutrition, inflammation, and atherosclerosis on the increased mortality observed in patients with ESRD [46, 70].

Yet, it should be noted that the exact pathomechanisms by which these nontraditional risk factors contribute to the development of CVD are still unclear, and various studies report contradictory results. In this regard, although the aforementioned studies demonstrated a positive association between elevated levels of CRP [60] and adverse CV outcomes, no such relationship was detected in the Irbesartan for Diabetic nephropathy trial [71]. Similarly, although coronary artery calcification, which is a frequent finding in CKD patients, has been linked to abnormalities in mineral-bone metabolism [72], studies evaluating the associations between parathyroid hormone, calcium, and phosphorus with coronary artery calcification report conflicting results [73, 74].

Characteristics of Dyslipidemia in CKD

Multiple lipoprotein abnormalities are detected in CKD patients caused by a profound dysregulation in their metabolism (Table 5.3). The primary characteristic of dyslipidemia in CKD is hypertriglyceridemia, with 40–50 % of CKD patients having fasting triglyceride levels greater than 200 mg/dL. Of note, the lipid profile of

Table 5.3 Features of lipid fractions and the enzymes implicated in their metabolism in CKD

	Predialysis CKD (stages I–IV)	Hemodialysis	Nephrotic syndrome	Peritoneal dialysis
Triglycerides	↔ or ↑	↑	↑	↑
Total cholesterol	↓ or ↔ or ↑	↔ or ↓	↑	↑
LDL cholesterol	↓ or ↔ or ↑	↔ or ↓	↑	↑
HDL cholesterol	↓ or ↔	↓	↓ or ↔ or ↑	↓
Small dense LDL	↑	↑	↑	↑
Lipoprotein a	↑	↑	↑	↑
LPL activity	↓	↓	↓	↓
Hepatic lipase activity	↓	↓	↓	↓
LCAT activity	↓	↓	↓	↓

CKD chronic kidney disease, *LDL* low-density lipoprotein, *HDL* high-density lipoprotein, *LPL* lipoprotein lipase, *LCAT* lecithin cholesterol acyltransferase, ↓ decrease, ↔ no change, ↑ increase

patients with CKD depends on CKD stage, the presence or not of nephrotic syndrome, and the dialysis modality for ESRD patients [75]. In this regard, apart from the increased triglycerides, in patients with stage 5 CKD total serum cholesterol and LDL are normal or low, whereas high-density lipoprotein (HDL) is decreased [76, 77]. Patients with stage 1–4 CKD might exhibit increased total cholesterol and LDL cholesterol, whereas nephrotic patients are usually characterized by a marked increase in total cholesterol and LDL levels with cholesterol being directly correlated with the degree of albuminuria and indirectly with serum albumin level [78]. Finally, peritoneal dialysis patients are characterized by increased protein losses in the peritoneal fluid effluent, a condition mimicking the nephrotic syndrome [79]. These losses might induce the hepatic production of albumin and lipoproteins, resulting in elevated concentrations of total cholesterol, LDL, and a modified highly atherogenic form of LDL, lipoprotein (a) (Lp(a)) [80, 81]. Moreover, increased insulin levels, which is a consequence of the absorption of glucose from the dialysis fluid, may induce the hepatic synthesis of very low-density lipoprotein (VLDL) and possibly Lp(a) [82].

It should be noted that in CKD, apart from lipoproteins assessed in every day clinical practice, a variety of not routinely measured highly atherogenic lipoprotein fragments accumulate. These include chylomicron remnants, VLDL remnants or intermediate-density lipoproteins (IDL), oxidized LDL, small dense-LDL (sd-LDL), and Lp(a) [75]. The former two are products of chylomicron and VLDL metabolism whose clearance is impaired in CKD. These lipoproteins are prone to oxidization, a process that further increases their atherogenic potential. In fact, Shoji et al. showed that among LDL, HDL, VLDL, IDL, and Lp(a), IDL was the lipoprotein fraction more closely associated with aortic sclerosis in hemodialysis patients [83]. Moreover, chylomicron remnants potentiated endothelium-dependent arterial contraction [84], whereas oxidized VLDL remnants significantly enhanced macrophage cholesterol ester accumulation compared to either VLDL remnants, or oxidized LDL in experimental models of atherosclerosis [85]. It is well known that most clinical trials evaluating the role of lipid-lowering treatments in CKD patients do not assess these lipoprotein fractions, and this might be an explanation for the reported negative results.

In CKD there is an impairment in the distribution of LDL subclasses favoring the predominance of sd-LDL particles [86, 87] (see Table 5.3). These electronegative particles penetrate the endothelial barrier easier than large LDL particles and interact with electropositive intimal proteoglycans [88]. This interaction prolongs their retention in the arterial wall, thus rendering them more susceptible to oxidization by ROS. Indeed, sd-LDL particles appear to be more atherogenic than larger LDL fragments [89, 90]. The effect of the routinely administered lipid-lowering agents, statins on sd-LDL in CKD patients, remains unclear. Of note, a recent study reported that statins decrease sd-LDL in peritoneal dialysis patients but not in hemodialysis patients [91]. Apart from oxidization, under the uremic milieu, LDL also undergoes protein carbamylation. This process has been reported to increase the atherogenic potential of LDL through multiple mechanisms, including the proliferation of smooth muscle cells [92].

Elevated plasma levels of Lp(a) have been detected in patients with CKD [93] (see Table 5.3). Moreover, Lp(a) is now recognized as a risk factor for CV morbidity and mortality in hemodialysis patients [94, 95]. Lp(a) is a modified form of LDL emerging from the covalent binding of apolipoprotein(a) to apolipoprotein B through disulfide linkage [96]. In the general population, elevated serum Lp(a), has been recognized as a risk factor for CVD, whereas the association between Lp(a) and CHD risk seem to be continuous [97, 98]. Lp(a) excess is frequently detected in patients with premature CHD [99], and its levels are also associated with cerebrovascular disease, especially in men [100]. Because of its structural similarity to plasminogen, it has been proposed that Lp(a) may promote thrombogenesis by inhibiting fibrinolysis [101]. Moreover, Lp(a) is capable of binding to macrophage receptors, thus promoting foam cell formation and accelerating atherosclerosis [102]. Lp(a) also enhances LDL susceptibility to oxidization [55] and promotes monocyte attachment to vascular endothelial cells by increasing endothelial ICAM-1 expression [103]. Serum Lp(a) levels are genetically determined and are mostly due to polymorphisms at the apo(a) gene (LPA gene) [104]. These polymorphisms account for a variety of sizes of apo(a) isoforms. An inverse association of the size of apo(a) isoforms and Lp(a) levels has been detected (i.e., subjects with low molecular weight isoforms have higher levels of Lp(a)) [104, 105]. Intriguingly, in dialysis patients, small apo(a) isoform size but not Lp(a) level has been identified as an independent predictor of total and CV mortality [106, 107]. There are no clinical trials evaluating the effects of therapeutic regimes targeting the reduction of Lp(a) on CV morbidity and mortality in the general population or in patients with CKD.

Disorders of VLDL and Chylomicron Metabolism in CKD

Hypertriglyceridemia in CKD is a consequence of impaired VLDL and chylomicron metabolism, which leads to diminished triglyceride clearance [108] (Fig. 5.1a, b). VLDL and chylomicrons are triglyceride-rich lipoproteins that deliver lipids to muscle and adipose tissue for energy production and storage, respectively. Nascent VLDL consists of a apoB100 lipoprotein core, to which cholesterol ester, triglycerides, and phospholipids are bound. Similarly, in nascent chylomicrons, these lipid fractions are packed in apo48. Both nascent VLDL and chylomicrons mature by receiving apoE and apoC from HDL-2. Endothelium-bound lipoprotein lipase (LPL) in the capillaries of skeletal muscle and adipose tissue is responsible for the hydrolysis of triglycerides of VLDL and chylomicron and the disposal of fatty acids to the adjacent myocytes and adipocytes. This process leads to the formation of VLDL remnants (IDL) and chylomicron remnants, which are subsequently cleared by the liver via LDL receptor-related protein (LRP) [109]. However, the bulk of IDL is converted to LDL after being enriched in cholesterol esters by cholesterol ester transfer protein (CETP) and then lysed by hepatic lipase. LDL is then removed by LDL receptor in the hepatic cells. Finally, the fraction of VLDL that has not been lysed by LPL is cleared entirely by VLDL receptor in adipocytes and myocytes [110].

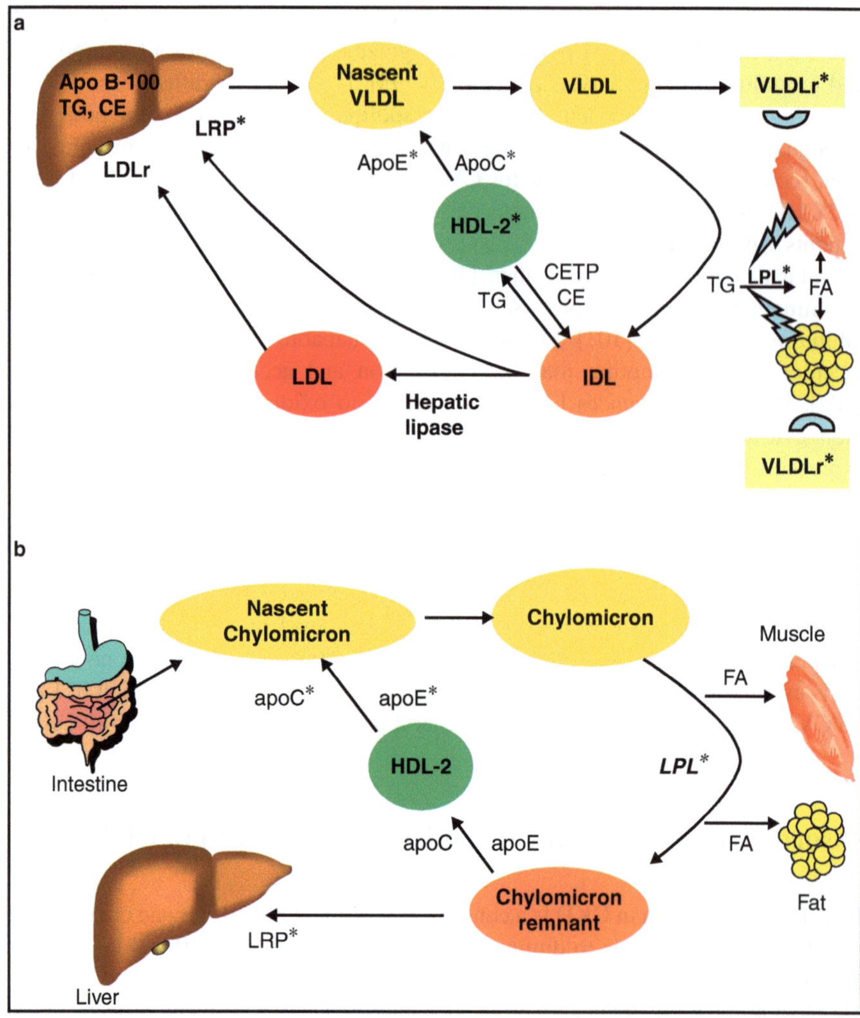

Fig. 5.1 VLDL (**a**) and chylomicron (**b**) metabolism. The *asterisk* (*) denotes downregulation. See text for details. Adapted from [108]

Impaired metabolism of VLDL in CKD is characterized by the downregulation of LPL, hepatic lipase, LPR, and VLDL receptor, leading to the accumulation of triglycerides, VLDL, and IDL and the triglyceride enrichment of LDL (see Fig. 5.1a, b and Table 5.3). In CKD an increase in plasma Apolipoprotein C-III (apoCIII), a potent inhibitor of LPL, has been reported [75]. ApoCIII and apo CII are important components of VLDL and chylomicrons, and apoCIII/apoCII ratio determines the ability of these lipoproteins to activate LPL. Moreover, in CKD-increased plasma levels of pre-β-HDL, an inhibitor of LPL has been reported [111]. Regular heparinization that occurs in dialysis patients might also result in the degradation of tissue-bound LPL [75].

Another mechanism involved in the impaired lipoprotein metabolism in CKD setting is the reduced expression and activity of hepatic lipase [112, 113]. As discussed earlier, hepatic lipase is responsible for the removal of almost all of the remaining triglycerides from IDL, a process crucial for its conversion to LDL. Therefore, hepatic lipase downregulation leads to the accumulation of IDL, triglyceride enrichment of LDL, and hypertriglyceridemia. Hepatic lipase as well as LPL activity might be diminished by calcium accumulation within liver and adipose tissue cells caused by secondary hyperparathyroidism, a common complication of CKD. Of note, parathyroidectomy can restore both hepatic lipase and LPL activity and plasma triglyceride levels in experimental animals and humans with CKD [114, 115]. Moreover, verapamil administration to rats with CKD prevented the development of hypertriglyceridemia and the reduction of hepatic lipase and LPL activity by reducing basal levels of cytosolic calcium [112].

CKD has also been reported to downregulate LRP, thus leading to the atherogenic chylomicron remnants and IDL accumulation [116]. The downregulation of VLDL receptors in the skeletal muscle, heart, and adipose tissue has also been reported in experimental animals with CKD, a condition leading to elevated VLDL and triglycerides [115, 117]. Finally, increased triglyceride synthesis might contribute to the hypertriglyceridemia observed in nephrotic patients and peritoneal dialysis patients but not in the remainder CKD population [118]. This is due to the upregulation of Acyl-CoA:diglycerol acyltransferase, an enzyme that catalyzes the conversion of diglyceride to triglyceride [119].

As discussed earlier, CKD is characterized by increased oxidative stress. In this environment chylomicron remnants, IDL, LDL, sd-LDL, and Lp(a) might undergo oxidization. These oxidized lipoproteins can bind to receptors on macrophages and trigger the release of pro-inflammatory cytokines thus amplifying the inflammatory status of CKD. The uptake of these lipoproteins by the scavenger receptors of arterial wall macrophages results in their transformation to foam cells, the hallmark of the atherosclerotic lesion. In this regard, increased scavenger receptor expression has been reported in CKD patients [120]. The formation of foam cells is also a consequence of impaired cholesterol export mechanisms (see section on "Disorders of HDL Metabolism in CKD"). LDL has also been reported to activate the renin–angiotensin system [121], leading to increased angiotensin II levels and the upregulation of the angiotensin type-I (AT1) receptor. Angiotensin II, in turn, acting through AT1 receptor, stimulates NAD(P)H oxidase and other enzymes, augmenting synthesis of the superoxide anion and proinflammatory mediators that result in endothelial dysfunction and atherosclerosis aggravation.

Disorders of HDL Metabolism in CKD

In CKD, impaired functionality and reduced levels of HDL have been reported [75]. Normally, HDL prevents atherosclerosis by various mechanisms [108, 122–125] (Fig. 5.2): (1) inhibits and reverses the oxidization of lipoproteins by its antioxidant enzyme constituents, paraoxonase-1 (PON-1) and glutathione peroxidase (GPX); (2)

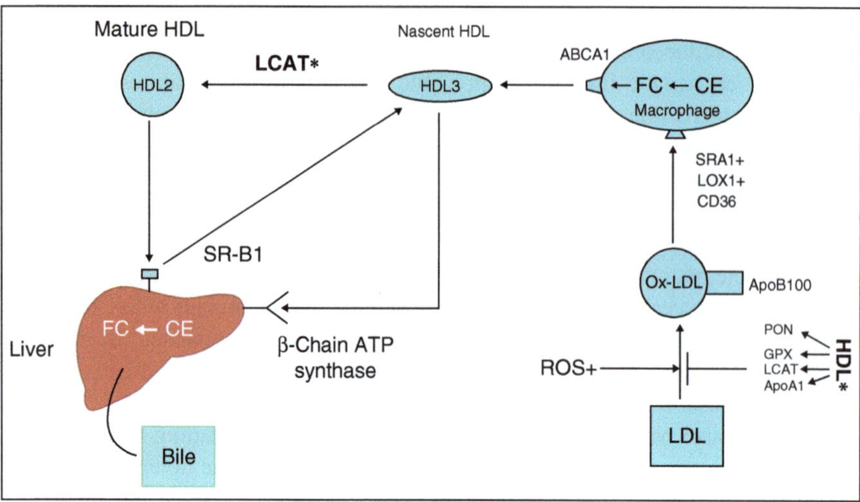

Fig. 5.2 Protective role of HDL against atherosclerosis. Reverse cholesterol pathway. The *asterisk* (*) denotes downregulation, whereas the *plus* (+) denotes elevation. See text for details. Adapted from [108]

removes oxidized phospholipids and endotoxins and disposes them to the liver via apoA1 and lecithin:cholesterol acyltransferase (LCAT); (3) improves endothelial function by inhibiting cellular adhesion molecule expression [126] and increasing eNOS production [127]; (4) reduces inflammation by alleviating oxidative stress and inhibiting cellular adhesion molecule expression; (5) transfers surplus cholesterol and phospholipids from the periphery to the liver (reverse cholesterol transport [RCT]); (6) contributes apoC and apoE to nascent VLDL and chylomicrons, thus facilitating their proper metabolism and removal; (7) facilitates the conversion of highly atherogenic oxidization-prone IDL to LDL via CETP-mediated exchange of cholesterol esters for triglycerides (indirect RCT); (8) exerts antithrombotic effects through its constituent platelet-activating factor (PAF) acetylhydrolase, which inactivates PAF, thus preventing platelet activation and thrombus formation.

RCT is a multiorgan, multistep process via which excess cholesterol is retrieved from lipid-laden macrophages in the peripheral tissue and then is transported to the liver, where it is processed and excreted in bile and intestine [108, 123, 128, 129] (see Fig. 5.2). Oxidized LDL and other atherogenic lipid fractions are internalized by vascular macrophages through scavenger receptors (SRA1 and LOX1). This leads to their transformation into foam cells and the acceleration of atherosclerosis. In RCT nascent (lipid-poor) HDL binds to ATP-binding cassette transporter type A1 (ABCA1) and ABCG1 on the macrophage cell membrane [123, 130]. Then free cholesterol is actively transferred to the surface of HDL where it is rapidly esterified by LCAT and then sequestered in the core of HDL (mature HDL). Of note, albumin has also been shown to play a role in transferring cellular-free cholesterol from peripheral tissues to the circulating nascent HDL via passive transportation [131]. Thereafter, mature HDL moves to the liver, where it binds to the HDL docking receptor SRB-1. SRB-1 facilitates the unloading of HDL's lipid content (cholesterol esters, triglycerides, and phospholipids) and subsequently HDL is released to the circulation as lipid-poor HDL to repeat the cycle [132].

CKD is associated with a reduction in serum apoA-I and apoA-II, which are mandatory components of the HDL particle [133, 134]. This mechanism might play a crucial role in the reduction of HDL levels detected in CKD patients. Hypoalbuminemia, which is a result of chronic inflammation, in CKD patients might also contribute to reduced HDL levels [77]. However, the main reason for the impaired HDL cholesterol enrichment and maturation in CKD is LCAT deficiency (see Fig. 5.2 and Table 5.3). LCAT deficiency is a result of decreased production by the liver [135]. LCAT deficiency, apart from preventing the maturation of HDL through the esterification of free cholesterol on its surface, also facilitates HDL degradation by the hepatic endocytic receptor (β-chain of ATP synthase). This receptor has higher affinity for the nascent HDL than the mature one, whereas SRB-1 has higher affinity for mature HDL and, as noted above, facilitates HDL cycle from the liver to peripheral tissues and does not degrade it. Apart from the reduced levels of HDL in CKD, there also seems to exist a decreased affinity to its ABCA-1 macrophage receptors due to its oxidization in the uremic milieu [136, 137]. Accumulating evidence also suggests that HDL under systemic oxidative and inflammatory conditions (as in CKD) might also transform and promote oxidative stress and inflammation [138, 139]. Thus, HDL oxidization might impair the maturation of HDL and RCT in general. As discussed earlier, by inhibiting the formation and increasing the disposal of oxidized lipids, HDL exerts both antioxidant and anti-inflammatory effects. It has been reported that in dialysis patients there is a significant reduction in paraoxonase and GPX [136]. Moreover, the expression of macrophage scavenger receptors SRA1 and LOX1 is upregulated in both experimental models and in patients with CKD, a process that seems to be induced by inflammatory cytokines and oxidized LDL [120, 140]. This, combined with apoA-1 reduction, limits the ability of HDL to prevent or reverse the oxidization of LDL and phospholipids, thus promoting an influx of oxidized LDL in macrophages in the artery wall and facilitating foam cell formation and atherosclerosis. In this context, HDL anti-inflammatory activity has been reported to decrease in the uremic plasma of dialysis patients [141]. Thus, it seems that HDL impaired anti-oxidant and anti-inflammatory properties are both a consequence and a cause of increased oxidative stress and inflammation observed in CKD.

Based on the evidence that HDL level is reduced in CKD patients, the design of treatment strategies targeted to increase HDL levels seems plausible. However, efforts to raise HDL in the clinical setting have unexpectedly resulted in unfavorable CV outcomes. CETP inhibitors are a novel class of compounds that are very effective in increasing plasma HDL [142]. However, despite a meaningful increase of plasma HDL, the administration of the CETP inhibitor torcetrapib was early terminated in patients at high risk of coronary events due to increased CV events and overall mortality [143]. This negative outcome was probably related to an off-target effect indicated by increased arterial blood pressure in the treatment group, although a possible torcetrapib adverse effect could not be ruled out. Moreover, in another RCT, torcetrapib failed to halt the progression of coronary atherosclerosis or improve carotid intimal thickness [144]. These discouragingly negative outcomes might be a result of the accumulation of the highly atherogenic IDL [145]. As discussed earlier, CETP plays a crucial role in the conversion of IDL to LDL by promoting the transfer of cholesterol esters from IDL to LDL in exchange of triglycerides [108]. Therefore, CETP inhibition might result in the accumulation of IDL and the acceleration of atherosclerosis, especially in CKD patients in whom IDL clearance is impaired due to LRP-1 and hepatic lipase deficiency. Moreover, neither low HDL nor high CETP activity was associated with CV events in hemodialysis patients over a 48-month observation period [146], implying that functional changes in HDL might play a more important role in atherosclerosis progression. Thus, in CKD, the absolute increase in HDL levels might not be enough to prevent CVD, as there also exist qualitative changes in the HDL molecule impairing its composition, maturation process, as well as its antioxidant and anti-inflammatory properties [136, 139, 147].

Pathophysiology of CVD in the General Population and in the CKD Setting

Atherosclerosis is a chronic, complex, and progressive inflammatory process of the vascular wall of large and medium-sized arteries. Although the exact pathomechanism of this process remains unclear, dyslipidemia and abnormal immune response to endothelial damage with inflammatory recruitment of monocytes and the formation of foam cells seem to play a central role in the development of the atherosclerotic lesions [148, 149]. The chronic inflammation of the vascular wall results in multifocal plaque development. Furthermore, intraplaque hemorrhage, lipid deposition, proliferation of neovessels, and plaque remodeling all contribute to atherosclerotic plaque formation [149, 150]. Although most plaques remain asymptomatic, some progress to luminal obstruction, whereas a few are vulnerable to thrombosis, leading to acute atherothrombotic events such as acute myocardial infarction and stroke [149, 151].

Intriguingly, the pathogenesis and, consequently, the pathologic findings of arterial lesions in CKD patients differ substantially from patients with preserved renal function with classic atherosclerotic disease. In the latter, arterial lesions consist of lipid-laden atheromatous or fibroatheromatous plaques, whereas in the former, atherosclerotic plaques are rich in calcium deposits and fibrous tissue and exhibit a prominent thickening of the intima and media of the vessel wall, resulting in lumen narrowing [152, 153]. Calcium deposition in CKD may occur in the intima (as in classic atherosclerotic plaques) or in the medial layer, where it increases vascular stiffness as well as in cardiac valves [154]. In fact, coronary artery calcification has been reported to be significantly more frequent in predialysis patients compared with matched control subjects with no renal impairment (40 % vs. 13 %) [155]. The calcium content of atherosclerotic lesions in advanced CKD stages is in some occasions so high that many of these patients' vessels can be readily delineated on simple plain radiograms. The most devastating demonstration of vascular calcification presented in dialysis patients is calciphylaxis or calcific uremic arteriopathy. This life-threatening condition is characterized by extensive microvascular calcification accompanied by intimal proliferation and thrombosis leading to non-healing skin ulcers, necrosis, secondary infection, and sepsis [156]. Although the exact pathomechanisms contributing to vascular calcification remain unclear, elevated calcium (Ca) × phosphate (P) product facilitating the precipitation of Ca and P along with the induction of calcification promoters and the reduction of calcification inhibitors seem to play a major role in this process [157, 158]. Under these conditions, vascular smooth muscle cells acquire an osteoblast phenotype, thus promoting hydroxyapatite formation in the media resulting in vascular calcification. Vascular calcification promotes vascular stiffening. Aortic stiffening combined with anemia and hypertension, which are common in CKD patients, result in the development of LVH. The combination of LVH and tissue calcification may result in myocardial fibrosis and conduction abnormalities that predispose to potentially lethal arrhythmias [152, 153, 159]. Indeed, arrhythmias or cardiac arrest seem to be more common death causes in CKD patients (they account for approximately 60 % of all cardiac deaths in dialysis patients) than myocardial infarction or stroke, which represent typical atherosclerotic diseases [160].

Conclusion

It is well established that reduced GFR and albuminuria predict CV event rates in a continuous and independent manner. This relation between CVD and CKD, apart from the presence of non-traditional CV risk factors such as oxidative stress and inflammation, which are prominent in CKD, has also been attributed to the substantial variations of lipid abnormalities and dyslipidemia characteristics in CKD. Indeed, hypertriglyceridemia is the hallmark of CKD dyslipidemia, whereas total and LDL cholesterol are normal or low. Moreover, a variety of highly atherogenic lipoprotein fragments, which are minimally affected by classic lipid-lowering treatments, such as chylomicron remnants, IDL, sd-LDL, oxidized LDL, and Lp(α), are present in CKD, further aggravating atherosclerotic lesions. Finally, the pathogenesis of arterial lesions in CKD differs substantially from the pathogenesis of classical atherosclerotic disease. In this regard, calcium-rich atherosclerotic plaques with prominent thickening of the intima and media of the vessel wall are the pathologic hallmarks of CKD atherosclerotic lesions, whereas lipid-laden atheromatous or fibroatheromatous plaques are detected in classic atherosclerotic disease. Therefore, it is not surprising that lipid-lowering strategies alone seem to have no meaningful effect in ameliorating CVD in CKD patients, especially in those with advanced renal failure [161, 162]. Thus, an adequately designed therapeutic regime apart from modifying lipoprotein levels (i.e., by the use of a statin) should also probably include agents that reduce oxidative stress, inflammation, and vascular calcification. Therefore, combined treatments targeted at inhibiting or reversing multilevel pathogenetic mechanisms responsible for CVD in CKD will pave the way for the effective management of dyslipidemia and CVD in this fragile population.

References

1. Coresh J, Selvin E, Stevens LA, Manzi J, Kusek JW, Eggers P, et al. Prevalence of chronic kidney disease in the United States. JAMA. 2007;298(17):2038–47. PubMed PMID: 17986697.
2. Foley RN, Collins AJ. End-stage renal disease in the United States: an update from the United States Renal Data System. J Am Soc Nephrol. 2007;18(10):2644–8. PubMed PMID: 17656472.
3. Leoncini G, Viazzi F, Pontremoli R. Overall health assessment: a renal perspective. Lancet. 2010;375(9731):2053–4. PubMed PMID: 20483450. Epub 2010/05/21.eng.
4. van der Velde M, Matsushita K, Coresh J, Astor BC, Woodward M, Levey A, et al. Lower estimated glomerular filtration rate and higher albuminuria are associated with all-cause and cardiovascular mortality. A collaborative meta-analysis of high-risk population cohorts. Kidney Int. 2011;79(12):1341–52. PubMed PMID: 21307840. Epub 2011/02/11.eng.
5. Levey AS, de Jong PE, Coresh J, El Nahas M, Astor BC, Matsushita K, et al. The definition, classification, and prognosis of chronic kidney disease: a KDIGO Controversies Conference report. Kidney Int. 2011;80(1):17–28. PubMed PMID: 21150873. Epub 2010/12/15.eng.
6. Sarnak MJ, Levey AS, Schoolwerth AC, Coresh J, Culleton B, Hamm LL, et al. Kidney disease as a risk factor for development of cardiovascular disease: a statement from the American Heart Association Councils on Kidney in Cardiovascular Disease, High Blood Pressure Research, Clinical Cardiology, and Epidemiology and Prevention. Hypertension. 2003;42(5):1050–65. PubMed PMID: 14604997.
7. Manjunath G, Tighiouart H, Coresh J, Macleod B, Salem DN, Griffith JL, et al. Level of kidney function as a risk factor for cardiovascular outcomes in the elderly. Kidney Int. 2003;63(3):1121–9. PubMed PMID: 12631096.
8. Cheung AK, Sarnak MJ, Yan G, Berkoben M, Heyka R, Kaufman A, et al. Cardiac diseases in maintenance hemodialysis patients: results of the HEMO Study. Kidney Int. 2004;65(6):2380–9. PubMed PMID: 15149351. Epub 2004/05/20.eng.
9. United States Renal Data System. Excerpts from USRDS 2009 Annual Data Report. U.S. Department of Health and Human Services. The National Institutes of Health, National Institute of Diabetes and Digestive and Kidney Diseases. Am J Kidney Dis. 2010;55(Suppl 1):S1.
10. Law MR, Wald NJ, Thompson SG. By how much and how quickly does reduction in serum cholesterol concentration lower risk of ischaemic heart disease? BMJ. 1994;308(6925): 367–72. PubMed PMID: 8043072.
11. Liu Y, Coresh J, Eustace JA, Longenecker JC, Jaar B, Fink NE, et al. Association between cholesterol level and mortality in dialysis patients: role of inflammation and malnutrition. JAMA. 2004;291(4):451–9. PubMed PMID: 14747502.
12. Stevens LA, Padala S, Levey AS. Advances in glomerular filtration rate-estimating equations. Curr Opin Nephrol Hypertens. 2010;19(3):298–307. PubMed PMID: 20393287. Epub 2010/04/16.eng.
13. National Kidney Foundation. K/DOQI clinical practice guidelines for chronic kidney disease: evaluation, classification, and stratification. Am J Kidney Dis. 2002;39(2 Suppl 1): S1–266. PubMed PMID: 11904577. Epub 2002/03/21.eng.
14. Levey AS, Eckardt KU, Tsukamoto Y, Levin A, Coresh J, Rossert J, et al. Definition and classification of chronic kidney disease: a position statement from Kidney Disease: Improving Global Outcomes (KDIGO). Kidney Int. 2005;67(6):2089–100. PubMed PMID: 15882252. Epub 2005/05/11.eng.
15. Kidney Disease: Improving Global Outcomes (KDIGO) CKD Work Group. KDIGO 2012 clinical practice guideline for the evaluation and management of chronic kidney disease. Kidney Int Suppl. 2013;3:1–150.
16. Tonelli M, Wiebe N, Culleton B, House A, Rabbat C, Fok M, et al. Chronic kidney disease and mortality risk: a systematic review. J Am Soc Nephrol. 2006;17(7):2034–47. PubMed PMID: 16738019.
17. Muntner P, He J, Hamm L, Loria C, Whelton PK. Renal insufficiency and subsequent death resulting from cardiovascular disease in the United States. J Am Soc Nephrol. 2002;13(3): 745–53. PubMed PMID: 11856780. Epub 2002/02/22.eng.

18. Sarnak MJ, Levey AS, Schoolwerth AC, Coresh J, Culleton B, Hamm LL, et al. Kidney disease as a risk factor for development of cardiovascular disease: a statement from the American Heart Association Councils on Kidney in Cardiovascular Disease, High Blood Pressure Research, Clinical Cardiology, and Epidemiology and Prevention. Circulation. 2003;108(17):2154–69. PubMed PMID: 14581387. Epub 2003/10/29.eng.
19. Matsushita K, van der Velde M, Astor BC, Woodward M, Levey AS, de Jong PE, et al. Association of estimated glomerular filtration rate and albuminuria with all-cause and cardiovascular mortality in general population cohorts: a collaborative meta-analysis. Lancet. 2010;375(9731):2073–81. PubMed PMID: 20483451. Epub 2010/05/21.eng.
20. Tonelli M, Muntner P, Lloyd A, Manns BJ, James MT, Klarenbach S, et al. Using proteinuria and estimated glomerular filtration rate to classify risk in patients with chronic kidney disease: a cohort study. Ann Intern Med. 2011;154(1):12–21. PubMed PMID: 21200034. Epub 2011/01/05.eng.
21. Weiner DE, Tighiouart H, Amin MG, Stark PC, MacLeod B, Griffith JL, et al. Chronic kidney disease as a risk factor for cardiovascular disease and all-cause mortality: a pooled analysis of community-based studies. J Am Soc Nephrol. 2004;15(5):1307–15. PubMed PMID: 15100371. Epub 2004/04/22.eng.
22. Go AS, Chertow GM, Fan D, McCulloch CE, Hsu CY. Chronic kidney disease and the risks of death, cardiovascular events, and hospitalization. N Engl J Med. 2004;351(13):1296–305. PubMed PMID: 15385656. Epub 2004/09/24.eng.
23. Rahman M, Pressel S, Davis BR, Nwachuku C, Wright Jr JT, Whelton PK, et al. Cardiovascular outcomes in high-risk hypertensive patients stratified by baseline glomerular filtration rate. Ann Intern Med. 2006;144(3):172–80. PubMed PMID: 16461961. Epub 2006/02/08.eng.
24. Perkovic V, Ninomiya T, Arima H, Gallagher M, Jardine M, Cass A, et al. Chronic kidney disease, cardiovascular events, and the effects of perindopril-based blood pressure lowering: data from the PROGRESS study. J Am Soc Nephrol. 2007;18(10):2766–72. PubMed PMID: 17804673. Epub 2007/09/07.eng.
25. Schneider CA, Ferrannini E, Defronzo R, Schernthaner G, Yates J, Erdmann E. Effect of pioglitazone on cardiovascular outcome in diabetes and chronic kidney disease. J Am Soc Nephrol. 2008;19(1):182–7. PubMed PMID: 18057215. Epub 2007/12/07.eng.
26. Segura J, Campo C, Gil P, Roldan C, Vigil L, Rodicio JL, et al. Development of chronic kidney disease and cardiovascular prognosis in essential hypertensive patients. J Am Soc Nephrol. 2004;15(6):1616–22. PubMed PMID: 15153573. Epub 2004/05/22.eng.
27. Knobler H, Zornitzki T, Vered S, Oettinger M, Levy R, Caspi A, et al. Reduced glomerular filtration rate in asymptomatic diabetic patients: predictor of increased risk for cardiac events independent of albuminuria. J Am Coll Cardiol. 2004;44(11):2142–8. PubMed PMID: 15582311. Epub 2004/12/08.eng.
28. Kong AP, So WY, Szeto CC, Chan NN, Luk A, Ma RC, et al. Assessment of glomerular filtration rate in addition to albuminuria is important in managing type II diabetes. Kidney Int. 2006;69(2):383–7. PubMed PMID: 16408130. Epub 2006/01/13.eng.
29. Mann JF, Gerstein HC, Pogue J, Bosch J, Yusuf S. Renal insufficiency as a predictor of cardiovascular outcomes and the impact of ramipril: the HOPE randomized trial. Ann Intern Med. 2001;134(8):629–36. PubMed PMID: 11304102. Epub 2001/04/17.eng.
30. Anavekar NS, Gans DJ, Berl T, Rohde RD, Cooper W, Bhaumik A, et al. Predictors of cardiovascular events in patients with type 2 diabetic nephropathy and hypertension: a case for albuminuria. Kidney Int Suppl. 2004;92:S50–5. PubMed PMID: 15485418.Epub 2004/10/16.eng.
31. Mann JF, Yi QL, Gerstein HC. Albuminuria as a predictor of cardiovascular and renal outcomes in people with known atherosclerotic cardiovascular disease. Kidney Int Suppl. 2004;92:S59–62. PubMed PMID: 15485420. Epub 2004/10/16.eng.
32. Weiner DE, Tighiouart H, Elsayed EF, Griffith JL, Salem DN, Levey AS, et al. The Framingham predictive instrument in chronic kidney disease. J Am Coll Cardiol. 2007;50(3):217–24. PubMed PMID: 17631213. Epub 2007/07/17.eng.
33. Muntner P, He J, Astor BC, Folsom AR, Coresh J. Traditional and nontraditional risk factors predict coronary heart disease in chronic kidney disease: results from the atherosclerosis risk in communities study. J Am Soc Nephrol. 2005;16(2):529–38. PubMed PMID: 15625072. Epub 2004/12/31.eng.

34. Shlipak MG, Fried LF, Cushman M, Manolio TA, Peterson D, Stehman-Breen C, et al. Cardiovascular mortality risk in chronic kidney disease: comparison of traditional and novel risk factors. JAMA. 2005;293(14):1737–45. PubMed PMID: 15827312. Epub 2005/04/14.eng.
35. Kobayashi S, Maesato K, Moriya H, Ohtake T, Ikeda T. Insulin resistance in patients with chronic kidney disease. Am J Kidney Dis. 2005;45(2):275–80. PubMed PMID: 15685504. Epub 2005/02/03.eng.
36. Sacks FM, Pfeffer MA, Moye LA, Rouleau JL, Rutherford JD, Cole TG, et al. The effect of pravastatin on coronary events after myocardial infarction in patients with average cholesterol levels. Cholesterol and Recurrent Events Trial investigators. N Engl J Med. 1996;335(14):1001–9. PubMed PMID: 8801446.
37. Heart Protection Study Collaborative Group. MRC/BHF Heart Protection Study of cholesterol lowering with simvastatin in 20,536 high-risk individuals: a randomised placebo-controlled trial. Lancet. 2002;360(9326):7–22. PubMed PMID: 12114036.
38. Sever PS, Dahlof B, Poulter NR, Wedel H, Beevers G, Caulfield M, et al. Prevention of coronary and stroke events with atorvastatin in hypertensive patients who have average or lower-than-average cholesterol concentrations, in the Anglo-Scandinavian Cardiac Outcomes Trial-Lipid Lowering Arm (ASCOT-LLA): a multicentre randomised controlled trial. Drugs. 2004;64 Suppl 2:43–60. PubMed PMID: 15765890.
39. Rossouw JE, Lewis B, Rifkind BM. The value of lowering cholesterol after myocardial infarction. N Engl J Med. 1990;323(16):1112–9. PubMed PMID: 2215579.
40. Kilpatrick RD, McAllister CJ, Kovesdy CP, Derose SF, Kopple JD, Kalantar-Zadeh K. Association between serum lipids and survival in hemodialysis patients and impact of race. J Am Soc Nephrol. 2007;18(1):293–303. PubMed PMID: 17167113. Epub 2006/12/15.eng.
41. Iseki K, Yamazato M, Tozawa M, Takishita S. Hypocholesterolemia is a significant predictor of death in a cohort of chronic hemodialysis patients. Kidney Int. 2002;61(5):1887–93. PubMed PMID: 11967041. Epub 2002/04/23.eng.
42. Chawla V, Greene T, Beck GJ, Kusek JW, Collins AJ, Sarnak MJ, et al. Hyperlipidemia and long-term outcomes in nondiabetic chronic kidney disease. Clin J Am Soc Nephrol. 2010;5(9):1582–7. PubMed PMID: 20558558. Epub 2010/06/19.eng.
43. Kalantar-Zadeh K, Block G, Humphreys MH, Kopple JD. Reverse epidemiology of cardiovascular risk factors in maintenance dialysis patients. Kidney Int. 2003;63(3):793–808. PubMed PMID: 12631061. Epub 2003/03/13.eng.
44. Schiffrin EL, Lipman ML, Mann JF. Chronic kidney disease: effects on the cardiovascular system. Circulation. 2007;116(1):85–97. PubMed PMID: 17606856. Epub 2007/07/04.eng.
45. Kaysen GA, Eiserich JP. The role of oxidative stress-altered lipoprotein structure and function and microinflammation on cardiovascular risk in patients with minor renal dysfunction. J Am Soc Nephrol. 2004;15(3):538–48. PubMed PMID: 14978155. Epub 2004/02/24.eng.
46. Weiner DE, Tighiouart H, Elsayed EF, Griffith JL, Salem DN, Levey AS, et al. The relationship between nontraditional risk factors and outcomes in individuals with stage 3 to 4 CKD. Am J Kidney Dis. 2008;51(2):212–23. PubMed PMID: 18215699. Epub 2008/01/25.eng.
47. Parekh RS, Plantinga LC, Kao WH, Meoni LA, Jaar BG, Fink NE, et al. The association of sudden cardiac death with inflammation and other traditional risk factors. Kidney Int. 2008;74(10):1335–42. PubMed PMID: 18769368. Epub 2008/09/05.eng.
48. Kendrick J, Chonchol MB. Nontraditional risk factors for cardiovascular disease in patients with chronic kidney disease. Nat Clin Pract Nephrol. 2008;4(12):672–81. PubMed PMID: 18825155. Epub 2008/10/01.eng.
49. Canaud B, Cristol J, Morena M, Leray-Moragues H, Bosc J, Vaussenat F. Imbalance of oxidants and antioxidants in haemodialysis patients. Blood Purif. 1999;17(2–3):99–106. PubMed PMID: 10449867. Epub 1999/08/18.eng.
50. Small DM, Coombes JS, Bennett N, Johnson DW, Gobe GC. Oxidative stress, anti-oxidant therapies and chronic kidney disease. Nephrology (Carlton). 2012;17(4):311–21. PubMed PMID: 22288610. Epub 2012/02/01.eng.
51. Himmelfarb J, Stenvinkel P, Ikizler TA, Hakim RM. The elephant in uremia: oxidant stress as a unifying concept of cardiovascular disease in uremia. Kidney Int. 2002;62(5):1524–38. PubMed PMID: 12371953. Epub 2002/10/10.eng.

52. Vaziri ND, Dicus M, Ho ND, Boroujerdi-Rad L, Sindhu RK. Oxidative stress and dysregulation of superoxide dismutase and NADPH oxidase in renal insufficiency. Kidney Int. 2003;63(1):179–85. PubMed PMID: 12472781. Epub 2002/12/11.eng.
53. Touyz RM, Yao G, Quinn MT, Pagano PJ, Schiffrin EL. p47phox associates with the cytoskeleton through cortactin in human vascular smooth muscle cells: role in NAD(P)H oxidase regulation by angiotensin II. Arterioscler Thromb Vasc Biol. 2005;25(3):512–8. PubMed PMID: 15618548. Epub 2004/12/25.eng.
54. Daugherty A, Dunn JL, Rateri DL, Heinecke JW. Myeloperoxidase, a catalyst for lipoprotein oxidation, is expressed in human atherosclerotic lesions. J Clin Invest. 1994;94(1):437–44. PubMed PMID: 8040285. Epub 1994/07/01.eng.
55. Tsimikas S, Brilakis ES, Miller ER, McConnell JP, Lennon RJ, Kornman KS, et al. Oxidized phospholipids, Lp(a) lipoprotein, and coronary artery disease. N Engl J Med. 2005;353(1):46–57. PubMed PMID: 16000355. Epub 2005/07/08.eng.
56. Maggi E, Bellazzi R, Falaschi F, Frattoni A, Perani G, Finardi G, et al. Enhanced LDL oxidation in uremic patients: an additional mechanism for accelerated atherosclerosis? Kidney Int. 1994;45(3):876–83. PubMed PMID: 8196291. Epub 1994/03/01.eng.
57. Rao M, Wong C, Kanetsky P, Girndt M, Stenvinkel P, Reilly M, et al. Cytokine gene polymorphism and progression of renal and cardiovascular diseases. Kidney Int. 2007;72(5):549–56. PubMed PMID: 17579660. Epub 2007/06/21.eng.
58. Jofre R, Rodriguez-Benitez P, Lopez-Gomez JM, Perez-Garcia R. Inflammatory syndrome in patients on hemodialysis. J Am Soc Nephrol. 2006;17(12 Suppl 3):S274–80. PubMed PMID: 17130274. Epub 2006/11/30.eng.
59. Vaziri ND, Oveisi F, Ding Y. Role of increased oxygen free radical activity in the pathogenesis of uremic hypertension. Kidney Int. 1998;53(6):1748–54. PubMed PMID: 9607208. Epub 1998/06/02.eng.
60. Menon V, Greene T, Wang X, Pereira AA, Marcovina SM, Beck GJ, et al. C-reactive protein and albumin as predictors of all-cause and cardiovascular mortality in chronic kidney disease. Kidney Int. 2005;68(2):766–72. PubMed PMID: 16014054. Epub 2005/07/15.eng.
61. Honda H, Qureshi AR, Heimburger O, Barany P, Wang K, Pecoits-Filho R, et al. Serum albumin, C-reactive protein, interleukin 6, and fetuin a as predictors of malnutrition, cardiovascular disease, and mortality in patients with ESRD. Am J Kidney Dis. 2006;47(1):139–48. PubMed PMID: 16377395. Epub 2005/12/27.eng.
62. Endemann DH, Schiffrin EL. Endothelial dysfunction. J Am Soc Nephrol. 2004;15(8):1983–92. PubMed PMID: 15284284. Epub 2004/07/31.eng.
63. Stehouwer CD, Smulders YM. Microalbuminuria and risk for cardiovascular disease: analysis of potential mechanisms. J Am Soc Nephrol. 2006;17(8):2106–11. PubMed PMID: 16825333. Epub 2006/07/11.eng.
64. Wever R, Boer P, Hijmering M, Stroes E, Verhaar M, Kastelein J, et al. Nitric oxide production is reduced in patients with chronic renal failure. Arterioscler Thromb Vasc Biol. 1999;19(5):1168–72. PubMed PMID: 10323766. Epub 1999/05/14.eng.
65. Passauer J, Pistrosch F, Bussemaker E, Lassig G, Herbrig K, Gross P. Reduced agonist-induced endothelium-dependent vasodilation in uremia is attributable to an impairment of vascular nitric oxide. J Am Soc Nephrol. 2005;16(4):959–65. PubMed PMID: 15728785. Epub 2005/02/25.eng.
66. Zoccali C, Bode-Boger S, Mallamaci F, Benedetto F, Tripepi G, Malatino L, et al. Plasma concentration of asymmetrical dimethylarginine and mortality in patients with end-stage renal disease: a prospective study. Lancet. 2001;358(9299):2113–7. PubMed PMID: 11784625. Epub 2002/01/11.eng.
67. Ravani P, Tripepi G, Malberti F, Testa S, Mallamaci F, Zoccali C. Asymmetrical dimethylarginine predicts progression to dialysis and death in patients with chronic kidney disease: a competing risks modeling approach. J Am Soc Nephrol. 2005;16(8):2449–55. PubMed PMID: 15944335. Epub 2005/06/10.eng.
68. Cooke JP. Asymmetrical dimethylarginine: the Uber marker? Circulation. 2004;109(15):1813–8. PubMed PMID: 15096461. Epub 2004/04/21.eng.

69. Antoniades C, Demosthenous M, Tousoulis D, Antonopoulos AS, Vlachopoulos C, Toutouza M, et al. Role of asymmetrical dimethylarginine in inflammation-induced endothelial dysfunction in human atherosclerosis. Hypertension. 2011;58(1):93–8. PubMed PMID: 21518967. Epub 2011/04/27.eng.
70. de Mutsert R, Grootendorst DC, Axelsson J, Boeschoten EW, Krediet RT, Dekker FW. Excess mortality due to interaction between protein-energy wasting, inflammation and cardiovascular disease in chronic dialysis patients. Nephrol Dial Transplant. 2008;23(9):2957–64. PubMed PMID: 18400817. Epub 2008/04/11.eng.
71. Friedman AN, Hunsicker LG, Selhub J, Bostom AG. C-reactive protein as a predictor of total arteriosclerotic outcomes in type 2 diabetic nephropathy. Kidney Int. 2005;68(2):773–8. PubMed PMID: 16014055. Epub 2005/07/15.eng.
72. Covic A, Kothawala P, Bernal M, Robbins S, Chalian A, Goldsmith D. Systematic review of the evidence underlying the association between mineral metabolism disturbances and risk of all-cause mortality, cardiovascular mortality and cardiovascular events in chronic kidney disease. Nephrol Dial Transplant. 2009;24(5):1506–23. PubMed PMID: 19001560. Epub 2008/11/13.eng.
73. Tomiyama C, Higa A, Dalboni MA, Cendoroglo M, Draibe SA, Cuppari L, et al. The impact of traditional and non-traditional risk factors on coronary calcification in pre-dialysis patients. Nephrol Dial Transplant. 2006;21(9):2464–71. PubMed PMID: 16735378. Epub 2006/06/01.eng.
74. Dellegrottaglie S, Saran R, Gillespie B, Zhang X, Chung S, Finkelstein F, et al. Prevalence and predictors of cardiovascular calcium in chronic kidney disease (from the Prospective Longitudinal RRI-CKD Study). Am J Cardiol. 2006;98(5):571–6. PubMed PMID: 16923438. Epub 2006/08/23.eng.
75. Vaziri ND. Dyslipidemia of chronic renal failure: the nature, mechanisms, and potential consequences. Am J Physiol Renal Physiol. 2006;290(2):F262–72. PubMed PMID: 16403839. Epub 2006/01/13.eng.
76. Attman PO, Alaupovic P. Lipid abnormalities in chronic renal insufficiency. Kidney Int Suppl. 1991;31:S16–23. PubMed PMID: 2046265.
77. Vaziri ND, Moradi H. Mechanisms of dyslipidemia of chronic renal failure. Hemodial Int. 2006;10(1):1–7. PubMed PMID: 16441821.
78. Kaysen GA, Gambertoglio J, Felts J, Hutchison FN. Albumin synthesis, albuminuria and hyperlipemia in nephrotic patients. Kidney Int. 1987;31(6):1368–76. PubMed PMID: 3613408.
79. Attman PO, Samuelsson O, Johansson AC, Moberly JB, Alaupovic P. Dialysis modalities and dyslipidemia. Kidney Int Suppl. 2003;84:S110–2. PubMed PMID: 12694322. Epub 2003/04/16.eng.
80. Heimburger O, Stenvinkel P, Berglund L, Tranoeus A, Lindholm B. Increased plasma lipoprotein(a) in continuous ambulatory peritoneal dialysis is related to peritoneal transport of proteins and glucose. Nephron. 1996;72(2):135–44. PubMed PMID: 8684516. Epub 1996/01/01.eng.
81. Wheeler DC. Abnormalities of lipoprotein metabolism in CAPD patients. Kidney Int Suppl. 1996;56:S41–6. PubMed PMID: 8914053. Epub 1996/11/01.eng.
82. Johansson AC, Samuelsson O, Attman PO, Haraldsson B, Moberly J, Knight-Gibson C, et al. Dyslipidemia in peritoneal dialysis—relation to dialytic variables. Perit Dial Int. 2000;20(3):306–14. PubMed PMID: 10898048. Epub 2000/07/18.eng.
83. Shoji T, Nishizawa Y, Kawagishi T, Kawasaki K, Taniwaki H, Tabata T, et al. Intermediate-density lipoprotein as an independent risk factor for aortic atherosclerosis in hemodialysis patients. J Am Soc Nephrol. 1998;9(7):1277–84. PubMed PMID: 9644639. Epub 1998/06/30.eng.
84. Grieve DJ, Avella MA, Botham KM, Elliott J. Chylomicron remnants potentiate phenylephrine-induced contractions of rat aorta by an endothelium-dependent mechanism. Atherosclerosis. 2000;151(2):471–80. PubMed PMID: 10924724. Epub 2000/08/05.eng.
85. Whitman SC, Sawyez CG, Miller DB, Wolfe BM, Huff MW. Oxidized type IV hypertriglyceridemic VLDL-remnants cause greater macrophage cholesteryl ester accumulation than oxidized LDL. J Lipid Res. 1998;39(5):1008–20. PubMed PMID: 9610767. Epub 1998/06/04.eng.

86. Rajman I, Harper L, McPake D, Kendall MJ, Wheeler DC. Low-density lipoprotein subfraction profiles in chronic renal failure. Nephrol Dial Transplant. 1998;13(9):2281–7. PubMed PMID: 9761510. Epub 1998/10/07.eng.
87. Quaschning T, Krane V, Metzger T, Wanner C. Abnormalities in uremic lipoprotein metabolism and its impact on cardiovascular disease. Am J Kidney Dis. 2001;38(4 Suppl 1):S14–9. PubMed PMID: 11576915. Epub 2001/09/29.eng.
88. de Graaf J, Hak-Lemmers HL, Hectors MP, Demacker PN, Hendriks JC, Stalenhoef AF. Enhanced susceptibility to in vitro oxidation of the dense low density lipoprotein subfraction in healthy subjects. Arterioscler Thromb. 1991;11(2):298–306. PubMed PMID: 1998647. Epub 1991/03/01.eng.
89. St-Pierre AC, Cantin B, Dagenais GR, Mauriege P, Bernard PM, Despres JP, et al. Low-density lipoprotein subfractions and the long-term risk of ischemic heart disease in men: 13-year follow-up data from the Quebec Cardiovascular Study. Arterioscler Thromb Vasc Biol. 2005;25(3):553–9. PubMed PMID: 15618542. Epub 2004/12/25.eng.
90. Austin MA, King MC, Vranizan KM, Krauss RM. Atherogenic lipoprotein phenotype. A proposed genetic marker for coronary heart disease risk. Circulation. 1990;82(2):495–506. PubMed PMID: 2372896. Epub 1990/08/01.eng.
91. Clementi A, Kim JC, Floris M, Cruz DN, Garzotto F, Zanella M, et al. Statin therapy is associated with decreased small, dense low-density lipoprotein levels in patients undergoing peritoneal dialysis. Contrib Nephrol. 2012;178:111–5. PubMed PMID: 22652726. Epub 2012/06/02.eng.
92. Ok E, Basnakian AG, Apostolov EO, Barri YM, Shah SV. Carbamylated low-density lipoprotein induces death of endothelial cells: a link to atherosclerosis in patients with kidney disease. Kidney Int. 2005;68(1):173–8. PubMed PMID: 15954906. Epub 2005/06/16.eng.
93. Kuboyama M, Ageta M, Ishihara T, Fujiura Y, Kashio N, Ikushima I. Serum lipoprotein(a) concentration and Apo(a) isoform under the condition of renal dysfunction. J Atheroscler Thromb. 2003;10(5):283–9. PubMed PMID: 14718745. Epub 2004/01/14.eng.
94. Cressman MD, Heyka RJ, Paganini EP, O'Neil J, Skibinski CI, Hoff HF. Lipoprotein(a) is an independent risk factor for cardiovascular disease in hemodialysis patients. Circulation. 1992;86(2):475–82. PubMed PMID: 1386292. Epub 1992/08/01.eng.
95. Koda Y, Nishi S, Suzuki M, Hirasawa Y. Lipoprotein(a) is a predictor for cardiovascular mortality of hemodialysis patients. Kidney Int Suppl. 1999;71:S251–3. PubMed PMID: 10412791. Epub 1999/07/21.eng.
96. Steyrer E, Durovic S, Frank S, Giessauf W, Burger A, Dieplinger H, et al. The role of lecithin: cholesterol acyltransferase for lipoprotein (a) assembly. Structural integrity of low density lipoproteins is a prerequisite for Lp(a) formation in human plasma. J Clin Invest. 1994;94(6):2330–40.
97. Erqou S, Kaptoge S, Perry PL, Di Angelantonio E, Thompson A, White IR, et al. Lipoprotein(a) concentration and the risk of coronary heart disease, stroke, and nonvascular mortality. JAMA. 2009;302(4):412–23. PubMed PMID: 19622820. Epub 2009/07/23.eng.
98. Bennet A, Di Angelantonio E, Erqou S, Eiriksdottir G, Sigurdsson G, Woodward M, et al. Lipoprotein(a) levels and risk of future coronary heart disease: large-scale prospective data. Arch Intern Med. 2008;168(6):598–608. PubMed PMID: 18362252. Epub 2008/03/26.eng.
99. Genest Jr JJ, Martin-Munley SS, McNamara JR, Ordovas JM, Jenner J, Myers RH, et al. Familial lipoprotein disorders in patients with premature coronary artery disease. Circulation. 1992;85(6):2025–33. PubMed PMID: 1534286. Epub 1992/06/11.eng.
100. Ohira T, Schreiner PJ, Morrisett JD, Chambless LE, Rosamond WD, Folsom AR. Lipoprotein(a) and incident ischemic stroke: the Atherosclerosis Risk in Communities (ARIC) study. Stroke. 2006;37(6):1407–12. PubMed PMID: 16675734. Epub 2006/05/06.eng.
101. Loscalzo J, Weinfeld M, Fless GM, Scanu AM. Lipoprotein(a), fibrin binding, and plasminogen activation. Arteriosclerosis. 1990;10(2):240–5. PubMed PMID: 2138452. Epub 1990/03/01.eng.
102. Zioncheck TF, Powell LM, Rice GC, Eaton DL, Lawn RM. Interaction of recombinant apolipoprotein(a) and lipoprotein(a) with macrophages. J Clin Invest. 1991;87(3):767–71. PubMed PMID: 1825665. Epub 1991/03/01.eng.

103. Takami S, Yamashita S, Kihara S, Ishigami M, Takemura K, Kume N, et al. Lipoprotein(a) enhances the expression of intercellular adhesion molecule-1 in cultured human umbilical vein endothelial cells. Circulation. 1998;97(8):721–8. PubMed PMID: 9498534. Epub 1998/03/14.eng.
104. Boerwinkle E, Leffert CC, Lin J, Lackner C, Chiesa G, Hobbs HH. Apolipoprotein(a) gene accounts for greater than 90% of the variation in plasma lipoprotein(a) concentrations. J Clin Invest. 1992;90(1):52–60. PubMed PMID: 1386087. Epub 1992/07/01.eng.
105. Bowden JF, Pritchard PH, Hill JS, Frohlich JJ. Lp(a) concentration and apo(a) isoform size. Relation to the presence of coronary artery disease in familial hypercholesterolemia. Arterioscler Thromb. 1994;14(10):1561–8. PubMed PMID: 7918305. Epub 1994/10/01.eng.
106. Kronenberg F, Neyer U, Lhotta K, Trenkwalder E, Auinger M, Pribasnig A, et al. The low molecular weight apo(a) phenotype is an independent predictor for coronary artery disease in hemodialysis patients: a prospective follow-up. J Am Soc Nephrol. 1999;10(5):1027–36. PubMed PMID: 10232689. Epub 1999/05/08.eng.
107. Longenecker JC, Klag MJ, Marcovina SM, Powe NR, Fink NE, Giaculli F, et al. Small apolipoprotein(a) size predicts mortality in end-stage renal disease: the CHOICE study. Circulation. 2002;106(22):2812–8. PubMed PMID: 12451008. Epub 2002/11/27.eng.
108. Vaziri ND, Norris K. Lipid disorders and their relevance to outcomes in chronic kidney disease. Blood Purif. 2011;31(1–3):189–96. PubMed PMID: 21228589. Epub 2011/01/14.eng.
109. Herz J, Strickland DK. LRP: a multifunctional scavenger and signaling receptor. J Clin Invest. 2001;108(6):779–84. PubMed PMID: 11560943. Epub 2001/09/19.eng.
110. Takahashi S, Kawarabayasi Y, Nakai T, Sakai J, Yamamoto T. Rabbit very low density lipoprotein receptor: a low density lipoprotein receptor-like protein with distinct ligand specificity. Proc Natl Acad Sci U S A. 1992;89(19):9252–6. PubMed PMID: 1384047. Epub 1992/10/01.eng.
111. Cheung AK, Parker CJ, Ren K, Iverius PH. Increased lipase inhibition in uremia: identification of pre-beta-HDL as a major inhibitor in normal and uremic plasma. Kidney Int. 1996;49(5):1360–71. PubMed PMID: 8731101. Epub 1996/05/01.eng.
112. Akmal M, Perkins S, Kasim SE, Oh HY, Smogorzewski M, Massry SG. Verapamil prevents chronic renal failure-induced abnormalities in lipid metabolism. Am J Kidney Dis. 1993;22(1):158–63. PubMed PMID: 8322779. Epub 1993/07/01.eng.
113. Sato T, Liang K, Vaziri ND. Protein restriction and AST-120 improve lipoprotein lipase and VLDL receptor in focal glomerulosclerosis. Kidney Int. 2003;64(5):1780–6. PubMed PMID: 14531811. Epub 2003/10/09.eng.
114. Lacour B, Roullet JB, Liagre AM, Jorgetti V, Beyne P, Dubost C, et al. Serum lipoprotein disturbances in primary and secondary hyperparathyroidism and effects of parathyroidectomy. Am J Kidney Dis. 1986;8(6):422–9. PubMed PMID: 3812471. Epub 1986/12/01.eng.
115. Liang K, Oveisi F, Vaziri ND. Role of secondary hyperparathyroidism in the genesis of hypertriglyceridemia and VLDL receptor deficiency in chronic renal failure. Kidney Int. 1998;53(3):626–30. PubMed PMID: 9507207. Epub 1998/03/21.eng.
116. Kim C, Vaziri ND. Down-regulation of hepatic LDL receptor-related protein (LRP) in chronic renal failure. Kidney Int. 2005;67(3):1028–32. PubMed PMID: 15698441. Epub 2005/02/09.eng.
117. Vaziri ND, Liang K. Down-regulation of VLDL receptor expression in chronic experimental renal failure. Kidney Int. 1997;51(3):913–9. PubMed PMID: 9067930. Epub 1997/03/01.eng.
118. Vaziri ND, Kim CH, Dang B, Zhan CD, Liang K. Downregulation of hepatic acyl-CoA:diglycerol acyltransferase in chronic renal failure. Am J Physiol Renal Physiol. 2004;287(1):F90–4. PubMed PMID: 15010358. Epub 2004/03/11.eng.
119. Vaziri ND, Kim CH, Phan D, Kim S, Liang K. Up-regulation of hepatic Acyl CoA: diacylglycerol acyltransferase-1 (DGAT-1) expression in nephrotic syndrome. Kidney Int. 2004;66(1):262–7. PubMed PMID: 15200432. Epub 2004/06/18.eng.
120. Chmielewski M, Bryl E, Marzec L, Aleksandrowicz E, Witkowski JM, Rutkowski B. Expression of scavenger receptor CD36 in chronic renal failure patients. Artif Organs. 2005;29(8):608–14. PubMed PMID: 16048476. Epub 2005/07/29.eng.

121. Park SY, Song CY, Kim BC, Hong HK, Lee HS. Angiotensin II mediates LDL-induced superoxide generation in mesangial cells. Am J Physiol Renal Physiol. 2003;285(5):F909–15. PubMed PMID: 12837686. Epub 2003/07/03.eng.
122. Rader DJ. Molecular regulation of HDL metabolism and function: implications for novel therapies. J Clin Invest. 2006;116(12):3090–100. PubMed PMID: 17143322. Epub 2006/12/05.eng.
123. Fielding CJ, Fielding PE. Cellular cholesterol efflux. Biochim Biophys Acta. 2001;1533(3):175–89. PubMed PMID: 11731329. Epub 2001/12/04.eng.
124. Kaysen GA. Hyperlipidemia in chronic kidney disease. Int J Artif Organs. 2007;30(11):987–92. PubMed PMID: 18067100. Epub 2007/12/11.eng.
125. Tsimihodimos V, Dounousi E, Siamopoulos KC. Dyslipidemia in chronic kidney disease: an approach to pathogenesis and treatment. Am J Nephrol. 2008;28(6):958–73. PubMed PMID: 18612199. Epub 2008/07/10.eng.
126. McGrath KC, Li XH, Puranik R, Liong EC, Tan JT, Dy VM, et al. Role of 3beta-hydroxysteroid-delta 24 reductase in mediating antiinflammatory effects of high-density lipoproteins in endothelial cells. Arterioscler Thromb Vasc Biol. 2009;29(6):877–82. PubMed PMID: 19325144. Epub 2009/03/28.eng.
127. Bisoendial RJ, Hovingh GK, Levels JH, Lerch PG, Andresen I, Hayden MR, et al. Restoration of endothelial function by increasing high-density lipoprotein in subjects with isolated low high-density lipoprotein. Circulation. 2003;107(23):2944–8. PubMed PMID: 12771001. Epub 2003/05/29.eng.
128. Wang X, Rader DJ. Molecular regulation of macrophage reverse cholesterol transport. Curr Opin Cardiol. 2007;22(4):368–72. PubMed PMID: 17556891. Epub 2007/06/09.eng.
129. Wang X, Collins HL, Ranalletta M, Fuki IV, Billheimer JT, Rothblat GH, et al. Macrophage ABCA1 and ABCG1, but not SR-BI, promote macrophage reverse cholesterol transport in vivo. J Clin Invest. 2007;117(8):2216–24. PubMed PMID: 17657311. Epub 2007/07/28.eng.
130. Oram JF, Vaughan AM. ATP-binding cassette cholesterol transporters and cardiovascular disease. Circ Res. 2006;99(10):1031–43. PubMed PMID: 17095732. Epub 2006/11/11.eng.
131. Zhao Y, Marcel YL. Serum albumin is a significant intermediate in cholesterol transfer between cells and lipoproteins. Biochemistry. 1996;35(22):7174–80. PubMed PMID: 8679545. Epub 1996/06/04.eng.
132. Acton S, Rigotti A, Landschulz KT, Xu S, Hobbs HH, Krieger M. Identification of scavenger receptor SR-BI as a high density lipoprotein receptor. Science. 1996;271(5248):518–20. PubMed PMID: 8560269. Epub 1996/01/26.eng.
133. Attman PO, Samuelsson O, Alaupovic P. Lipoprotein metabolism and renal failure. Am J Kidney Dis. 1993;21(6):573–92. PubMed PMID: 8503411. Epub 1993/06/01.eng.
134. Vaziri ND, Deng G, Liang K. Hepatic HDL receptor, SR-B1 and Apo A-I expression in chronic renal failure. Nephrol Dial Transplant. 1999;14(6):1462–6. PubMed PMID: 10383008. Epub 1999/06/26.eng.
135. Liang K, Kim CH, Vaziri ND. HMG-CoA reductase inhibition reverses LCAT and LDL receptor deficiencies and improves HDL in rats with chronic renal failure. Am J Physiol Renal Physiol. 2005;288(3):F539–44. PubMed PMID: 15507547. Epub 2004/10/28.eng.
136. Moradi H, Pahl MV, Elahimehr R, Vaziri ND. Impaired antioxidant activity of high-density lipoprotein in chronic kidney disease. Transl Res. 2009;153(2):77–85. PubMed PMID: 19138652. Epub 2009/01/14.eng.
137. Shao B, Oda MN, Oram JF, Heinecke JW. Myeloperoxidase: an inflammatory enzyme for generating dysfunctional high density lipoprotein. Curr Opin Cardiol. 2006;21(4):322–8. PubMed PMID: 16755201. Epub 2006/06/07.eng.
138. Van Lenten BJ, Reddy ST, Navab M, Fogelman AM. Understanding changes in high density lipoproteins during the acute phase response. Arterioscler Thromb Vasc Biol. 2006;26(8):1687–8. PubMed PMID: 16857958. Epub 2006/07/22.eng.
139. Ansell BJ, Navab M, Hama S, Kamranpour N, Fonarow G, Hough G, et al. Inflammatory/antiinflammatory properties of high-density lipoprotein distinguish patients from control subjects better than high-density lipoprotein cholesterol levels and are favorably affected by simvastatin treatment. Circulation. 2003;108(22):2751–6. PubMed PMID: 14638544. Epub 2003/11/26.eng.

140. Moradi H, Yuan J, Ni Z, Norris K, Vaziri ND. Reverse cholesterol transport pathway in experimental chronic renal failure. Am J Nephrol. 2009;30(2):147–54. PubMed PMID: 19321994. Epub 2009/03/27.eng.
141. Vaziri ND, Moradi H, Pahl MV, Fogelman AM, Navab M. In vitro stimulation of HDL anti-inflammatory activity and inhibition of LDL pro-inflammatory activity in the plasma of patients with end-stage renal disease by an apoA-1 mimetic peptide. Kidney Int. 2009;76(4):437–44. PubMed PMID: 19471321. Epub 2009/05/28.eng.
142. van der Steeg WA, Kuivenhoven JA, Klerkx AH, Boekholdt SM, Hovingh GK, Kastelein JJ. Role of CETP inhibitors in the treatment of dyslipidemia. Curr Opin Lipidol. 2004;15(6):631–6. PubMed PMID: 15529021. Epub 2004/11/06.eng.
143. Barter PJ, Caulfield M, Eriksson M, Grundy SM, Kastelein JJ, Komajda M, et al. Effects of torcetrapib in patients at high risk for coronary events. N Engl J Med. 2007;357(21):2109–22. PubMed PMID: 17984165. Epub 2007/11/07.eng.
144. Bots ML, Visseren FL, Evans GW, Riley WA, Revkin JH, Tegeler CH, et al. Torcetrapib and carotid intima-media thickness in mixed dyslipidaemia (RADIANCE 2 study): a randomised, double-blind trial. Lancet. 2007;370(9582):153–60. PubMed PMID: 17630038. Epub 2007/07/17.eng.
145. Vaziri ND, Navab M, Fogelman AM. HDL metabolism and activity in chronic kidney disease. Nat Rev Nephrol. 2010;6(5):287–96. PubMed PMID: 20308998. Epub 2010/03/24.eng.
146. Seiler S, Schlitt A, Jiang XC, Ulrich C, Blankenberg S, Lackner KJ, et al. Cholesteryl ester transfer protein activity and cardiovascular events in patients with chronic kidney disease stage V. Nephrol Dial Transplant. 2008;23(11):3599–604. PubMed PMID: 18503096. Epub 2008/05/27.eng.
147. Navab M, Reddy ST, Van Lenten BJ, Anantharamaiah GM, Fogelman AM. The role of dysfunctional HDL in atherosclerosis. J Lipid Res. 2009;50(Suppl):S145–9. PubMed PMID: 18955731. Epub 2008/10/29.eng.
148. Libby P. Inflammation in atherosclerosis. Nature. 2002;420(6917):868–74. PubMed PMID: 12490960. Epub 2002/12/20.eng.
149. Falk E. Pathogenesis of atherosclerosis. J Am Coll Cardiol. 2006;47(8 Suppl):C7–12. PubMed PMID: 16631513. Epub 2006/04/25.eng.
150. Hansson GK. Inflammation, atherosclerosis, and coronary artery disease. N Engl J Med. 2005;352(16):1685–95. PubMed PMID: 15843671. Epub 2005/04/22.eng.
151. Davies MJ. The pathophysiology of acute coronary syndromes. Heart. 2000;83(3):361–6. PubMed PMID: 10677422. Epub 2000/03/04.eng.
152. Schwarz U, Buzello M, Ritz E, Stein G, Raabe G, Wiest G, et al. Morphology of coronary atherosclerotic lesions in patients with end-stage renal failure. Nephrol Dial Transplant. 2000;15(2):218–23. PubMed PMID: 10648668. Epub 2000/01/29.eng.
153. London GM, Parfrey PS. Cardiac disease in chronic uremia: pathogenesis. Adv Ren Replace Ther. 1997;4(3):194–211. PubMed PMID: 9239425. Epub 1997/07/01.eng.
154. Qunibi WY. Reducing the burden of cardiovascular calcification in patients with chronic kidney disease. J Am Soc Nephrol. 2005;16 Suppl 2:S95–102. PubMed PMID: 16251249. Epub 2005/10/28.eng.
155. Russo D, Palmiero G, De Blasio AP, Balletta MM, Andreucci VE. Coronary artery calcification in patients with CRF not undergoing dialysis. Am J Kidney Dis. 2004;44(6):1024–30. PubMed PMID: 15558523. Epub 2004/11/24.eng.
156. Budisavljevic MN, Cheek D, Ploth DW. Calciphylaxis in chronic renal failure. J Am Soc Nephrol. 1996;7(7):978–82. PubMed PMID: 8829111. Epub 1996/07/01.eng.
157. Ketteler M, Schlieper G, Floege J. Calcification and cardiovascular health: new insights into an old phenomenon. Hypertension. 2006;47(6):1027–34. PubMed PMID: 16618842. Epub 2006/04/19.eng.
158. Covic A, Kanbay M, Voroneanu L, Turgut F, Serban DN, Serban IL, et al. Vascular calcification in chronic kidney disease. Clin Sci (Lond). 2010;119(3):111–21. PubMed PMID: 20443781. Epub 2010/05/07.eng.

159. Parfrey PS, Foley RN. The clinical epidemiology of cardiac disease in chronic renal failure. J Am Soc Nephrol. 1999;10(7):1606–15. PubMed PMID: 10405218. Epub 1999/07/15.eng.
160. United States Rena Data System 2007. Mortality and cause of death. www.usrds.org/2007/ref/H_morte_07.pdf.
161. Heymann EP, Kassimatis TI, Goldsmith DJ. Dyslipidemia, statins, and CKD patients' outcomes—review of the evidence in the post-sharp era. J Nephrol. 2012;25(4):460–72. PubMed PMID: 22641572. Epub 2012/05/30.eng.
162. Kassimatis TI, Konstantinopoulos PA. Rosuvastatin in patients undergoing hemodialysis. N Engl J Med. 2009;361(1):93; author reply 4–5. PubMed PMID: 19579277. Epub 2009/07/07.eng.

Chapter 6
The CKD Patient with Dyslipidemia

Valentina Batini and Stefano Bianchi

Introduction

Dyslipidemia in patients with CKD shows a unique profile, different from general population. All stages of CKD are involved [1–3], with significant variations depending on worsening of renal function [4, 5], dialysis dependency, and on associated diseases such as diabetes [6] and nephrotic syndrome [7], and, finally, on whether the patient is a kidney transplant patient [8].

This chapter will review the pathogenesis and epidemiology of lipid abnormalities in CKD stages 1–5 not requiring dialysis and without nephrotic syndrome. In order to understand alterations of dyslipidemia in CKD a concise overview of lipid metabolism is necessary.

Lipoproteins

Human plasma contains nucleic acids, proteins, carbohydrates, and lipids. While much is known about the first three biological molecules, efforts are being made to perform a wide-scale lipid profiling analysis hosted by their structural diversities and the utter number of molecular species, apparently in an order of hundreds of thousands [9]. A first human plasma lipidome has been recently lined out by the LIPID MAPS consortium (www.lipidmaps.org) [10], which quantified almost 600 molecular species.

V. Batini, M.D. • S. Bianchi, M.D. (✉)
Department of Nephrology and Dialysis, Hospital of Livorno,
Viale Afieri 36, Livorno 57100, Tuscany, Italy
e-mail: valentina.batini@gmail.com; s.bianchi@usl6.toscana.it

A. Covic et al. (eds.), *Dyslipidemias in Kidney Disease*, DOI 10.1007/978-1-4939-0515-7_6,

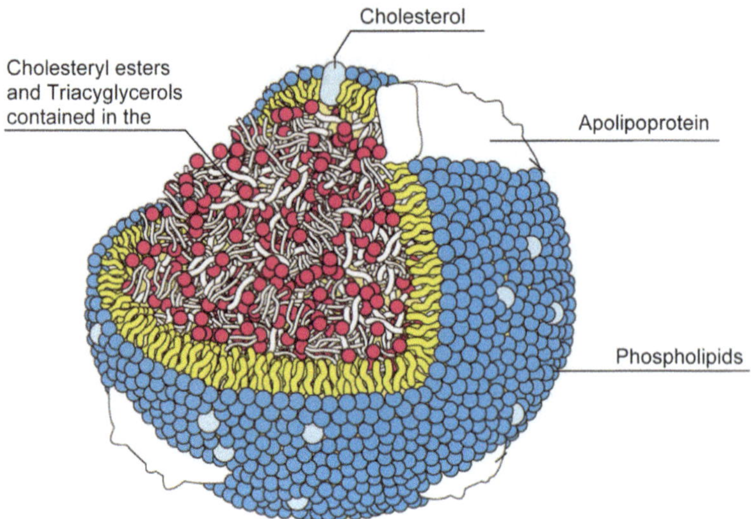

Fig. 6.1 Representation of the typical structure of apolipoprotein

Most of the fat found in food is in the form of triglycerides, cholesterol, and phospholipids. Lipids, such as cholesterol and triglycerides, are insoluble in plasma and, in order to be able to circulate in plasma, they need a proteic carrier, so forming lipoproteins that, through various functions, choreograph the transport of lipid from sites of absorption or synthesis to sites of utilization or storage. More precisely, this system cycles tryglicerides for distribution to muscles for energy use, or to adipose tissue, for storage; and cycles cholesterol for distribution throughout the body for cell membranes, bile acids, and steroid hormone synthesis. A complementary cycle, called "reverse cholesterol transport," completes the system.

The lipoprotein consists of esterified and unesterified cholesterol, triglycerides, phospholipids, and proteins. The protein components of the lipoprotein are known as apolipoproteins or apoproteins. The different apolipoproteins serve as cofactors for enzymes and ligands for receptors.

The lipoprotein's core is composed of lipid, primarily triacylglycerol and cholesterol ester. The envelope (plasma membrane) is composed of phospholipids, a small amount of free cholesterol, and apolipoproteins (Fig. 6.1). The apolipoproteins may be integral components of the plasma membrane, or they may be peripheral to the plasma membrane.

The density of a lipoprotein particle is determined by the relative amounts of lipid and protein contained in the particle (Table 6.1). Lipoproteins not only change the density of each particle throughout the metabolic pathway but also interact with lipid transfer proteins and receptor molecules, therefore controlling lipid structure and metabolism. These properties are on behalf of the protein component, the apolipoprotein. Therefore, ideally, the lipoprotein aggregates should be described in terms of the different apoproteins.

Table 6.1 Different types of circulating lipoproteins in normal plasma

		Relative content (%) in plasma lipoproteins				
Lipoprotein	Function	TG	Chol	Pl	Pr	Apolipoproteins
Chylomicron	Carry dietary TG to liver or peripheral tissues	90	5	3	2	B-48, C-II, C-III, A-IV, E
VLDL	Carry endogenous TG from liver to peripheral tissues	60	20	14	6	B-100, C-II, C-III, E
IDL	Intermediate metabolite of VLDL, among the most atherogenous (↑ in CKD)	20	40	22	18	B-100, E
LDL	Carry cholesterol from liver to peripheral tissue	7	50	22	21	B-100
HDL	Reverse cholesterol transport from peripheral tissues to liver	5	25	26	44	A-I, A-II, A-IV
Lp(a)	Unknown	5	45	20	26	apo(a), B-100

Modified from [3]

Chol cholesterol, *TG* triglycerides, *Pl* phospholipids, *Pr* proteins, *CKD* chronic kidney disease, *VLDL* very low-density lipoprotein, *IDL* intermediate-density lipoprotein, *LDL* low-density lipoprotein, *HDL* high-density lipoprotein, *Lp(a)* lipoprotein (a)

However, the practical methods that have been used to segregate different lipoprotein classes have determined the nomenclature. So the main groups are classified as chylomicrons, very low-density lipoproteins (VLDLs), low-density lipoproteins (LDLs), and high-density lipoproteins (HDLs), based on the relative densities of the aggregates on ultracentrifugation. Moreover, these classes can be further refined by improved separation procedures, defining intermediate-density lipoproteins (IDLs) and subdivisions of the HDL (e.g., HDL1, HDL2, HDL3).

Based on the apolipoprotein compositions, there are two major groups of lipoprotein subclasses. One group consists of apoA-containing lipoprotein subclasses and the other group of apoB-containing lipoprotein subclasses. The individual apoA-containing lipoproteins are almost exclusively found in HDL as Lp-A-I, Lp-A-I:A-II, and Lp-A-II. The apoB-containing lipoproteins, also called non-HDL, are distributed throughout VLDL, IDL, and LDL ranges. The five distinct apoB-containing lipoprotein subclasses are Lp-B, Lp-B:E, Lp-B:C:E, Lp-B:C, and Lp-A-II:B:C:D:E.

Several studies in patients without renal disease have clearly shown that apoB-containing lipoproteins are atherogenic [11–13]. Recent studies strongly indicate that lipoproteins, that in addition to apoB also contain apoC-III, could be particularly damaging [14, 15].

ApoB-containing lipoproteins comprise the lipid delivery pathway, while apoA1-containing lipoproteins participate in reverse cholesterol transport.

ApoB-containing lipoproteins originate from two sources: an intestinal apoB-48 lineage (see exogenous pathway) and hepatic apoB-100 lineage (see endogenous pathway). Travelling along similar pathways, apoB particles are remodelled into smaller and smaller cholesterol-rich remnants as triglycerides are released in the form of fatty acids to peripheral tissues.

Lipoprotein Metabolic Pathways

There are two main pathways involved in lipoproteins metabolism depending mainly on the source of lipoproteins: the exogenous pathway (dietary lipids) and the endogenous one (lipids originate in the liver) (Fig. 6.2).

In the exogenous pathway, lipids (triglycerides and cholesterol) are absorbed from the diet in the small intestine and assembled with apolipoproteins B-48 into chylomicrons, which reach the systemic circulation.

In the bloodstream, HDL particles donate apolipoprotein C-II, C-III, and apolipoprotein E to the nascent chylomicrons, which become mature. With attachment to proteoglycans on capillary endothelium, mature chylomicrons, triglyceride-rich, start the lipoprotein-remodelling process. Here apoC-II activates lipoprotein lipase (LPL), which hydrolyzes the lipoprotein's core triglycerides into free fatty acids that diffuse through the capillaries to muscles and adipose cells for energy and storage. During this catabolic process, chylomicrons shrink and become chylomicron remnants (CMRs), which continue circulating until they bind to CMR receptors or LDL receptor-related protein (LRP) entering the liver.

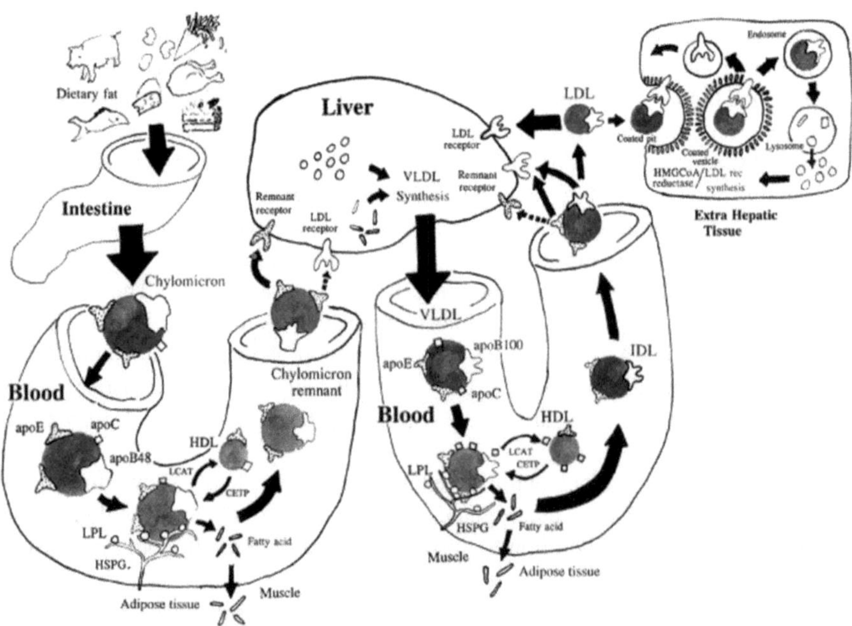

Fig. 6.2 Schematic representation of lipoprotein metabolism. See text for explanation. *Apo* apolipoprotein, *CETP* cholesteryl ester transfer protein, *HSPG* heparan sulfate proteoglycans, *LCAT* lecithin cholesterol acyltransferase, *LPL* lipoprotein lipase; *open circle*, cholesterol; *open square*, proteins. Reprinted with permission from Advanced Drug Delivery Reviews, 47, Rensen PCN, de Vrueh RLA, Kulper J, Bijsterbosch MK, Biessen EAL, Van Berkel TJC, Recombinant lipoproteins: lipoprotein-like lipid particles for drug targeting, 251-276, Copyright 2001, with permission from Elsevier

In the endogenous pathway, the liver assembles triacylglycerol and cholesterol, with apolipoprotein B-100 forming VLDL particles which are then released in the bloodstream, transporting triglycerides from the liver to peripheral tissues.

Nascent VLDL get apoE and apoC from HDL2 particles, once released into the circulation. ApoE proteins allow attachment of VLDL particles to endothelial cells and lipoprotein removal by the liver. ApoC-II activates LPL; apoC-I and C-III have inhibitor activity.

Like chylomicrons, VLDL particles circulate and encounter LPL expressed on endothelial cells, undergoing hydrolysis and the release of glycerol and fatty acids. These products can be absorbed from the blood by peripheral tissues, principally adipose and muscle. The hydrolyzed VLDL particles are now called VLDL remnants or IDLs, which can be taken up by the liver via LRP or, the majority, can be further hydrolyzed, through an enzyme called hepatic lipase (HL) to IDL remnants, called LDL particles, which have lost most triglycerides but preserve large amounts of cholesterol [16]. LDL particles contain cholesterol, triglycerides, phospholipids, and apolipoproteins B-100 and C-III. As already mentioned, all LDL particles contain one copy of apolipoproteins B-100, whereas 10–20 % of LDL particles contain apolipoprotein C-III. Thus, there is a direct relationship between apolipoprotein B-100 and LDL levels. In general, we can say that apolipoprotein B-100 is the major apolipoprotein component of the atherogenic lipoproteins (VLDL, LDL, IDL).

LDL circulates and transports cholesterol primarily to hepatocytes but also to peripheral tissues. Binding of LDL to its target tissue occurs through an interaction between the LDL receptor and apolipoprotein B-100 or E on the LDL particle, this way clearing approximately 60–80 % of LDL in adults. Remaining LDL can also be removed by other receptors, as LRP or scavenger receptors (the most important of these receptors being CD36, also called scavenger receptor B) [17]. Uptake by these receptors requires chemical modification of the LDL particle including oxidation. Oxidation of LDL can occur in any of the cells within the artery, including the endothelial cells, macrophages, smooth muscle cells, and T lymphocytes. When these macrophages become overloaded with cholesterol, foam cells are formed that contribute to the formation of atheromatous plaques. When LDL reach its target, absorption occurs through endocytosis, and the internalized LDL particles are hydrolyzed within lysosomes, releasing lipids, chiefly cholesterol. Once LDL becomes lipid-depleted, small dense LDL (sdLDL) is generated, which has lower affinity for the LDL receptor but more susceptibility to oxidative modification.

Finally, there is a pathway of reverse cholesterol transport that allows removal of cholesterol from the tissues and its return to the liver. HDL (or apoA1), which is the smallest and most dense of the lipoprotein particles, is the key lipoprotein involved in reverse cholesterol transport. The other major implications of HDL regard preventing LDL oxidation, that together with the reverse cholesterol transport give HDL a fundamental atheroprotective role.

HDL is formed through a maturation process whereby precursor particles (nascent HDL) secreted by the liver and intestine proceed through a series of conversions (known as the "HDL cycle") to attract cholesterol from cell membranes and free cholesterol to the core of the HDL particle, by interaction with numerous proteins and receptors. By such changes HDL particles increase in size as they circulate through the bloodstream.

Poorly lipidated apoA1 is secreted from the liver and intestine and released into the plasma for circulation to peripheral cells where it removes excess cholesterol forming nascent HDL. HDL's removal of cholesterol from cells comprises several mechanisms. Excess cholesterol in the macrophage triggers up-regulation of the ATP-binding cassette transporter A1 (ABCA1) and a hydrolase that converts cholesteryl ester in the lipid pool to free cholesterol. The ABCA1 transporter operates to harvest this free cholesterol and deliver it to the cell membrane, where it is acquired by apoA-I to create nascent HDL. The transporter shuttles back and forth, transferring cholesterol from the macrophage to HDL. Next the free cholesterol on HDL's surface is esterified by lecithin cholesterol acyltransferase (LCAT). The cholesterol ester then moves to the lipoprotein's core, forming the more spherical mature HDL3. Further cholesterol removal by HDL3 occurs through scavenger receptor class B type 1 receptors (SRB-1 receptors) in membrane cholesterol pools. As HDL3 collects more cholesterol and is acted on by LCAT, it expands to HDL2.

ABCA1 and SRB-1 are, therefore, key devices for cholesterol efflux. However, HDL also collects cholesterol from both lipid rafts and caveolae within the cell membrane. In these ways, HDL facilitates cholesterol efflux from the macrophage.

At this point, rich in cholesteryl esters, HDL2 engages in an exchange with triglyceride-rich lipoproteins mediated by cholesteryl ester transfer protein (CETP). Cholesteryl ester from HDL2 is transferred to apoB-containing lipoproteins in a one-to-one exchange for triglycerides. The result is further cholesterol enrichment of apoB lipoproteins and triglyceride enrichment of HDL.

HDL may now have one of the three fates: HDL's triglycerides may be hydrolyzed by hepatic lipase, converting it back to HDL3. Alternatively, HDL2 can return to the liver and interact with SRB-1, which removes cholesterol, converting it back to HDL3. Finally, HDL2 may be catabolized by the liver.

Lipid Abnormalities in Patients with CKD

CKD results in significant alteration of the plasma lipid profile and profound dysregulation of lipid and lipoprotein metabolism [18, 19]. Hallmarks of CKD-induced dyslipidemia are hypertriglyceridemia, increased concentrations of intact and partially metabolized apolipoprotein B- and apoC-III-containing triglyceride-rich lipoproteins in VLDL and IDLs, accumulation of atherogenic sdLDL, CMRs, reduction of plasmatic HDL with impaired maturation of HDL3 to cardioprotective HDL2, and depressed HDL antioxidant, anti-inflammatory, and reverse cholesterol transport capacities [20–23].

In CKD there are both quantitative and qualitative alterations of lipoproteins, the latter being predominant and responsible for the constitution of more atherogenic particles. The most common feature of dyslipidemia in CKD, among the upper cited, is hypertriglyceridemia, while total cholesterol is usually normal or low, partly due to malnutrition [24].

Table 6.2 Trend of changes in lipids and lipoproteins, in different stages of CKD, including those on renal replacement therapy

Parameter	CKD 1–5	CKD 1–5 with nephrotic proteinuria	Hemodialysis	Peritoneal dialysis
Total cholesterol	↔↑	↑↑	↔↓	↑
LDL cholesterol	↔↑	↑↑	↔↓	↑
HDL cholesterol	↓	↓	↓	↓
Non-HDL cholesterol	↔↑	↑↑	↔↓	↑
TG	↔↑	↑↑	↑	↑
Lp(a)	↔↑	↑↑	↑	↑↑

Modified from [3]

LDL low-density lipoprotein, *HDL* high-density lipoprotein, *TG triglycerides*, *Lp*(*a*) lipoprotein (a). Non-HDL cholesterol includes cholesterol in LDL, VLDL, IDL (intermediate-density lipoprotein), chylomicron, and its remnant. Explanation of arrows: normal or slightly increased (↔↑), normal or slightly decreased (↔↓), increased (↑), markedly increased (↑ ↑), and decreased (↓), compared with plasma levels of individuals without kidney disease

Such alterations, however, are typical of moderate CKD (stage III–V NKF). Little data are available in earlier stages. de Boer et al. examined cross-sectional associations of serum cystatin C with conventional lipid measurements and detailed nuclear magnetic resonance lipoprotein measurements in a population with estimated glomerular filtration rate (eGFR) > 60 mL/min per 1.73 m^2, recruited from the community-based Multi-Ethnic Study of Atherosclerosis Lipoprotein, and it resulted that abnormalities are present with milder degrees of renal impairment than usually recognized, and that alterations in LDL particle distribution may not be appreciated using conventional lipid measurements [25].

Also, Attman et al. showed how renal dyslipidemia is already present at mildly reduced renal function. The alterations are primarily seen in a characteristic apolipoproteins pattern but are not necessarily manifested as hyperlipidemia [26]. In a recent interesting study, Attman et al. also measured individual lipoprotein subclasses in CKD patients and related them to the degree of renal functional impairment. This study showed that reduced renal function is associated with a complex dyslipoproteinemia primarily characterized by increased concentrations of apoC-III-containing triglyceride-rich lipoproteins. Main finding was that when GFR is reduced to <75 mL/min, there is an increase in atherogenic lipoprotein subclasses, which in addition to apoB also have apoC-III as their protein moieties [27].

The main features of dyslipidemia of CKD are summarized in Table 6.2.

Hypertriglyceridemia

As described above, there are two types of lipoproteins that carry triglycerides: chylomicrons and VLDL. Both an increased production and reduced clearance of such lipoproteins lead to hypertriglyceridemia.

As far as increased production is concerned, contradictory results emerge from humans and experimental studies conducted on triglyceride and VLDL production. Only some studies have shown increased triglyceride production [28–30], while others have found no such increases [31, 32].

Hypotheses that stand for increased production correlate it to impaired carbohydrate tolerance, which induces increased hepatic synthesis of VLDL [1].

It is of note that fatty acid production and expression of the relative enzymes implied are reportedly increased in the adipose tissues of rats with chronic renal failure [33–35]. This fact may represent a compensatory response to diminished fatty acid entry into the adipose tissue consequent to LPL and VLDL receptor deficiencies, as demonstrated in LPL-deficient mice [36].

In this context, the diacylglycerol acyltransferase (DGAT) enzyme deserves to be mentioned.

DGAT is the final step in triglyceride biosynthesis. In an elegant study, Vaziri et al. found down-regulation of hepatic DGAT expression and activity in rats with chronic renal failure and minimal proteinuria induced by 5/6 nephrectomy, suggesting decreased hepatic triglyceride biosynthetic capacity in this model [37]. This study excludes increased production as a contributing factor to uremic hypertriglyceridemia and explains the reduction in VLDL triglyceride content in CKD. It should be pointed out that, on the contrary, heavy proteinuria results in significant up-regulation of hepatic DGAT and, hence, triglyceride synthetic capacity [38]. Thus, nephrotic proteinuria, when associated with CKD, can produce opposite results in the affected animals and, presumably, humans.

The diminished catabolism is attributed, in the first place, to decreased activity of LPL and hepatic triglyceride lipase, which are involved in triglyceride removal [39–41]. Several studies have shown that LPL activity is reduced in end-stage renal disease (ESRD) patients [20, 42, 43]. This glycoprotein enzyme is a member of the lipase gene family that includes pancreatic and hepatic lipases. It is copiously secreted as an inactive enzyme mainly by myocytes and adipocytes, after which it is translocated through the extracellular matrix and across endothelial cells to the capillary lumen. After translation, the inactive enzyme undergoes sequential glycation and cleavage of a 27-amino acid peptide, so becoming catalytically active. Once secreted, the enzyme binds to the heparan sulfate proteoglycans on the surface of the original cell and, eventually, the adjacent capillary endothelium. The endothelium-bound pool of LPL is relevant to lipolysis of VLDL and chylomicrons. Soluble heparin can displace and release LPL from binding sites on endothelial cells. Accordingly, measurement of lipolytic activity in plasma obtained after intravenous injection of soluble heparin can be used to assess LPL activity in humans and animals [20].

The main reason why lipase activity is decreased is thought to be an enhanced inhibitor activity [40] due to increase in the plasma apoC-III/apoC-II ratio [39] (apoC-II being an activator of LPL and apoC-III an inhibitor) and retention of other circulating inhibitors such as pre-β-HDL [44], which is a form of apolipoprotein A-I. The first abnormality seems to be primarily caused by the defective maturation of HDL3 to HDL2, which serves as an apoC and apoE donor to the nascent VLDL and chylomicrons. Animal studies demonstrated that the reduction in LPL activity is associated with marked down-regulation of both LPL gene expression and protein abundance in adipose tissue, skeletal muscle, as well as myocardium [45]. These observations clearly demonstrated that in addition to limiting LPL activity, CKD causes a true LPL deficiency [20].

Moreover, other factors, such as insulin depletion and secondary hyperparathyroidism, seem to play important role in inhibiting LPL activity; the latter may be mediated by intracellular accumulation of calcium in liver and adipose cells. Studies in humans and experimental animals demonstrated that parathyroidectomy can normalize serum triglyceride and hepatic lipase activity [46, 47]. Also verapamil has been showed to have similar effects on experimental animals sharing analogous mechanism [48], but there are no data on humans.

As far as hepatic lipase is concerned, this is another member of the lipase gene family with structural similarity with LPL.

Hepatic lipase is a lipolytic enzyme, synthesized by hepatocytes and found localized at the surface of liver sinusoid capillaries. In humans, the enzyme is mostly bound onto heparan sulfate proteoglycans at the surface of hepatocytes and also of sinusoid endothelial cells. Hepatic lipase plays a major role in lipoprotein metabolism. Unlike LPL, hepatic lipase activity is independent of apoC-II and as such can catalyze hydrolysis of triglycerides in IDL particles (which normally do not contain apoC-II) and their conversion to LDL. Moreover, hepatic lipase is responsible for hydrolysis of triglycerides and phospholipids in HDL and CMRs. CKD is associated with impaired clearance and elevated plasma concentration of IDL as well as the triglyceride enrichment of IDL, LDL, CMRs, and HDL, events that are indicative of hepatic lipase deficiency.

In CKD, studies conducted in experimental animals demonstrated a marked down-regulation of hepatic lipase expression and activity. It has been postulated that the CKD-associated hepatic lipase deficiency may be caused, in part, by secondary hyperparathyroidism and dysregulation of cytosolic calcium [49].

In addition to LPL and hepatic lipase abnormalities, decreased LRP, LDL, and VLDL receptor activities demonstrated in animal studies may contribute to reduced removal of these lipoproteins. In nephrectomized rats with CKD, expression of LRP is down-regulated [50] as well as VLDL receptor mRNA in adipose tissue, skeletal muscle, and myocardium of rats with CKD [47, 51].

Deficient catabolism results in accumulation of CMRs and IDL, predisposing to atherogenesis. It has also been suggested that such accumulation may limit the delivery of energy-derived lipid, to adipocytes and myocytes, predisposing ESRD patients to cachexia and decreased exercise capacity [43].

High-Density Lipoprotein

Plasma HDL cholesterol is reduced in patients affected by CKD, and the HDL cycle is impaired in these patients. Numerous mechanisms are implied.

HDL fails to mature normally as a result of reduced apoA1 level and, thereby, reduced activity of the enzyme LCAT, normally activated by the apoA1. Consequently, the packaging of the cholesterol for reverse transport is spoiled. Cholesterol cannot get back to the liver and so loads the circulation, promoting atherosclerosis. Such evidence is also shown in animal models: in 5/6 nephrectomy rats, hepatic apoA1 synthesis is reduced and its catabolism increased [52].

Apart from the indirect lack of activity of LCAT induced by diminished apoA1, LCAT is also deficient itself in CKD, which contributes to diminished plasma HDL cholesterol and impaired HDL maturation. It is demonstrated that plasma LCAT activity is consistently diminished in patients with ESRD [53–55]. This leads to a significant rise of plasma free cholesterol and to a marked reduction in plasma esterified cholesterol concentration, providing functional evidence for diminished LCAT-dependent cholesterol esterification. Doubts were addressed as to whether such deficiency was attributable to reduction in its hepatic production and plasma concentration or to its inhibition by an unknown uremic toxin. Only recently a series of studies demonstrated that the reduction in plasma LCAT activity in uremic rats is associated with a parallel reduction in plasma concentration of immunodetectable LCAT and down-regulation of hepatic LCAT gene expression [56–58].

As detailed in section "Lipoprotein Metabolic Pathways," apoA1 serves not only as LCAT activator but also as ligand for the SRB-1 and HDL binding protein (ABCA1 transporter), whereas apoA-II (the other major structural component of HDL together with apoA1) serves as hepatic lipase activator. Hepatic SRB-1 is a key device for HDL transport into the liver. Therefore, potential dysregulation of this protein can impact HDL metabolism. Heavy glomerular proteinuria has been shown to significantly reduce hepatic SRB-1 protein expression in experimental animals [59]. In contrast, CKD per se, without heavy proteinuria, induced by 5/6 nephrectomy, does not significantly change SRB-1 mRNA or protein abundance in the liver [52]. However, concomitant heavy proteinuria and renal insufficiency may affect SRB-1 expression and, hence, HDL-mediated reverse cholesterol transport.

Reviewing HDL dysregulation in CKD, it is of importance to cite a few interesting studies which have investigated the role of acyl-CoA:cholesterol acyltransferase (ACAT). To more efficiently transport both dietary and synthesized cholesterol, this has to be converted to cholesteryl esters. Free cholesterol can be taken up by lipoproteins, but is confined to the outer surface of the particle. By converting cholesterol to cholesteryl esters, more cholesterol can be packaged into the interior of lipoproteins. This vastly increases the capacity of lipoproteins, allowing for more efficient cholesterol transport through the blood stream.

While in the peripheral tissue LCAT is responsible for esterification of cholesterol to cholesteryl ester, in the lumen, dietary cholesterol absorbed by enterocytes is esterified by ACAT2, which is found in both the intestine and liver. ACAT1 is found in all tissues.

In the reverse cholesterol transport system, cholesterol esters contained in the intracellular vesicles must undergo deesterification to free cholesterol in order to be uptaken by HDL from extrahepatic tissues. This process is opposed by ACAT.

Therefore, a relative increase in ACAT activity can potentially limit HDL-mediated cholesterol uptake and, hence, contribute to the reduction in plasma HDL cholesterol and impaired maturation of HDL. Although the effect of CKD on ACAT expression and activity in the extrahepatic tissues is not known, CKD has been recently shown to up-regulate hepatic ACAT2 mRNA with consequent protein abundance, as well as total ACAT activity [60]. A subsequent interesting study confirmed the potential contribution of ACAT to the CRF-induced dysregulation of HDL metabolism, by demonstrating that inhibition of ACAT results in a dramatic shift in plasma cholesterol from apoB-containing lipoproteins to HDL with virtually no change in plasma total cholesterol in CKD animals [61]. It also revealed that the improvement in the lipid profile with an ACAT inhibitor was accompanied by a significantly higher creatinine clearance both in the treated than in the untreated animals. This phenomenon may be due to amelioration of dyslipidemia and enhanced HDL-mediated reverse cholesterol transport, leading to attenuation of glomerulosclerosis.

Also, as noted earlier, CKD results in pronounced hepatic lipase deficiency in humans and experimental animals [49]. Hepatic lipase, as already said, catalyzes hydrolysis and removal of the triglyceride content of HDL. Thus, hepatic lipase deficiency can potentially contribute to increased HDL triglyceride content.

The role of HDL in CKD goes beyond trafficking of lipids. It is well known that mortality in CKD is highly associated with chronic inflammation. Normal HDL possesses potent antioxidant, anti-inflammatory, and antithrombotic properties that are critical for the protection against atherosclerosis.

Such properties are mediated by its constituent antioxidant enzymes, paraoxonase and glutathione peroxidase, which help reverse or prevent peroxidation of lipids and/or lipoproteins. Much evidence, however, suggests that systemic oxidative stress and inflammation, as it happens in patients and animals with CKD, reduce the antioxidant and anti-inflammatory capabilities of HDL and even convert HDL into a prooxidant and proinflammatory agent [62, 63]. Vaziri et al. conducted many studies on impairment of HDL antioxidant activity. They also demonstrated how the reduction in antioxidant activity of HDL induced by CKD is associated with a reduction of HDL anti-inflammatory activity, as measured by a monocyte chemotactic activity assay in cultured human aortic endothelial cells [23].

Given that systemic inflammation is known to reduce HDL antioxidant and anti-inflammatory activity, and that oxidative stress and inflammation are prevalent features of advanced CKD, it is not surprising that HDL anti-inflammatory activity is reduced in patients with ESRD. This phenomenon creates a vicious cycle in which the underlying inflammation and oxidative stress promote HDL dysfunction, which consequently aggravates the oxidative stress and inflammation. This is also underlined by an intrigant study of Meier et al. that demonstrated that oxidized LDL modulates apoptosis of regulatory T cells mediated by proteosome inhibition in patients with CKD that is both dialysis-dependent and not dialysis-dependent. Such effects block the cellular defense system against micro-inflammation, atherogenesis, and immune dysfunction [64].

Moreover, increase in plasma CETP, which mediates transfer of cholesterol ester from HDL to IDL, has been demonstrated in dialysis-dependent CKD patients [65] and, therefore, postulated in CKD late stages. The effect seems to be amplified by proteinuria, which has been shown to increase synthesis and markedly raise plasma concentration of CETP [66]. The mechanism responsible for the reported elevation of CETP in patients with ESRD is unknown and requires future investigation. Such alteration can contribute to the reduction in HDL cholesterol ester and the rise in HDL triglycerides found in ESRD.

Low-Density Lipoprotein

Plasma total cholesterol is usually normal or reduced in CKD patients, when measured with conventional methods.

Plasma cholesterol concentration is the result of its synthesis, catabolism, and tissue uptake. A paucity of studies have investigated the effect of CKD on these pathways.

CKD in the absence of heavy proteinuria does not significantly affect gene expressions of either hydroxyl-3-methylglutaryl-CoA reductase (HMG-CoA reductase), which is the rate-limiting enzyme for cholesterol biosynthesis, or that of cholesterol 7a-hydroxylase, which is the rate-limiting enzyme for cholesterol catabolism and conversion to bile acids [67]. Also, hepatic LDL receptor gene expression, which controls cholesterol uptake, is not altered in CKD without heavy proteinuria [67, 68].

The levels of LDL cholesterol remain normal or are only slightly elevated in uremic dyslipidemia [69, 70]. Kastarinen et al., in a recent study, assessed LDL clearance in non-dialyzed patients with various degrees of CKD. The major finding of the study was that LDL clearance is related to the renal function. LDL clearance was shown to be significantly decreased in severe renal impairment, whereas in patients with mild to moderate kidney failure, LDL metabolism remained comparable to that of control subjects [71]. Studies regarding LDL metabolism, conducted in experimental animal models with CKD, lead to analogue conclusions [72, 73]. All these findings suggest that in CKD both LDL receptor and LDL particle itself are defective.

There are, however, important qualitative changes in LDL of patients with CKD. The proportions of sdLDL and IDL, which are among the most atherogenic particles, are increased [74, 75]. sdLDL is a subtype of LDL that has high propensity to penetrate the vessel wall, becomes oxidized, and triggers the atherosclerotic process.

IDL is an intermediate metabolite of VLDL that undergoes further triglyceride hydrolysis by lipases. Especially in HD patients, but also in predialysis ones, hepatic triglyceride lipase activities are reduced, which limits IDL conversion to LDL with accumulation of plasmatic IDL [76].

IDL and sdLDL promote the growth of atheroma by inducing macrophages to become foam cells, while LDL requires oxidation in order to do so.

Lipoprotein (a)

Increased levels of lipoprotein (a) [Lp(a)] are a risk factor for cardiovascular disease (CVD) [77, 78]. Lp(a) is an LDL-like particle made of an apolipoprotein (a) [apo(a)] attached to the LDL by a disulfide linkage [79].

Studies in healthy individuals and in patients with CKD have shown that serum Lp(a) levels are strongly and negatively associated with apo(a) isoform size [80]. The molecular weight is inversely related to the plasma Lp(a) concentration. So individuals with small apo(a) isoforms have on average higher Lp(a) concentrations and vice versa [81]. This explains the high variability in plasma Lp(a) levels.

In patients with renal disease, GFR also contributes to change in plasma Lp(a) levels. In patients with high molecular weight (HMW) Lp(a) isoforms, but not those with low molecular weight (LMW) apo(a) isoforms, plasma Lp(a) levels start rising in stage 1 CKD even when GFR is still in normal range. Thus, predialysis CKD patients with HMW apo(a) isoforms tend to have much higher Lp(a) values than apo(a) phenotype-matched healthy controls, whereas patients with kidney diseases and LMW apo(a) isoforms have similar Lp(a) concentrations with phenotype-matched healthy individuals, who already have high Lp(a) levels [4, 79]. Prospective studies identified small apo(a) isoform size and not Lp(a) level as an independent predictor of total and cardiovascular mortality in patients with CKD [82, 83].

Apolipoprotein A-IV

ApolipoproteinA-IV (apoA-IV) is a 46-kDa glycoprotein mainly synthesized in intestinal enterocytes and incorporated in the nascent chylomicrons [84]. In vitro studies show that apoA-IV plays an important role in reverse cholesterol transport [85–88] and, thus, in protecting against arteriosclerosis. Because the reverse cholesterol transport is notoriously altered in patients with CKD [89], apoA-IV was investigated and found to be markedly increased in hemodialysis and peritoneal dialysis patients [90, 91]. It was identified as a marker of kidney impairment that starts increasing in the earliest stages of kidney disease [5], and high apoA-IV concentrations predict the progression of primary nondiabetic kidney disease [92]. Finally, some data demonstrate that the increase in apoA-IV caused by renal impairment is significantly modulated by low levels of serum albumin as a measure for the severity of the nephrotic syndrome [93].

Conclusion

CKD is a clinical condition characterized, in all stages of the natural history of the disease, by profound and complex alteration of lipid and lipoprotein metabolism. These abnormalities include both quantitative and qualitative modifications of the circulating lipoproteins. The main quantitative alterations are represented by an increase of triglycerides, apolipoprotein B- and apoC-III, VLDL, CMRs, and reduction of plasmatic HDL. The main qualitative alterations regard LDL with accumulation of its proportions of sdLDL and IDL and alterations in HDL cholesterol subfractions. The overall result is a complex unique alteration of the lipid profile compared to that normally described in healthy individuals, with accumulation of atherogenic particles and lack of the atheroprotective fractions, resulting in a notorious very high risk of CVD in CKD. However, the ideal target for plasma lipid in CKD is unknown, so as poorly described are the abnormalities present with milder degrees of renal impairment, since the conventional lipid measurements do not allow to appreciate them. Further investigations are, therefore, required in order to unmask the underworld of dyslipidemia in CKD stages I–V.

References

1. Appel G. Lipid abnormalities in renal disease. Kidney Int. 1991;39:169.
2. Sechi LA, Zingaro L, De Carli S, Sechi G, Catena C, Falleti E, et al. Increased serum lipoprotein(a) levels in patients with early renal failure. Ann Intern Med. 1998;129:457.
3. Kwan BC, Kronenberg F, Beddhu S, Cheung AK. Lipoprotein metabolism and lipid management in chronic kidney disease. J Am Soc Nephrol. 2007;18:1246.
4. Kronenberg F, Kuen E, Ritz E, Junker R, Konig P, Kraatz G, et al. Lipoprotein(a) serum concentrations and apolipoprotein(a) phenotypes in mild and moderate renal failure. J Am Soc Nephrol. 2000;11:105–15.
5. Kronenberg F, Kuen E, Ritz E, Konig P, Kraatz G, Lhotta K, et al. Apolipoprotein A-IV serum concentrations are elevated in patients with mild and moderate renal failure. J Am Soc Nephrol. 2002;13:461–9.
6. Krentz AJ. Lipoprotein abnormalities and their consequences for patients with type 2 diabetes. Diabetes Obes Metab. 2003;5 Suppl 1:S19–27.
7. Kronenberg F. Dyslipidemia and nephrotic syndrome: recent advances. J Ren Nutr. 2005;15:195–203.
8. Moore R, Thomas D, Morgan E, Wheeler D, Griffin P, Salaman J, et al. Abnormal lipid and lipoprotein profiles following renal transplantation. Transplant Proc. 1993;25:1060.
9. Dennis EA. Lipidomics joins the omics evolution. Proc Natl Acad Sci U S A. 2009;106: 2089–90.
10. Quehenberger O, Dennis EA. The human plasma lipidome. N Engl J Med. 2011;365: 1812–23.
11. Thompson A, Danesh J. Associations between apolipoprotein B, apolipoproteins AI, the apolipoprotein B/AI ratio and coronary heart disease: a literature-based meta-analysis of prospective studies. J Intern Med. 2006;259:481–92.
12. Benn M. Apolipoprotein B, levels, APOB alleles, and risk of ischemic cardiovascular disease in the general population, a review. Atherosclerosis. 2009;206:17–30.
13. Barter PJ, Ballantyne CM, Carmena R, Castro Cabezas M, Chapman BJ, Couture P, et al. Apo B versus cholesterol in estimating cardiovascular risk and in guiding therapy: report of the thirty-person/ten-country panel. J Intern Med. 2006;259:247–8.
14. Sacks F. The apolipoproteins story. Atherosclerosis. 2006;7(Suppl):23–7.
15. Bobik A. Apolipoprotein C-III and atherosclerosis. Circulation. 2008;118:702–4.
16. Eisenberg S, Bilheimer DW, Levy RI, Lindgren FT. On the metabolic conversion of human plasma very low density lipoprotein to low density lipoprotein. Biochim Biophys Acta. 1973;326:361–77.

17. Brown MS, Goldstein JL. Lipoprotein metabolism in the macrophage: implications for cholesterol deposition in atherosclerosis. Annu Rev Biochem. 1983;52:223–61.
18. Abrass CK. Cellular lipid metabolism and the role of lipids in progressive renal disease. Am J Nephrol. 2004;24:46–53.
19. Kaysen GA. New insights into lipid metabolism in chronic kidney disease. J Ren Nutr. 2011;21:120–3.
20. Vaziri ND. Dyslipidemia of chronic renal failure: the nature, mechanisms, and potential consequences. Am J Physiol Renal Physiol. 2006;290:F262–72.
21. Vaziri ND, Moradi H. Mechanisms of dyslipidemia of chronic renal failure. Hemodial Int. 2006;10:1–7.
22. Moradi H, Pahl MV, Elahimehr R, Vaziri ND. Impaired antioxidant activity of high-density lipoprotein in chronic kidney disease. Transl Res. 2009;153:77–85.
23. Vaziri ND, Moradi H, Pahl MV, Fogelman AM, Navab M. In vitro stimulation of HDL anti-inflammatory activity and inhibition of LDL pro-inflammatory activity in the plasma of patients with end-stage renal disease by an apoA-1 mimetic peptide. Kidney Int. 2009;76: 437–44.
24. Weiner DE, Sarnak MJ. Managing dyslipidemia in chronic kidney disease. J Gen Intern Med. 2004;19:1045.
25. de Boer IH, Astor BC, Kramer H, Palmas W, Seliger SL, Shlipak MG, et al. Lipoprotein abnormalities associated with mild impairment of kidney function in the multi-ethnic study of atherosclerosis. Clin J Am Soc Nephrol. 2008;3:125–32.
26. Samuelsson O, Attman PO, Knight-Gibson C, Kron B, Larsson R, Mulec H, et al. Lipoprotein abnormalities without hyperlipidaemia in moderate renal insufficiency. Nephrol Dial Transplant. 1994;9:1580–5.
27. Attman PO, Samuelsson O, Alaupovic P. The effect of decreasing renal function on lipoprotein profiles. Nephrol Dial Transplant. 2011;26:2572–5.
28. Chan MK, Varghese Z, Persaud JW, Baillod RA, Moorhead JF. Hyperlipidemia in patients on maintenance hemo- and peritoneal dialysis: the relative pathogenetic roles of triglyceride production and triglyceride removal. Clin Nephrol. 1983;17:183–90.
29. Cramp DG, Tickner TR, Beale DJ, Moorhead JF, Wills MR. Plasma triglyceride secretion and metabolism in chronic renal failure. Clin Chim Acta. 1977;76:237–41.
30. Verschoor L, Lammers R, Birkenhager JC. Triglyceride turnover in severe chronic non-nephrotic renal failure. Metabolism. 1978;27:879–83.
31. Bagdade JD, Yee E, Wilson D, Shafrir E. Hyperlipidemia in renal failure: studies of plasma lipoproteins, hepatic triglyceride production, and tissue lipoprotein lipase in a chronically uremic rat model. J Lab Clin Med. 1978;91:176–86.
32. Gregg RC, Diamond A, Mondon CE, Reaven GM. The effects of chronic uremia and dexamethasone on triglyceride kinetics in the rat. Metabolism. 1977;26:875–82.
33. Korczynska J, Stelmanska E, Nogalska A, Szolkiewicz M, Goyke E, Swierczynski J, et al. Upregulation of lipogenic enzymes genes expression in white adipose tissue of rats with chronic renal failure is associated with higher level of sterol regulatory element binding protein-1. Metabolism. 2004;53:1060–5.
34. Rutkowski B, Szolkiewicz M, Korczynska J, Sucajtys E, Stelmanska E, Nieweglowski T, et al. The role of lipogenesis in the development of uremic hyperlipidemia. Am J Kidney Dis. 2003;41:S84–8.
35. Szolkiewicz M, Nieweglowski T, Korczynska J, Sucajtys E, Stelmanska E, Goyke E, et al. Upregulation of fatty acid synthase gene expression in experimental chronic renal failure. Metabolism. 2002;51:1605–10.
36. Weinstock PH, Levak-Frank S, Hudgins LC, Radner H, Friedman JM, Zechner R, et al. Lipoprotein lipase controls fatty acid entry into adipose tissue, but fat mass is preserved by endogenous synthesis in mice deficient in adipose tissue lipoprotein lipase. Proc Natl Acad Sci U S A. 1997;94:10261–6.
37. Vaziri ND, Dang B, Zhan CD, Liang K. Downregulation of hepatic acyl-CoA: diglycerol acyltransferase (DGAT) in chronic renal failure. Am J Physiol Renal Physiol. 2004;287:F90–4.

38. Vaziri ND, Kim CH, Phan D, Kim S, Liang K. Upregulation of acyl-CoA: diacylglycerol acyltransferase (DGAT) expression in nephrotic syndrome. Kidney Int. 2004;66:262–7.
39. Sentí M, Romero R, Pedro-Botet J, Pelegrí A, Nogués X, Rubiés-Prat J. Lipoprotein abnormalities in hyperlipidemic and normolipidemic men on hemodialysis with chronic renal failure. Kidney Int. 1992;41:1394–9.
40. Attman PO, Samuelsson O, Alaupovic P. Lipoprotein metabolism and renal failure. Am J Kidney Dis. 1993;21:573.
41. Arnadottir M, Thysell H, Dallongeville J, Fruchart JC, Nilsson-Ehle P. Evidence that reduced lipoprotein lipase activity is not a primary pathogenetic factor for hypertriglyceridemia in renal failure. Kidney Int. 1995;48:779.
42. Kaysen GA. Lipid and lipoprotein metabolism in chronic kidney disease. J Ren Nutr. 2009;19:73–7.
43. Vaziri ND, Norris K. Lipid disorders and their relevance to outcomes in chronic kidney disease. Blood Purif. 2011;31:189–96.
44. Cheung AK, Parker CJ, Ren K, Iverius PH. Increased lipase inhibition in uremia: identification of pre-beta-HDL as a major inhibitor in normal and uremic plasma. Kidney Int. 1996;49:1360.
45. Vaziri ND, Liang K. Down-regulation of tissue lipoprotein lipase expression in experimental chronic renal failure. Kidney Int. 1996;50:1928–35.
46. Lacour B, Roullet JB, Liagre AM, Jorgetti V, Beyne P, Dubost C, et al. Serum lipoprotein disturbances in primary and secondary hyperparathyroidism and effects of parathyroidectomy. Am J Kidney Dis. 1986;8:422.
47. Liang K, Oveisi F, Vaziri ND. Role of secondary hyperparathyroidism in the genesis of hypertriglyceridemia and VLDL receptor deficiency in chronic renal failure. Kidney Int. 1998;53:626–30.
48. Akmal M, Perkins S, Kasim SE, Oh HY, Smogorzewski M, Massry SG. Verapamil prevents chronic renal failure-induced abnormalities in lipid metabolism. Am J Kidney Dis. 1993;22:158.
49. Klin M, Smogorzewski M, Ni Z, Zhang G, Massry SG. Abnormalities in hepatic lipase in chronic renal failure: role of excess parathyroid hormone. J Clin Invest. 1996;97:2167–73.
50. Kim C, Vaziri ND. Down-regulation of hepatic LDL receptor-related protein (LRP) in chronic renal failure. Kidney Int. 2005;67:1028–32.
51. Vaziri ND, Liang K. Down-regulation of VLDL receptor expression in chronic experimental renal failure. Kidney Int. 1997;51:913–9.
52. Vaziri ND, Deng G, Liang K. Hepatic HDL receptor, SR-B1 and Apo AI expression in chronic renal failure. Nephrol Dial Transplant. 1999;14:1462–6.
53. Guarnieri GF, Moracchiello M, Campanacci L, Ursini F, Ferri L, Valente M, et al. Lecithin-cholesterol acyltransferase (LCAT) activity in chronic uremia. Kidney Int Suppl. 1978;13: S26–30.
54. McLeod R, Reeve CE, Frohlich J. Plasma lipoproteins and lecithin: cholesterol acyltransferase distribution in patients on dialysis. Kidney Int. 1984;25:683–8.
55. Shoji T, Nishizawa Y, Nishitani H, Billheimer JT, Sturley SL. Impaired metabolism of high density lipoprotein in uremic patients. Kidney Int. 1992;41:1653–61.
56. Liang K, Kim C, Vaziri ND. HMG-CoA reductase inhibition reverses LCAT and LDL receptor deficiencies and improves HDL in rats with chronic renal failure. Am J Physiol Renal Physiol. 2005;288:F539–44.
57. Vaziri ND, Liang K, Parks JS. Downregulation of lecithin: cholesterol acyltransferase (LCAT) in chronic renal failure. Kidney Int. 2001;59:2192–6.
58. Vaziri ND, Sato T, Liang K. Molecular mechanism of altered cholesterol metabolism in focal glomerulosclerosis. Kidney Int. 2003;63:1756–63.
59. Liang K, Vaziri ND. Downregulation of hepatic high-density lipoprotein receptor, SR-B1 in nephrotic syndrome. Kidney Int. 1999;56:621–6.
60. Liang K, Vaziri ND. Upregulation of acyl-CoA: cholesterol acyltransferase in chronic renal failure. Am J Physiol Endocrinol Metab. 2002;283:E676–81.

61. Vaziri ND, Liang K. ACAT inhibition reverses LCAT deficiency and improves plasma HDL in chronic renal failure. Am J Physiol Renal Physiol. 2004;287:F1038–43.
62. Ansell BJ, Navab M, Hama S, Kamranpour N, Fonarow G, Hough G, et al. Inflammatory/anti-inflammatory properties of high density lipoprotein distinguish patients from control subjects better than high density lipoprotein cholesterol levels and are favourably affected by simvastatin treatment. Circulation. 2003;108:2751–6.
63. Van Lenten BJ, Reddy ST, Navab M, Fogelman AM. Understanding changes in high density lipoproteins during the acute phase response. Arterioscler Thromb Vasc Biol. 2006;26:1687–8.
64. Meier P, Golshayan D, Blanc E, Pascual M, Burnier M. Oxidized LDL modulates apoptosis of regulatory T cells in patients with ESRD. J Am Soc Nephrol. 2009;20:1368–84.
65. Kimura H, Miyazaki R, Imura T, Masunaga S, Suzuki S, Gejyo F, et al. Hepatic lipase mutation may reduce vascular disease prevalence in haemodialysis patients with high CETP levels. Kidney Int. 2003;64:1829–37.
66. De Sain-van der Velden MG, Rabelink TJ, Reijngoud DJ, Gadellaa MM, Voorbij HA, Stellaard F, et al. Plasma α2 macroglobulin is increased in nephrotic patients as a result of increased synthesis alone. Kidney Int. 1998;54:530–5.
67. Liang K, Vaziri ND. Gene expression of LDL receptor, HMG-CoA reductase, and cholesterol-7 alpha-hydroxylase in chronic renal failure. Nephrol Dial Transplant. 1997;12:1381–6.
68. Pandak WM, Vlahcevic ZR, Heuman DM, Krieg RJ, Hanna JD, Chan JC. Post transcriptional regulation of 3-hydroxy-3-methylglutaryl coenzyme A reductase and cholesterol 7α-hydroxylase in rats with subtotal nephrectomy. Kidney Int. 1994;46:358–64.
69. Attman PO, Alaupovic P. Lipid and apolipoprotein profiles of uremic dyslipoproteinemia—relation to renal function and dialysis. Nephron. 1991;57:401–10.
70. Hörkkö S, Huttunen K, Korhonen T, Kesäniemi YA. Decreased clearance of low-density lipoprotein in patients with chronic renal failure. Kidney Int. 1994;45:561–70.
71. Kastarinen H, Hörkkö S, Kauma H, Karjalainen A, Savolainen MJ, Kesäniemi YA. Low-density lipoprotein clearance in patients with chronic renal failure. Nephrol Dial Transplant. 2009;24:2131–5.
72. Shapiro RJ. Catabolism of low-density lipoprotein is altered in experimental chronic renal failure. Metabolism. 1993;42:162–9.
73. Hörkkö S, Huttunen K, Kervinen K, Kesäniemi YA. Decreased clearance of uraemic and mildly carbamylated low-density lipoprotein. Eur J Clin Invest. 1994;24:105–13.
74. Rajman I, Harper L, McPake D, Kendall MJ, Wheeler DC. Low density lipoprotein subfraction profiles in chronic renal failure. Nephrol Dial Transplant. 1998;13:2281–7.
75. Deighan CJ, Caslake MJ, McConnell M, Boulton-Jones JM, Packard CJ. Atherogenic lipoprotein phenotype in end-stage renal failure: origin and extent of small dense low-density lipoprotein formation. Am J Kidney Dis. 2000;35:852–62.
76. Oi K, Hirano T, Sakai S, Kawaguchi Y, Hosoya T. Role of hepatic lipase in intermediate-density lipoprotein and small, dense low-density lipoprotein formation in hemodialysis patients. Kidney Int Suppl. 1999;71:S227–8.
77. Craig WY, Neveux LM, Palomaki GE, Cleveland MM, Haddow JE. Lipoprotein(a) as a risk factor for ischemic heart disease: metaanalysis of prospective studies. Clin Chem. 1998;44:2301–6.
78. Dieplinger H, Kronenberg F. Genetics and metabolism of lipoprotein(a) and their clinical implications (Part 1). Wien Klin Wochenschr. 1999;111:5–20.
79. Milionis HJ, Elisaf MS, Tselepis A, Bairaktari E, Karabina SA, Siamopoulos KC. Apolipoprotein(a) phenotypes and lipoprotein(a) concentrations in patients with renal failure. Am J Kidney Dis. 1999;33:1100–6.
80. Tsimihodimos V, Mitrogianni Z, Elisaf M. Dyslipidemia associated with chronic kidney disease. Open Cardiovasc Med J. 2011;5:41–8.
81. Utermann G, Menzel HJ, Kraft HG, Duba HC, Kemmler HG, Seitz C. Lp(a) glycoprotein phenotypes. Inheritance and relation to Lp(a)-lipoprotein concentrations in plasma. J Clin Invest. 1987;80:458–65.

82. Kronenberg F, Neyer U, Lhotta K, Trenkwalder E, Auinger M, Pribasnig A, et al. The low molecular weight apo(a) phenotype is an independent predictor for coronary artery disease in hemodialysis patients: a prospective follow-up. J Am Soc Nephrol. 1999;10:1027–36.
83. Longenecker JC, Klag MJ, Marcovina SM, Powe NR, Fink NE, Giaculli F, et al. Small apolipoprotein(a) size predicts mortality in end-stage renal disease: the CHOICE study. Circulation. 2002;106:2812–8.
84. Green PHR, Glickman RM, Riley JW, Qinet E. Human apolipoprotein A-IV. Intestinal origin and distribution in plasma. J Clin Invest. 1980;65:911–9.
85. Stein O, Stein Y, Lefevre M, Roheim PS. The role of apolipoprotein A-IV in reverse cholesterol transport studied with cultured cells and liposomes derived from another analogue of phosphatidylcholine. Biochim Biophys Acta. 1986;878:7–13.
86. Steinmetz A, Utermann G. Activation of lecithin: cholesterol acyltransferase by human apolipoprotein A-IV. J Biol Chem. 1985;260:2258–64.
87. Chen CH, Albers JJ. Activation of lecithin: cholesterol acyltransferase by apolipoproteins E-2, E-3 and A-IV isolated from human plasma. Biochim Biophys Acta. 1985;836:279–85.
88. Guyard-Dangremont V, Lagrost L, Gambert P. Comparative effects of purified apolipoproteins A-I, A-II, and A-IV on cholesteryl ester transfer protein activity. J Lipid Res. 1994;35:982–92.
89. Fielding CJ. Lipoprotein receptors, plasma cholesterol metabolism, and the regulation of cellular free cholesterol concentration. FASEB J. 1992;6:3162–8.
90. Nestel PJ, Fide NH, Tan MH. Increased lipoprotein-remnant formation in chronic renal failure. N Engl J Med. 1982;307:329–33.
91. Kronenberg F, König P, Neyer U, Auinger M, Pribasnig A, Lang U, et al. Multicenter study of lipoprotein(a) and apolipoprotein(a) phenotypes in patients with end-stage renal disease treated by hemodialysis or continuous ambulatory peritoneal dialysis. J Am Soc Nephrol. 1995;6:110–20.
92. Boes E, Fliser D, Ritz E, König P, Lhotta K, Mann JFE, et al.; for the MMKD Study Group. Apolipoprotein A-IV predicts progression of chronic kidney disease: the Mild to Moderate Kidney Disease Study. J Am Soc Nephrol. 2006;17:528–36.
93. Lingenhel A, Lhotta K, Neyer U, Heid IM, Rantner B, Kronenberg MF, et al. Role of the kidney in the metabolism of apolipoproteins A-IV: influence of the type of proteinuria. J Lipid Res. 2006;47:2071–9.

Chapter 7
Review of Clinical Trials Pertaining to Dyslipidemias in CKD

Markus P. Schneider and Kai-Uwe Eckardt

Introduction

Patients with early stages of chronic kidney disease (CKD) are already at high risk for cardiovascular (CV) events, such as myocardial infarction or stroke. This risk is similar in magnitude to the risk in subjects who have established coronary artery disease [1]. In patients with advanced, dialysis-dependent CKD, the risk of a CV event is 40–50 times greater than the risk in the general population [2]. In part, this increased CV risk is due to the high prevalence of "classical" cardiovascular risk factors in this patient cohort, such as arterial hypertension and diabetes mellitus. In addition, a number of risk factors are of particular relevance to patients with CKD. This includes derangements in electrolyte and mineral metabolism (e.g., hyperphosphatemia), oxidative stress, chronic inflammation, nitric oxide deficiency/endothelial dysfunction, vascular calcifications, left ventricular hypertrophy, and chronic hemodynamic stress (e.g., due to high fistula blood flows and the hemodialysis procedure itself).

There are also profound disturbances in the lipid profile of patients with CKD. The alterations in lipids are complex, and a more precise description of these alterations is beyond the scope of this chapter. In the context of clinical decision making, it is important to note, however, that a standard lipid profile in a CKD patient often shows only a mild increase in triglyceride levels and a decrease in high density lipoprotein (HDL) cholesterol levels, while low density lipoprotein (LDL) and total cholesterol levels are commonly within the normal range. The more complex alterations associated with CKD (e.g., in the specific lipoprotein content, or the increase in small dense LDL particles, which is strongly linked with atherosclerosis) are not detected by standard clinical chemistry.

M.P. Schneider, M.D. (✉) • K.-U. Eckardt, M.D.
Department of Nephrology and Hypertension, University Hospital Erlangen and Community Hospital Nuremberg, Ulmenweg 18, Erlangen 91054, Bavaria, Germany
e-mail: markus.schneider@uk-erlangen.de; kai-uwe.eckardt@uk-erlangen.de

A. Covic et al. (eds.), *Dyslipidemias in Kidney Disease*, DOI 10.1007/978-1-4939-0515-7_7,

In patients on dialysis and in patients with a kidney transplant, this dyslipidemia, in particular the increase in non-HDL cholesterol, has been associated with increased CV mortality [3, 4]. However, the relationship between altered lipid levels and outcome is strongly confounded by the presence of inflammation and malnutrition in CKD. Statin therapy has been demonstrated to reduce cardiovascular events and lower mortality in a number of diverse patient populations at increased cardiovascular risk [5, 6]. Statin therapy can safely reduce major coronary events, coronary revascularization, and stroke by about one-fifth per millimole per liter reduction in LDL cholesterol [5]. Of note, a meta-analysis has shown that the absolute benefit of statin therapy relates chiefly to an individual's absolute CV risk, and to the absolute reduction in LDL cholesterol achieved, while it is largely independent of the initial lipid profile [5].

Most patients with CKD stages 1–2 have proteinuria and normal or only slightly reduced glomerular filtration rate (GFR), and a substantial number of these patients have been included in statin trials of the "general" population (e.g., because proteinuria was not assessed at baseline). The available evidence from these trials suggests that the subset of patients with CKD stages 1–2 have a similar benefit from statin therapy compared to subjects without CKD [7, 8].

In patients with more advanced forms of CKD (≥stage 3), observational studies [9, 10] and post hoc analyses of large-scale intervention trials [11, 12] have also suggested that statin therapy may improve survival. Until a few years ago, there was consequently great enthusiasm for the use of statins in all stages of CKD [13], even though evidence for this recommendation was very limited. It is only recently that large-scale randomized controlled trials have become available in patients with more advanced CKD.

In part because of the overall "negative" outcomes of some of these studies, and because of the financial risks involved, we consider it rather unlikely that more resources will be allocated in the future to lipid-lowering trials in patients with CKD. A critical review of the available studies is therefore particularly important. In this chapter, we will review the design and the results of the few large-scale studies that are available in this area, aiming to highlight similarities and discrepancies between these trials, and trying to identify those patients who are likely to benefit from this therapy. For a brief overview of the trials to be discussed in the following, please see Table 7.1.

The 4D Study

The "Deutsche Diabetes Dialyse Studie" (4D) was a multicenter, randomized, double-blind prospective trial comparing the effects of treatment with 20 mg of atorvastatin per day versus matching placebo [14]. A total number of 1,255 subjects were enrolled at 178 participating centers between March 1998 and October 2002 and were followed until their final visit in March 2004. The primary endpoint was a composite of death from cardiac causes, nonfatal myocardial infarction, and fatal or

Table 7.1 Overview of major randomized clinical trials on statin therapy in CKD patients

	4D	AURORA	SHARP	ALERT
Intervention	Atorvastatin 20 mg/day	Rosuvastatin 10 mg/day	Simvastatin 20 mg/day + ezetimibe 10 mg/day	Fluvastatin 40 mg/day (dose increase permitted)
Sample size	1,255	2,776	9,270	2,102
Major inclusion criteria	Age 18–80 years, with type 2 diabetes, on HD for <2 years LDL 80–190 mg/dL	Age 50–80 years, on HD for >3 months	Age > 40 years	Age 30–75 years, at least 6 months time from kidney transplantation, stable transplant function
Major exclusion criteria	LDL > 190 mg/dL	Any statin treatment in the prior 6 months	Prior MI or coronary revascularization Creatinine ≥ 1.7 mg/dL (men) Creatinine ≥ 1.5 mg/dL (women)	Recent MI
LDL cholesterol at baseline	3.13 mmol/L (121 mg/dL) in the atorvastatin group versus 3.23 mmol/L (125 mg/dL) in the placebo group	2.59 mmol/L (100 mg/dL) in the rosuvastatin versus 2.56 mmol/L (99 mg/dL) in the placebo group	2.77 mmol/L (107 mg/dL) in the simvastatin/ezetimibe group versus 2.78 mmol/L (108 mg/dL) in the placebo group	4.1 mmol/L (156 mg/dL) in the fluvastatin versus 4.1 mmol/L (156 mg/dL) in the placebo group
LDL cholesterol lowering (%)	42	43	31	32
Median follow-up (years)	4.0	3.8	4.9	5.4
Hemodialysis	100 %	100 %	33 %	NA
Diabetes mellitus (%)	100	26	23	19
Primary composite endpoint	Composite of death from cardiac causes, nonfatal MI, and fatal or nonfatal stroke	Composite of death from cardiovascular causes, nonfatal MI, or nonfatal stroke	Composite of coronary death, nonfatal MI, ischemic stroke, or any arterial revascularization procedure	Major adverse cardiac event, defined as cardiac death, nonfatal MI, or coronary revascularization procedure
Number of events: active therapy versus placebo group	226 (36.5 %) versus 243 (38.2 %)	396 (28.5 %) versus 408 (29.5 %)	526 (11.3 %) versus 619 (13.4 %)	112 (10.7 %) versus 134 (12.7 %)
Statistical significance for primary endpoint	RR, 0.92; 95 % confidence interval, 0.77–1.10; *P* = 0.37	HR, 0.96; 95 % confidence interval, 0.84–1.11; *P* = 0.59	RR, 0.83; 95 % confidence interval, 0.74–0.94; *P* = 0.0021	RR, 0.83; 95 % confidence interval, 0.64–1.06; *P* = 0.139
Effect on overall mortality	No	No	No	No

nonfatal stroke. Death from cardiac causes comprised fatal myocardial infarction (death within 28 days after a myocardial infarction), sudden death, death due to congestive heart failure, death due to coronary heart disease during or within 28 days after an intervention, and all other deaths ascribed to coronary heart disease. Those patients who died unexpectedly and did not present with a potassium level greater than 7.5 mmol/L before the start of the three most recent hemodialysis sessions were considered to have died from sudden cardiac death. Myocardial infarction was diagnosed when two of the following three criteria were met: typical symptoms, elevated levels of cardiac enzymes, or diagnostic changes on the electrocardiogram. A resting electrocardiogram was recorded every 6 months and evaluated by independent cardiologists from the electrocardiographic monitoring board. An electrocardiogram that documented silent myocardial infarction was considered evidence of a primary endpoint. Stroke was defined as a neurologic deficit lasting longer than 24 h, and computed-tomographic or magnetic resonance imaging of the brain was recommended to confirm the diagnosis. Secondary endpoints included death from all causes, all cardiac events combined, and all cerebrovascular events combined.

The choice of the primary composite endpoint in such studies is to some extent arbitrary. In order to demonstrate efficacy of an intervention, a sufficient number of endpoints must be reached. To increase the number of events, clinical endpoints that presumably share similar pathogenic mechanisms are often included into a single *composite* endpoint. It is interesting to note that stroke was included in the primary composite endpoint by the steering committee of 4D only just before the trial was unblinded (i.e., before treatment allocation was revealed and the study analyzed). Presumably, the investigators had concerns that there may not be a sufficiently large number of cardiac events to demonstrate significant differences in event rates between the two treatment groups.

The results of the trial were published in July 2005. The median level of LDL cholesterol was 121 mg/dL (3.13 mmol/L) in the atorvastatin group and 125 mg/dL (3.23 mmol/L) in the placebo group at the time of randomization. Four weeks after randomization, the median level of LDL cholesterol fell to 72 mg/dL in the atorvastatin group (1.86 mmol/L; median change from baseline, –42 %), while there was no significant change in the placebo group. There is no good evidence for a particular target level of LDL cholesterol in maintenance hemodialysis patients. However, the degree of LDL cholesterol lowering with atorvastatin in 4D would be well in keeping with the National Cholesterol Education Program Adult Treatment Panel (ATP) III guidelines from the American National Heart, Lung and Blood Institute, where an LDL cholesterol target of <100 mg/dL has been recommended for subjects with established coronary artery disease (≈30 % of subjects included in 4D had a history of coronary artery disease). A substantial number of subjects in the active treatment arm in 4D even reached the lower LDL cholesterol target of <70 mg/dL, recommended for subjects with a risk for a cardiovascular event rate of >20 % over the next 10 years [15].

During a median follow-up period of 4 years, a total of 469 patients (37 %) reached the primary composite endpoint, of which 226 were assigned to atorvastatin and 243 to placebo (relative risk [RR], 0.92; 95 % confidence interval [CI],

0.77–1.10; $P=0.37$). In addition to the primary composite endpoint, there were also no significant differences in the components of the primary endpoint, except for the relative risk of fatal stroke among those receiving atorvastatin, which was increased to 2.03 compared to the placebo group (95 % confidence interval, 1.05–3.93; $P=0.04$). However, the overall number of fatal strokes was low (13 in the placebo versus 27 in the atorvastatin group, $P=0.04$), and the apparent excess of fatal strokes in the atorvastatin groups was considered a chance finding.

Among the predefined secondary endpoints, atorvastatin had no effect on all cerebrovascular events combined (relative risk, 1.12; 95 % confidence interval, 0.81–1.55; $P=0.49$) or on total mortality (relative risk, 0.93; 95 % confidence interval, 0.79–1.08; $P=0.33$). The only "positive" finding for atorvastatin treatment in 4D, which was based on a predefined secondary endpoint, was that atorvastatin reduced cardiac events (205 in the atorvastatin group versus 246 in the placebo group; relative risk, 0.82; 95 % confidence interval, 0.68–0.99; $P=0.03$). Although the 4D study is widely perceived as a "negative" outcome trial, it was the first randomized controlled study to demonstrate some benefit of statin treatment in maintenance hemodialysis patients. Of note, 4D was also the first larger study providing information about the safety profile of statins in patients on hemodialysis. Prior to this study, some concerns were raised in view of potential safety issues with statin treatment in hemodialysis patients. In particular, there was concern of an increased rate of severe cases of rhabdomyolysis [16]. However, no cases of rhabdomyolysis or serious liver abnormalities were noted in 4D, providing reassurance that statin treatment should be safe in this patient population.

The AURORA Study

"A Study to Evaluate the Use of Rosuvastatin in Subjects on Regular Hemodialysis: An Assessment of Survival and Cardiovascular Events" (AURORA) included subjects on maintenance hemodialysis with diabetes mellitus and, in contrast to 4D, also hemodialysis patients without diabetes mellitus [17]. Recruitment took place from January 2003 through December 2004, and a total of 2,776 patients were randomly assigned to double-blind treatment with rosuvastatin at a dose of 10 mg or matched placebo. AURORA included more than twice as many subjects as the 4D study.

The primary endpoint was time to a major cardiovascular event, defined as a nonfatal myocardial infarction, nonfatal stroke, or death from cardiovascular causes. All myocardial infarctions, strokes, and deaths were reviewed and adjudicated by a clinical endpoint committee whose members were unaware of the randomized treatment assignments. Secondary endpoints included all-cause mortality, cardiovascular event-free survival (i.e., freedom from nonfatal myocardial infarction, nonfatal stroke, death from cardiovascular causes, and death from any other cause), procedures performed for stenosis or thrombosis of the vascular access for long-term hemodialysis (arteriovenous fistulas and grafts only), and coronary or peripheral revascularization, death from cardiovascular causes, and death from non-cardiovascular causes.

A 19.5 % decrease in major cardiovascular events was predicted with active treatment. It was estimated that at least 805 major cardiovascular events would occur, yielding a power of 87 % to demonstrate the predicted difference in events (at a *P*-value of <0.05).

The results of the trial were published in April 2009. Baseline LDL cholesterol levels were even lower than in the 4D study: 100±35 mg/dL (2.59±0.9 mmol/L) in subjects randomized to rosuvastatin and 99±34 mg/dL (2.56±0.9 mmol/L) in subjects randomized to placebo (n.s. between the groups). Three months after randomization, the LDL cholesterol level in the rosuvastatin group was 42.9 % lower than the baseline level, as compared with a 1.9 % reduction in the placebo group ($P<0.001$ for the between-group comparison). Total cholesterol levels were reduced by 27 %, and HDL cholesterol levels showed an increase of 2 % with active treatment. Again, LDL cholesterol levels were reached by many subjects in the active treatment group that would be in line with even stringent treatment goals in subjects with coronary artery disease [15]. Furthermore, after 3 months, high-sensitivity C-reactive protein (CRP) levels decreased by 14 % with active treatment compared with a 4 % increase in subjects allocated to placebo.

During a median follow-up period of 3.8 years, 396 patients in the rosuvastatin group and 408 patients in the placebo group reached the primary endpoint (hazard ratio [HR] for the combined endpoint in the rosuvastatin group versus the placebo group, 0.96; 95 % confidence interval, 0.84–1.11; $P=0.59$) by intention-to-treat analysis. Results were similar for the per-protocol analysis. Rosuvastatin also had no effect on individual components of the primary endpoint, and there was no significant effect on all-cause mortality (13.5 versus 14.0 events per 100 patient-years; hazard ratio, 0.96; 95 % confidence interval, 0.86–1.07; $P=0.51$). The lack of an effect of rosuvastatin therapy on the primary endpoint was consistent in all prespecified subgroups, including patients with diabetes, preexisting cardiovascular disease, hypertension, a high baseline LDL cholesterol level, or an elevated baseline high-sensitivity CRP level. Further, there was no relationship between the primary cardiovascular endpoint and baseline LDL cholesterol levels or LDL cholesterol levels at 3 months.

In terms of safety, a few cases of rhabdomyolysis were noted in this larger study, but there was no difference in the incidence between subjects randomized to rosuvastatin versus those randomized to placebo (3 out of 1,389 in the atorvastatin group versus 2 out of 1,378 in the placebo group, $P=0.66$). Again, statin therapy appears to be safe in hemodialysis patients.

Post Hoc Analysis of AURORA Limited to the Diabetic Subpopulation

More recently, a further analysis of the AURORA database was published, limited to the 731 subjects with type 2 diabetes mellitus that were included in the trial [18]. For the primary endpoint chosen in the overall AURORA trial (cardiac death, nonfatal myocardial infarction, fatal or nonfatal stroke), there was no reduction for rosuvastatin compared to placebo in the diabetes subpopulation (HR, 0.838; 95 % confidence interval, 0.654–1.074; $P=0.163$). However, a post hoc defined (i.e., not pre-specified), composite cardiac endpoint of cardiac death or nonfatal myocardial infarction occurred in 85 diabetic patients allocated to rosuvastatin and in 104 diabetic patients allocated to placebo (hazard ratio, 0.68; 95 % confidence interval, 0.51–0.90; $P=0.008$). The number needed to treat for this composite cardiac endpoint was 11.9 per 100 treated patients for 2.8 years. A key similarity between 4D and AURORA, therefore, is that both trials appear to suggest that statins are able to lower the risk of cardiac events in diabetic patients on maintenance hemodialysis (reduction of 32 % in AURORA and reduction of 18 % in 4D).

There was no difference in overall stroke rate in the diabetes subpopulation of AURORA, but subjects allocated to rosuvastatin had more hemorrhagic strokes than those allocated to placebo (12 versus two strokes, respectively; hazard ratio, 5.21; 95 % confidence interval, 1.17–23.27). Similar to 4D, which reported a small increase in the number of fatal stroke (but mostly of the ischemic subtype), it was argued by the authors that this may also have been a chance finding, considering the small number of fatal stroke events.

Although this analysis of AURORA suggests some benefit of statins on cardiac outcomes in diabetic hemodialysis patients, it needs to be emphasized that this was a post hoc analysis with an endpoint that was not pre-specified. We believe that the results of this post hoc analysis should therefore only be regarded as hypothesis-generating.

Potential Reasons for the Overall Negative Outcomes of 4D and AURORA

Table 7.2 shows a list of potential reasons for the overall negative outcomes of 4D and AURORA. LDL cholesterol levels were already low at baseline (≈120 mg/dL in 4D, ≈100 mg/dL in AURORA). In 4D, subjects with elevated LDL cholesterol levels (>4.9 mmol/L, corresponding to >189 mg/dL) were excluded from the trial, whereas in AURORA, subjects were included irrespective of their baseline LDL cholesterol levels. The low baseline LDL cholesterol levels may be related with the lack of effect of statin treatment in these trials, although meta-analysis (in subjects not on hemodialysis) suggests that the benefit of statin treatment mainly relates to the overall cardiovascular risk of the patient and the absolute reduction in LDL cholesterol level achieved during treatment, but does not relate to baseline LDL cholesterol levels [5].

Further, relatively few patients had coronary artery disease at baseline: less than one-third had coronary artery disease at baseline in 4D, and only ≈40 % had cardiovascular disease at baseline in AURORA. In AURORA, patients who had received a statin within the previous 6 months were excluded from participation. As a consequence, those subjects who had been deemed to benefit from statin therapy by the

Table 7.2 Potential reasons for the overall negative outcome of 4D and AURORA

Low baseline LDL cholesterol levels in both studies
In AURORA, exclusion of subjects who were treated with a statin in the previous 6 months → potential selection bias to include subjects which have been deemed NOT to benefit from statin therapy by their treating physician prior to the study
Relatively few patients with coronary artery disease at baseline (less than one-third in 4D and only ≈40 % of patients had cardiovascular disease at baseline in AURORA)
Deaths in hemodialysis patients largely due to non-atherosclerotic events (sepsis, sudden cardiac death, cancer)
Choice of primary composite endpoints included events not amenable to statin therapy (in particular sudden cardiac death)
Too small sample sizes to detect smaller effects of statins on atherosclerotic events in the hemodialysis population
Large number of drop-outs in active treatment arms (in 4D: 17 % of patients discontinued their statin after 2 years; in AURORA: 50 % discontinued their statin treatment)
Large number of "drop-ins" of non-study statin treatment (in 4D: 15 % of patients in the placebo-assigned group; not reported in AURORA)
Small difference in LDL cholesterol levels towards end of study (in 4D: –0.78 mmol/L, in AURORA: –0.5 mmol/L)

treating physician were not eligible for randomization, whereas those not deemed to benefit were more likely to be randomized. Thus, the low baseline LDL cholesterol levels, the inclusion of a large number of subjects without clinical evidence of cardiovascular disease, and the exclusion of subjects pretreated with statins might have introduced a bias to include subjects with lower cardiovascular risk.

Perhaps more important for the interpretation of these two studies are the specific endpoints that were chosen in 4D and AURORA. These included a number of clinical events that are not thought to be due to atherosclerotic disease, and therefore unlikely to be affected by statin therapy. In particular this should be the case for sudden cardiac death, which in 4D constituted 13 % of deaths in the placebo group and 12 % of deaths in the atorvastatin group. In contrast, coronary artery disease as an endpoint was less likely to occur in 4D: fatal myocardial infarctions occurred in 5 % in the placebo group versus in 4 % in the atorvastatin group. Further, deaths after interventions to treat coronary artery disease occurred in 0.6 % in the placebo group versus in 0.5 % in the atorvastatin group. Other deaths due to coronary artery disease were 0.8 % in the placebo versus 0.2 % in the atorvastatin group. Adding up all coronary events, there were a total of 6.4 % in the placebo versus 4.7 % in the atorvastatin group, significantly less than the rates of sudden cardiac death (13 and 12 %). In AURORA, sudden cardiac death was part of the endpoint "death from cardiovascular causes," which occurred in 324 subjects in the atorvastatin group compared with 324 subjects in the placebo group. Numbers for sudden cardiac death alone were not reported. Nonetheless, coronary events were also much less common in AURORA: definite death from coronary artery disease occurred in 143 patients in the atorvastatin group compared with 156 patients in the placebo group, and suspected death from coronary artery disease in 61 patients in the atorvastatin group compared with 53 patients in the placebo group. Thus, by including sudden cardiac death in their primary composite endpoints, the power to detect significant effects on atherosclerotic events was diminished in 4D and AURORA. The inclusion of stroke into the primary composite endpoint (in 4D just before the trial was unblinded) also contributed to the overall lack of an effect of statins in these two trials.

Last but not least, in 4D about 17 % of patients and in AURORA even 50 % of patients in each treatment arm discontinued their study medication before study completion. This occurred after an adverse event, after receiving a kidney transplant, or for other reasons. Furthermore, in addition to the drop-out of active treatment, a large number of "drop-ins" of non-study statin treatment occurred: in 4D, 15 % of patients assigned to placebo took a statin towards the end of the study. Numbers for drop-ins were not reported in AURORA, but were probably substantial as well. As a consequence, the difference in LDL cholesterol values between active treatment and placebo treatment arms diminished during the course of the study: LDL cholesterol levels towards the end of 4D and the AURORA study differed only by 0.78 and 0.5 mmol/L, respectively. It is likely that this affected the ability of these studies to demonstrate a beneficial effect of active treatment.

Of further interest is the comparison of the results of AURORA with those of the non-CKD studies JUPITER (Justification for the Use of Statins in Prevention: an Intervention Trial Evaluating Rosuvastatin) [19] and CORONA (Controlled Rosuvastatin Multinational Trial in Heart Failure) [20], in particular since all three studies measured CRP levels as a marker of inflammation.

In JUPITER, the rational was that rosuvastatin would reduce inflammation and cardiovascular events in subjects with normal cholesterol levels and without clinically apparent cardiovascular disease, but increased inflammatory burden (high sensitive CRP level of 2.0 mg/L or more was a key inclusion criterion). The primary endpoint was the occurrence of a first major cardiovascular event, defined as nonfatal myocardial infarction, nonfatal stroke, hospitalization for unstable angina, an arterial revascularization procedure, or confirmed death from cardiovascular causes. Rosuvastatin reduced CRP levels and reduced the primary endpoint in these apparently healthy subjects and, in contrast to AURORA, there was a significant reduction of coronary events and revascularization procedures.

CORONA (Controlled Rosuvastatin Multinational Trial in Heart Failure) randomly allocated patients with heart failure, but without kidney disease, to treatment with 10 mg rosuvastatin versus placebo [20]. The results were strikingly similar to those of AURORA. There was no reduction in deaths from cardiovascular disease, nonfatal myocardial infarctions, or strokes despite a decrease in LDL cholesterol of 45 %. Statin treatment did reduce the risk of coronary events, but similar to AURORA, these events accounted for the minority of the combined primary outcome (only 10 % of patients in CORONA had a coronary event and only 2 % of deaths were due to myocardial infarction). Similar to the situation in hemodialysis patients, a substantial number of patients with heart failure succumb to clinical events not directly related to atherosclerosis, and in particular to sudden cardiac death. This lack of effect of rosuvastatin on mortality in heart failure patients was also shown in the Italian GISSI-HF (Gruppo Italiano per lo Studio della Sopravvivenza nell'Infarto miocardico) trial [21], although CRP levels were not reported in this study.

The SHARP Study

The Study of Heart and Renal Protection (SHARP) is the largest of all available randomized controlled intervention trials in the CKD population [22]. A total of 9,270 patients with CKD, of which 3,023 were on dialysis (>80 % hemodialysis, <20 % peritoneal dialysis) and 6,247 were not, with no known history of myocardial infarction or coronary revascularization were randomized to treatment with simvastatin 20 mg plus ezetimibe 10 mg daily versus matching placebo.

Patients were eligible to participate if they were 40 years or older and if they had CKD with plasma creatinine of at least 150 μmol/L (1.7 mg/dL) in men or 130 μmol/L (1.5 mg/dL) in women or were receiving dialysis treatment. Randomization took place between August 2003 and August 2006.

The study was initially designed with the pre-specified primary endpoint being first major *vascular* event, i.e., cardiovascular death (including presumed sudden cardiac death), nonfatal myocardial infarction, hemorrhagic and non-hemorrhagic stroke, and any arterial revascularization procedure, but excluding dialysis access procedures. Before unblinding of SHARP, the results of 4D and AURORA were available. These studies, as discussed, have demonstrated that the majority of deaths in patients with advanced CKD are caused by non-atherosclerotic events such as sudden cardiac death, endpoints not considered amenable to cholesterol-lowering therapy. On the other hand, 4D and AURORA did suggest to some degree that statins might be effective in reducing atherosclerotic events. Thus, before unblinding of SHARP, hemorrhagic strokes and presumed sudden cardiac death were removed from the composite primary endpoint to increase the power of the study to detect a significant effect of active treatment on atherosclerotic events. Therefore, the primary endpoint of the study was changed from first major *vascular* event to first major *atherosclerotic* event, including nonfatal myocardial infarction or coronary death, non-hemorrhagic stroke, or any arterial revascularization procedure, but excluding dialysis access procedures [23]. SHARP also included pre-specified secondary endpoints related to the progression of kidney disease in the non-dialysis subpopulation of the study.

The results of the trial were published in June 2011. The publication provides a relatively detailed description on the number of drop-ins and drop-outs of therapy. As in the other trials, compliance with statin therapy in the active treatment group declined over the study duration such that at the midpoint of the study after 2.5 years, 71 % of the active treatment group took the study statin or a non-study statin. Conversely, in subjects allocated to placebo, the average use of a non-study statin was 9 % at study midpoint. This means that the intention-to-treat analysis actually assessed the effects of a difference in statin use of two-thirds of the subjects (rather than 100 % versus 0 %). LDL cholesterol at baseline was 2.77 ± 0.88 mmol/L (107 ± 34 mg/dL) in those randomized to simvastatin and ezetimibe versus 2.78 ± 0.87 mmol/L (108 ± 34 mg/dL) in those randomized to placebo. The average reduction of LDL cholesterol during the study with active treatment compared to placebo was 0.85 mmol/L (33 mg/dL). Again, this is less than expected if there were no drop-outs and drop-ins. Statin use was even lower in the subpopulation on dialysis, yielding an average reduction of LDL cholesterol of 0.6 mmol/L. The proportion of subjects with diabetes mellitus was 23 %, which was similar to AURORA with 26 % and much less of course than in 4D (100 %). The mean estimated GFR of the subjects not on dialysis was 26.6 mL/min, with 79 % of these subjects in CKD stage 3 or 4.

There were 526 (11.3 %) first major atherosclerotic events (nonfatal myocardial infarction or coronary death, non-hemorrhagic stroke, or arterial revascularization) among the 4,650 participants allocated to simvastatin plus ezetimibe compared with 619 (13.4 %) among the 4,620 allocated to placebo. This corresponded to a 17 % reduction in the primary endpoint with active treatment (RR 0.83, 95 % confidence interval, 0.74–0.94; $P=0.0021$). Allocation to simvastatin plus ezetimibe was not associated with a difference in first major coronary events (213 [4.6 %] versus 230 [5.0 %]; RR 0.92, 95 % confidence interval, 0.76–1.11; $P=0.37$), but there was a slight trend towards fewer nonfatal myocardial infarctions (134 [2.9 %] versus 159 [3.4 %]; RR 0.84, 0.66–1.05; $P=0.12$). Death from a coronary event was not significantly affected by active treatment (91 [2.0 %] versus 90 [1.9 %]; RR 1.01, 0.75–1.35; $P=0.95$). The authors of SHARP pointed out that the trial lacked power for separate assessment of components of the primary endpoint, but the confidence intervals (e.g., for nonfatal myocardial infarction or coronary death [RR 0.92, 95 % confidence interval, 0.76–1.11]) were consistent with the results of the Cholesterol Treatment Trialists' (CTT) Collaboration meta-analysis, and suggest a reduction in these endpoints of a similar magnitude as in non-CKD patients [5].

Further, simvastatin plus ezetimibe significantly reduced the incidence of any arterial revascularization (284 [6.1 %] versus 352 [7.6 %]; RR 0.79, 95 % confidence interval, 0.68–0.93; $P=0.0036$), including both coronary and non-coronary revascularization procedures (i.e., carotid, aortic, or leg, but not hemodialysis access procedures). The significant one-quarter reduction in coronary revascularization procedures ($P=0.0027$) in SHARP would also be in keeping with a reduction in coronary disease.

In SHARP, allocation to simvastatin plus ezetimibe produced a significant reduction in non-hemorrhagic stroke (131 [2.8 %] versus 174 [3.8 %]; RR 0.75, 95 % confidence interval, 0.60–0.94; $P=0.01$), mainly due to a reduction in strokes that were definitely ischemic (114 [2.5 %] versus 157 [3.4 %]; RR 0.72, 0.57–0.92; $P=0.0073$). Of note, the significant one-quarter reduction in ischemic strokes was consistent with the one-fifth reduction reported in previous statin trials [24]. There was no difference in hemorrhagic strokes between the two groups (45 [1.0 %] versus 37 [0.8 %]; RR 1.21, 95 % CI 0.78–1.86; $P=0.4$).

The authors emphasize in their publication that SHARP was not expected to have sufficient power for subgroup analyses (e.g., separate analyses in the dialysis or the non-dialysis subgroups of the study population). However, a statement was included that there was "no good evidence" that the effects on major atherosclerotic events differed between patients on dialysis and those not on dialysis ($P=0.25$), nor were there trends towards smaller reductions in patients not on dialysis with lower versus higher estimated GFR ($P=0.73$) or higher versus lower urinary albumin excretion rates ($P=0.54$).

Similar to 4D and AURORA, active treatment was safe. There were very few cases of myopathy of any severity, of more severe cases with rhabdomyolysis or cases with severe liver abnormalities. Among the 6,247 patients not on dialysis at randomization, allocation to active treatment did not produce reductions in any of the pre-specified measures of renal disease progression: end-stage renal disease defined as commencement of maintenance dialysis or transplantation (1,057 [33.9 %] versus 1,084 [34.6 %]; RR 0.97, 95 % confidence interval, 0.89–1.05; $P=0.41$); end-stage renal disease or death (1,477 [47.4 %] versus 1,513 [48.3 %]; RR 0.97, 0.90–1.04; $P=0.34$); and end-stage renal disease or doubling of baseline serum creatinine (1,190 [38.2 %] versus 1,257 [40.2 %]; RR 0.93, 0.86–1.01; $P=0.09$).

In summary, the SHARP trial was able to demonstrate that lowering of LDL cholesterol with simvastatin plus ezetimibe safely reduces the risk of major atherosclerotic events in a wide range of patients with CKD. Again, only about 8 % of deaths were definitely attributable to coronary artery disease, and although SHARP was much larger than AURORA and 4D, it was also not able to detect effects on coronary mortality. The authors argue that SHARP was still too small, since the confidence interval of the reduction of myocardial infarction fits with the effect size in patients without kidney disease as shown in the CTT meta-analysis, and that the profound reduction in coronary revascularization procedures strongly suggests effects on coronary disease. Perhaps the exclusion of subjects with prior myocardial infarction or coronary revascularization, resulting in the inclusion of subjects with relatively low CV risk, and making SHARP in this regard a primary prevention trial, also contributed to the lack of demonstrable effects on coronary events. SHARP did however demonstrate clearly that there is a significant reduction in ischemic strokes with statin therapy in patients with CKD. This is particularly reassuring, considering the uncertainty created by 4D and AURORA showing trends towards higher stroke rates. In view of the high morbidity and severe quality of life implications of stroke, treatment with a statin therefore seems worthwhile, independent of whether there is an additional reduction in coronary events.

Considering the results of 4D and AURORA, and even after SHARP, there is still some uncertainty regarding the effects of statins in patients on dialysis. There was no evidence for statistical heterogeneity between the non-dialysis and dialysis subgroups, but a separate analysis of the dialysis-dependent subgroups revealed no benefit, whereas an analysis in the non-dialysis subgroups did. It should be emphasized again, however, that the study was not powered to analyze these subgroups separately. It might be helpful in this context to remember that approximately one-third of the subjects in the initially non-dialysis subgroup progressed to end-stage kidney disease during the trial. It could be therefore argued that patients with CKD, including those who will progress to end-stage renal disease, should receive a statin to prevent atherosclerotic events. Whether statin treatment should be started in those patients already on dialysis remains uncertain.

ALERT

“The Assessment of Lescol in Renal Transplantation” (ALERT) study is the largest randomized study on outcomes of statin therapy in patients with a kidney transplant [25]. Subjects who had received a renal, or a combined renal and pancreas transplant more than 6 months ago, and who had stable renal graft function, were randomized to treatment with fluvastatin 40 mg or matching placebo. After around 2 years, and if the individual study participant consented, the dose of study drug could be doubled by the investigator. All patients received a cyclosporine-based immunosuppressive regime.

The primary endpoint was the first occurrence of a major adverse cardiac event, defined as cardiac death, nonfatal myocardial infarction verified by hospital records, or a coronary revascularization procedure, including coronary artery bypass graft or percutaneous coronary intervention. It is important to emphasize that both *definite* and *probable* myocardial infarctions were originally included, since it was argued that the occurrence of myocardial infarction is difficult to establish in renal transplant recipients in view of the high prevalence of resting electrocardiographic abnormalities and potentially spurious increases in creatinine kinase levels in this patient population. A myocardial infarction was adjudicated as *definite* if a new Q-wave developed in the presence of abnormal cardiac markers plus symptoms, or pathological ST elevations and T-wave changes developed in the presence of abnormal cardiac markers *plus* symptoms. A myocardial infarction was classified as *probable* in case of pathological ST elevations and T-wave changes with the presence of abnormal cardiac markers *or* symptoms consistent with myocardial infarction.

Predefined secondary endpoints were individual cardiac events, combined cardiac death or nonfatal myocardial infarction, combined cerebrovascular events, non-cardiovascular death, all-cause mortality, and the composite renal endpoint of graft loss or doubling of serum creatinine.

The results of the study were published in June 2003. One thousand and fifty subjects were randomized to fluvastatin and 1,052 to placebo. The dose of study medication was doubled in 65 % of patients in both groups. In terms of "drop-in" of non-study lipid-lowering therapy, 77 (7 %) patients in the fluvastatin and 145 (14 %) in the placebo group started taking other lipid-lowering treatments, mainly statins, in the course of the study. Subjects randomized to fluvastatin had an LDL cholesterol that was on average 32 % lower than in subjects randomized to placebo at the end of the study, with an average difference of 1.0 mmol/L (39 mg/dL) between groups throughout the study.

The occurrence of the primary endpoint, total major adverse cardiac event, was not significantly different between the two groups despite a slightly favorable result for those randomized to fluvastatin (risk ratio 0.83 [95 % confidence interval, 0.64–1.06], $P=0.139$). Treatment with fluvastatin also reduced the risk of two secondary endpoints: cardiac death by 38 % (0.62 [0.40–0.96], $P=0.031$) and definite nonfatal myocardial infarction by 32 % (0.68 [0.47–1.00], $P=0.050$). The combined endpoint of cardiac death or definite nonfatal myocardial infarction was reduced by 35 % (0.65 [0.48–0.88], $P=0.005$). Rates of probable nonfatal myocardial infarction or coronary interventions did not differ significantly between groups. Further, there was no difference in cerebrovascular events, non-cardiovascular death, all-cause mortality, and the renal composite endpoint of graft loss or doubling of serum creatinine.

Of note, in ALERT, there was a relationship between LDL cholesterol levels and occurrence of the primary endpoint, such that an increase in 1 mmol/L in LDL cholesterol was associated with a 41 % increase in risk for the primary endpoint and the composite endpoint of cardiac death and nonfatal myocardial infarction. No association was noted between LDL cholesterol and non-cardiovascular death or any renal endpoint. In terms of safety, 155 (15 %) patients randomized to fluvastatin and 172 (17 %) patients randomized to placebo discontinued their study medication because of laboratory or clinical adverse events. One patient in each group developed nonfatal rhabdomyolysis, which in both cases was due to severe trauma.

In the discussion, the authors argued that the cardiac event rate in the placebo group was lower than expected, and therefore the trial lacked power to detect a reduction in the primary combined endpoint. The reduction in the secondary endpoint of cardiac death and nonfatal myocardial infarction was consisted with reductions observed in other populations. However, the authors pointed out that since the combined primary endpoint did not reach statistical significance, these secondary analyses should to be treated with caution. Similar to SHARP, ALERT was essentially a primary prevention study since subjects with recent myocardial infarction were excluded from randomization.

ALERT Secondary Analysis

Subsequently, a further analysis of the ALERT database was published [26]. As discussed, the original combined primary endpoint in ALERT did not reach statistical significance, and therefore analysis of secondary endpoints needed to be interpreted cautiously. The authors therefore reanalyzed the study using a different post hoc-defined primary endpoint, consisting of cardiac death or *definite* nonfatal myocardial infarction. Probable myocardial infarction was excluded from the primary endpoint in this post hoc analysis. This new primary endpoint was reached in significantly less subjects randomized to fluvastatin compared to those randomized to placebo (70 versus 104; RR 0.65; 95 % confidence interval, 0.48, 0.88; $P=0.005$). This permitted analyses in a variety of subgroups. In most subgroups (e.g., subjects with lower or higher cardiovascular risk, in those who were younger or older, had or had not diabetes), the results were similar to the analysis in the overall study population, meaning that the reduction in the risk for the primary endpoint was of a similar magnitude. Further, it was estimated that 31 patients would need to be treated with fluvastatin for a duration of 5 years to prevent the occurrence of one cardiac death or nonfatal myocardial infarction. Therefore, a "narrower" endpoint, by excluding probable myocardial infarctions, led to a statistically significant difference in outcomes between fluvastatin and placebo. Similar to 4D and AURORA, this is likely because *probable* myocardial infarctions consisted of a larger number of subjects that experienced sudden cardiac death, which is not amenable to statin therapy.

ALERT Extension Trial

After completion of the blinded study, subjects were followed in an extension trial for the duration of 2 years [27]. All subjects were offered active statin therapy in this extension phase of ALERT. Since the clinical effects of statins usually take 1–2 years to become apparent, it was argued that any differences in clinical outcomes observed 2 years after the end of the core study should be the result of randomization *during* the core study. The original primary outcome of ALERT, major adverse cardiac event defined as cardiac death, nonfatal myocardial infarction (*definite* or *probable*), or coronary revascularization procedure, occurred in significantly less subjects originally randomized to fluvastatin compared to those originally randomized to placebo (HR 0.79, 95 % confidence interval, 0.63–0.99; $P=0.036$). The reduction of cardiac death or definite myocardial infarction was similar in magnitude to the aforementioned *post hoc* analysis of the ALERT core study (HR 0.71, 95 % confidence interval, 0.55–0.93; $P=0.014$). A further conclusion from the ALERT extension trial could be that longer follow-up durations are required to detect benefits of statin treatment. Unfortunately, this manuscript does not report the results for the endpoint *probable* myocardial infarctions (i.e., whether longer treatment duration has any noticeable effects on sudden cardiac death rates).

In summary, the ALERT trial, the largest randomized study on the effects of statin therapy in kidney transplant recipients, was able to show that statin treatment significantly reduces cardiac death and *definite* cases of nonfatal myocardial infarction. The magnitude in the benefit of statin therapy on these outcomes in kidney transplant recipients appears similar to that in non-CKD populations.

Conclusion

Many subjects with CKD stages 1–2 were included in large-scale non-CKD studies, and post hoc analyses of these trials suggest that the benefit of statin therapy in patients with these milder forms of CKD is comparable to the benefit achieved in non-CKD populations. In CKD stages 3–5, the SHARP trial strongly suggests that statin therapy should be initiated in the majority of patients, in particular when there are additional CV risk factors present such as diabetes mellitus, or established CV disease as documented by a history of myocardial infarction or stroke. We have also good evidence from SHARP that CKD patients already taking a statin do not need to stop this therapy once dialysis has been commenced (i.e., when progressing to dialysis-dependent renal failure). The area of greatest uncertainty is whether to initiate statin treatment in patients who are already on dialysis. Current evidence (4D, AURORA) does not suggest that substantial benefit can generally be derived from statin therapy in this patient population, although decisions should be tailored to the individual patient. Although statin therapy is not of general benefit it may have a positive impact in those at particularly high risk for atherosclerotic events. Finally, the ALERT trial has demonstrated that patients with a kidney transplant clearly benefit from statin therapy.

References

1. Foley RN, Parfrey PS, Sarnak MJ. Clinical epidemiology of cardiovascular disease in chronic renal disease. Am J Kidney Dis. 1998;32(5 Suppl 3):S112–9. Epub 1998/11/20.
2. de Jager DJ, Grootendorst DC, Jager KJ, van Dijk PC, Tomas LM, Ansell D, et al. Cardiovascular and noncardiovascular mortality among patients starting dialysis. JAMA. 2009;302(16):1782–9. Epub 2009/10/29.
3. Belani SS, Goldberg AC, Coyne DW. Ability of non-high-density lipoprotein cholesterol and calculated intermediate-density lipoprotein to identify nontraditional lipoprotein subclass risk factors in dialysis patients. Am J Kidney Dis. 2004;43(2):320–9. Epub 2004/01/30.
4. Holme I, Fellstrom B, Jardine A, Holdaas H. Comparison of predictive ability of lipoprotein components to that of traditional risk factors of coronary events in renal transplant recipients. Atherosclerosis. 2010;208(1):234–9. Epub 2009/07/15.
5. Baigent C, Keech A, Kearney PM, Blackwell L, Buck G, Pollicino C, et al. Efficacy and safety of cholesterol-lowering treatment: prospective meta-analysis of data from 90,056 participants in 14 randomised trials of statins. Lancet. 2005;366(9493):1267–78. Epub 2005/10/11.
6. Thavendiranathan P, Bagai A, Brookhart MA, Choudhry NK. Primary prevention of cardiovascular diseases with statin therapy: a meta-analysis of randomized controlled trials. Arch Intern Med. 2006;166(21):2307–13. Epub 2006/11/30.
7. Colhoun HM, Betteridge DJ, Durrington PN, Hitman GA, Neil HA, Livingstone SJ, et al. Effects of atorvastatin on kidney outcomes and cardiovascular disease in patients with diabetes: an analysis from the Collaborative Atorvastatin Diabetes Study (CARDS). Am J Kidney Dis. 2009;54(5):810–9. Epub 2009/06/23.
8. Tonelli M, Jose P, Curhan G, Sacks F, Braunwald E, Pfeffer M. Proteinuria, impaired kidney function, and adverse outcomes in people with coronary disease: analysis of a previously conducted randomised trial. BMJ. 2006;332(7555):1426. Epub 2006/05/23.
9. Mason NA, Bailie GR, Satayathum S, Bragg-Gresham JL, Akiba T, Akizawa T, et al. HMG-coenzyme a reductase inhibitor use is associated with mortality reduction in hemodialysis patients. Am J Kidney Dis. 2005;45(1):119–26. Epub 2005/02/08.
10. Seliger SL, Weiss NS, Gillen DL, Kestenbaum B, Ball A, Sherrard DJ, et al. HMG-CoA reductase inhibitors are associated with reduced mortality in ESRD patients. Kidney Int. 2002;61(1):297–304. Epub 2002/01/12.
11. Tonelli M, Isles C, Curhan GC, Tonkin A, Pfeffer MA, Shepherd J, et al. Effect of pravastatin on cardiovascular events in people with chronic kidney disease. Circulation. 2004;110(12):1557–63. Epub 2004/09/15.
12. Shepherd J, Kastelein JJ, Bittner V, Deedwania P, Breazna A, Dobson S, et al. Intensive lipid lowering with atorvastatin in patients with coronary heart disease and chronic kidney disease: the TNT (Treating to New Targets) study. J Am Coll Cardiol. 2008;51(15):1448–54. Epub 2008/04/12.
13. Molitch ME. Management of dyslipidemias in patients with diabetes and chronic kidney disease. Clin J Am Soc Nephrol. 2006;1(5):1090–9. Epub 2007/08/19.
14. Wanner C, Krane V, Marz W, Olschewski M, Mann JF, Ruf G, et al. Atorvastatin in patients with type 2 diabetes mellitus undergoing hemodialysis. N Engl J Med. 2005;353(3):238–48. Epub 2005/07/22.
15. Grundy SM, Cleeman JI, Merz CN, Brewer Jr HB, Clark LT, Hunninghake DB, et al. Implications of recent clinical trials for the National Cholesterol Education Program Adult Treatment Panel III guidelines. Circulation. 2004;110(2):227–39. Epub 2004/07/14.
16. Baigent C, Burbury K, Wheeler D. Premature cardiovascular disease in chronic renal failure. Lancet. 2000;356(9224):147–52. Epub 2000/08/30.
17. Fellstrom BC, Jardine AG, Schmieder RE, Holdaas H, Bannister K, Beutler J, et al. Rosuvastatin and cardiovascular events in patients undergoing hemodialysis. N Engl J Med. 2009;360(14):1395–407. Epub 2009/04/01.

18. Holdaas H, Holme I, Schmieder RE, Jardine AG, Zannad F, Norby GE, et al. Rosuvastatin in diabetic hemodialysis patients. J Am Soc Nephrol. 2011;22(7):1335–41. Epub 2011/05/14.
19. Ridker PM, Danielson E, Fonseca FA, Genest J, Gotto Jr AM, Kastelein JJ, et al. Rosuvastatin to prevent vascular events in men and women with elevated C-reactive protein. N Engl J Med. 2008;359(21):2195–207. Epub 2008/11/11.
20. Kjekshus J, Apetrei E, Barrios V, Bohm M, Cleland JG, Cornel JH, et al. Rosuvastatin in older patients with systolic heart failure. N Engl J Med. 2007;357(22):2248–61. Epub 2007/11/07.
21. Tavazzi L, Maggioni AP, Marchioli R, Barlera S, Franzosi MG, Latini R, et al. Effect of rosuvastatin in patients with chronic heart failure (the GISSI-HF trial): a randomised, double-blind, placebo-controlled trial. Lancet. 2008;372(9645):1231–9. Epub 2008/09/02.
22. Baigent C, Landray MJ, Reith C, Emberson J, Wheeler DC, Tomson C, et al. The effects of lowering LDL cholesterol with simvastatin plus ezetimibe in patients with chronic kidney disease (Study of Heart and Renal Protection): a randomised placebo-controlled trial. Lancet. 2011;377(9784):2181–92. Epub 2011/06/15.
23. Sharp Collaborative G. Study of Heart and Renal Protection (SHARP): randomized trial to assess the effects of lowering low-density lipoprotein cholesterol among 9,438 patients with chronic kidney disease. Am Heart J. 2010;160(5):785–94.e10. Epub 2010/11/26.
24. Baigent C, Blackwell L, Emberson J, Holland LE, Reith C, Bhala N, et al. Efficacy and safety of more intensive lowering of LDL cholesterol: a meta-analysis of data from 170,000 participants in 26 randomised trials. Lancet. 2010;376(9753):1670–81. Epub 2010/11/12.
25. Holdaas H, Fellstrom B, Jardine AG, Holme I, Nyberg G, Fauchald P, et al. Effect of fluvastatin on cardiac outcomes in renal transplant recipients: a multicentre, randomised, placebo-controlled trial. Lancet. 2003;361(9374):2024–31. Epub 2003/06/20.
26. Jardine AG, Holdaas H, Fellstrom B, Cole E, Nyberg G, Gronhagen-Riska C, et al. Fluvastatin prevents cardiac death and myocardial infarction in renal transplant recipients: post-hoc subgroup analyses of the ALERT Study. Am J Transplant. 2004;4(6):988–95. Epub 2004/05/19.
27. Holdaas H, Fellstrom B, Cole E, Nyberg G, Olsson AG, Pedersen TR, et al. Long-term cardiac outcomes in renal transplant recipients receiving fluvastatin: the ALERT extension study. Am J Transplant. 2005;5(12):2929–36. Epub 2005/11/24.

Chapter 8
Pharmacokinetics of Lipid-Lowering Medications in Chronic Kidney Disease

Ali Olyaei, Jessica Lassiter, and Edgar V. Lerma

Introduction

Coronary heart disease (CHD) and other forms of cardiovascular disease (CVD) are among the leading causes of death in the Western world, including the United States and Europe [1] Hyperlipidemia is a well-established contributor to the formation of atherosclerotic plaques and a known risk for CVD in the general population [2, 3]. However, in patients with advanced stages of chronic kidney disease (CKD) and those on dialysis, the relationship between lipid abnormalities and CVD are less clear and require further study, although there have been several well-done studies recently which do shed some light on this issue [4–7]. The goal of this chapter is to discuss the pharmacokinetic and pharmacodynamic properties of lipid-lowering drugs in patients with advanced CKD (stage IIIb, IV, and V), those on dialysis, and patients following renal transplantation. This chapter will also discuss the safety, drug dosing, and drug interactions that are important in this group of patients.

A. Olyaei, Pharm.D. (✉)
Department of Nephrology and Hypertension, Oregon Health and Sciences University, 3303 SW Bond Avenue, CH12C, Portland, OR 97239, USA
e-mail: olyaeia@ohsu.edu

J. Lassiter, Pharm.D.
Department of Pharmacy, University of Michigan Health System, Ann Arbor, MI, USA

E.V. Lerma, M.D., F.A.C.P., F.A.S.N., F.A.H.A., F.A.S.H., F.N.L.A., F.N.K.F.
Section of Nephrology, Advocate Christ Medical Center, University of Illinois at Chicago College of Medicine, Oak Lawn, IL, USA

A. Covic et al. (eds.), *Dyslipidemias in Kidney Disease*, DOI 10.1007/978-1-4939-0515-7_8

Table 8.1 Classification of chronic kidney disease

Chronic kidney disease: a clinical action plan			
Stage	Description	GFR (mL/min/1.73 m^2)	Action
	At increased risk	≥90 (with CKD risk factors)	Screening CKD risk reduction
1.	Kidney damage with normal or ↑ GFR	≥90	Diagnosis and treatment Treatment of comorbid conditions, slowing progression, CVD risk reduction
2.	Kidney damage with mild ↓ GFR	60–89	Estimating progression
3.	Moderate ↓ GFR	30–59	Evaluating and treating complications
4.	Severe ↓ GFR	15–29	Preparation for kidney replacement therapy
5.	Kidney failure	<15 (or dialysis)	Replacement (if uremia present)

Chronic Kidney Disease Staging

The Kidney Disease Outcomes Quality Initiative (K/DOQI) developed a system of staging of CKD in 2002 [8, 9]. The staging system is based on estimated glomerular filtration rate (eGFR or GFR) and is divided into stages 1–5 (Table 8.1). Many of the deleterious effects of CKD are seen as patients progress into stage 3b CKD (eGFR 30–44 mL/min), and drug dosing becomes more important with increasing impairment of GFR. Not many studies have been done in the advanced CKD population, and even fewer in the stage 5D (dialysis) population. Our chapter will discuss the studies that have been done looking at lipid management in patients with advanced CKD and on dialysis.

Pharmacology

The first HMG-CoA reductase inhibitor, mevastatin, was isolated from Penicillium citrinum and P. brevicompactum by Japanese and British researchers in 1976 [10]. It served as the lead compound from which lovastatin was later synthesized. The choice of a specific lipid-lowering agents depends on the individual patient's clinical presentation, the LDL predicted response, the potential for drug interactions of specific lipid-lowering agent, and, finally, side-effect profile of the agent. Bile acid sequestrants represent the first generation of lipid-lowering agent with acceptable clinical outcome but significant risk of drug interactions. The use of niacin was associated with high risk of adverse drug reactions such as flushing, diabetes, gout, or peptic ulcer disease. This led to the development and introduction of a new class of drugs, HMG-CoA reductase inhibitors [statins], that have excellent clinical outcome, are better tolerated, and have a lower potential risk of drug interactions. In contrast to other lipid-lowering agents, statins are easier to initiate, monitor, and do not require careful dose escalation when starting the treatment. Statins competitively inhibit the activity of HMG-CoA reductase, the rate-limiting enzyme and step in cholesterol biosynthesis. Inhibition of this enzyme results in both reduction in cholesterol biosynthesis and a significant reduction on plasma LDL levels [11, 12]. Statins inhibit HMG-CoA reductase, the enzyme that converts HMG-CoA into mevalonic acid, a cholesterol precursor in the liver. The liver plays a vital role in LDL receptor expression and hemostases of LDL receptors. Approximately 70 % of LDL receptors are expressed by hepatocytes. A reduction of intracellular cholesterol activates a protease enzyme cascade of sterol regulatory element-binding protein (SREBP), which regulates binding proteins from the endoplasmic reticulum [13]. These proteins increase the gene expression for LDL receptors and, as a result, decrease plasma LDL-cholesterol concentration. Compared to other lipid-lowering agents, the absolute risk reduction for CVD cannot be explained solely relative to the absolute reduction in cholesterol level [14, 15]. The other explanation is that statins are also involved in the alteration of the isoprenoid pathway, which accounts for their pleiotropic effects [16–18]. Currently, the drugs of this class that are available in the US market are atorvastatin, fluvastatin, lovastatin, pitavastatin, pravastatin, rosuvastatin, and simvastatin. Lovastatin, pravastatin, and simvastatin are derived from fungal precursors; the other statins are fully synthetic [19].

Molecular Structure and Chemical Properties (Fig. 8.1)

To understand the pharmacokinetic differences between the various statins, it is necessary to examine the structural differences. In general, the structure of a statin can be reduced to three constituents: an HMG-CoA analog; a central, aromatic ring structure; and one or more side chains. Modifications to these components are responsible for changes in solubility, potency, and metabolism [20].

The majority of statins are lipophilic; however, pravastatin and rosuvastatin are relatively hydrophilic due to the addition of polar side groups. Lipophilicity (in decreasing order): simvastatin > lovastatin ≈ fluvastatin ≈ atorvastatin ≈ pitavastatin >> rosuvastatin ≈ pravastatin. Simvastatin and lovastatin are administered as highly lipophilic lactone prodrugs, while the other statins are administered as the active, hydroxy-acid forms [21–24].

Pharmacokinetics

All statins are rapidly absorbed following oral administration, with peak plasma concentrations (Tmax) occurring within 4 h. The effect of food on statin absorption is variable and, with the exception of lovastatin, not clinically significant. Co-administration with food decreases the rate (Cmax) and/or extent (AUC) of absorption for atorvastatin, fluvastatin instant-release (IR), lovastatin extended-release (ER), and pitavastatin [25]. Conversely, food increases the AUC for lovastatin IR and fluvastatin ER [20]. Simvastatin and rosuvastatin are not affected [21]. It is recommended to administer lovastatin IR with food; other statins may be given without regard to meals (Table 8.2) [26, 27].

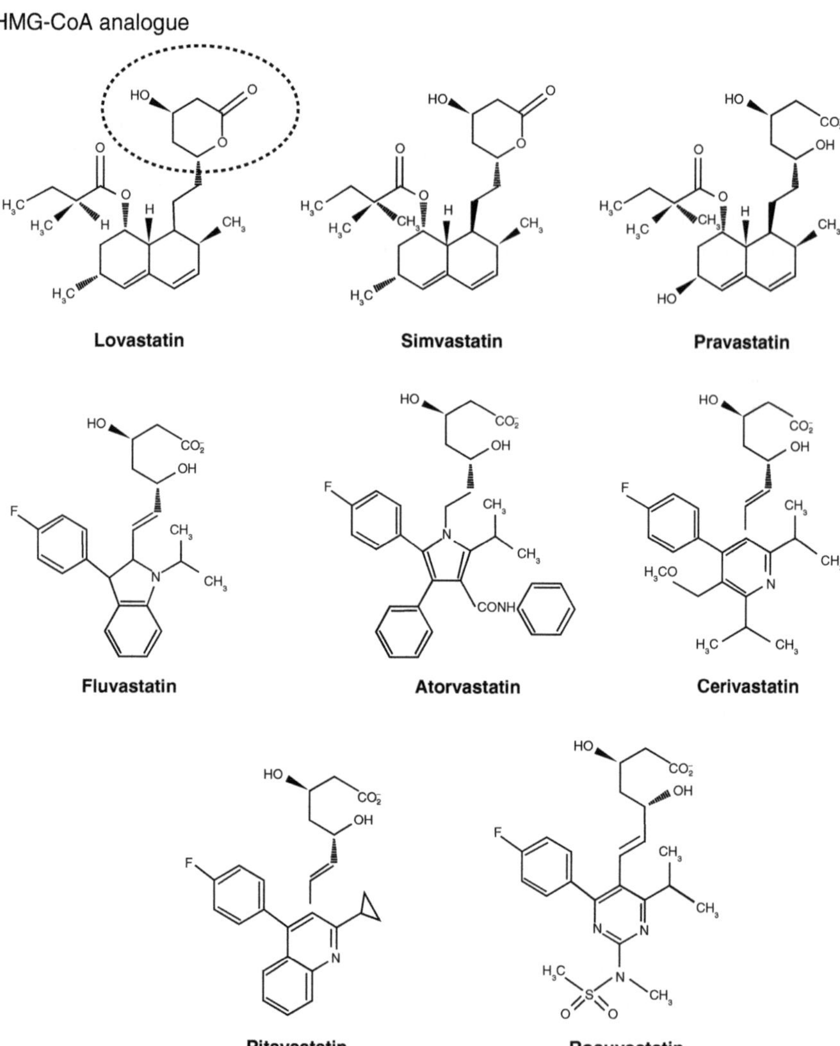

Fig. 8.1 Chemical structures of the statins. Reprinted from Schachter M. Chemical, pharmacokinetic and pharmacodynamic properties of statins: an update. Fundam Clin Pharmacol 2005 Feb;19(1):117–25, with permission from John Wiley and Sons

With the exception of pravastatin, the statins are highly bound to plasma proteins, further limiting extrahepatic tissue exposure. The hydrophilic nature of pravastatin prevents extensive tissue uptake, despite decreased protein binding [28].

Following absorption, simvastatin and lovastatin are rapidly metabolized via ester hydrolysis to their active hydroxy-acid form. In general, the statins exhibit low systemic bioavailability due to significant hepatic extraction and first-pass metabolism. Pitavastatin exhibits the highest bioavailability at ~51 %. Because the liver is the target organ, however, a high first-pass extraction is likely more relevant than absolute systemic bioavailability [12].

Table 8.2 Summary of statin pharmacokinetics

	Atorvastatin	Fluvastatin	Lovastatin	Pitavastatin	Pravastatin	Rosuvastatin	Simvastatin
Administration	Any time of day; with or without food	Bedtime; with or without food	Evening meal	Any time of day; with or without food	Bedtime; with or without food	Any time of day; with or without food	Bedtime; with or without food
Lipophilicity (Log P)							
Lactone prodrug	No	No	Yes	No	No	No	Yes
Bioavailability (%)	14	24 (IR)	<5	51	17	20	<5
Time to peak (Tmax) (h)	1–2	<1 (IR); 3(ER)	2–4	1	~1	3–5	1–2.5
Effect of food	Decreased rate and extent of absorption	Decreased rate, but not extent of absorption (IR); Decreased rate, increased bioavailability (ER)	Increased bioavailability (IR); decreased bioavailability (ER)	Decreased rate of absorption	Decreased bioavailability	No effect	No effect
Protein binding (%)	98	98	>95	>99	~50	88	95
Half-life ($t_{1/2}$) (h)	14	<3 (IR); 9 (ER)	3–4 (IR)	12	~2	19	3
Metabolism	CYP 3A4; CYP 2C8 (minor)	CYP 2C9 (major); CYP 3A4 (minor)	CYP 3A4; CYP 2C8	CYP 2C9 (minor)	Limited	Limited	CYP 3A4; CYP 2C8
Renal elimination (%)	<2	5	10	15	20	10	13
Effect of renal impairment	No effect	AUC and Cmax increased 20 % with GFR <40 mL/min; increased 50 % in patients on hemodialysis	Plasma concentration increased twofold with GFR <30 mL/min	AUC increased 102 % with GFR <60 mL/min	AUC increased 69 % and Cmax increased 37 % with GFR <30 mL/min	Plasma concentration increased threefold with GFR <30 mL/min	Increased systemic exposure with GFR <30 mL/min
Renal dosing adjustment	Dosage adjustment not required	Max 40 mg/day with GFR <30 mL/min	10 mg/day initial dose with GFR <30 mL/min	1 mg/day initial dose and 2 mg/day max dose with GFR <60 mL/min	10 mg/day initial dose with GFR <30 mL/min	5 mg/day initial dose and 10 mg max dose with GFR <30 mL/min	5 mg/day initial dose with GFR <30 mL/min

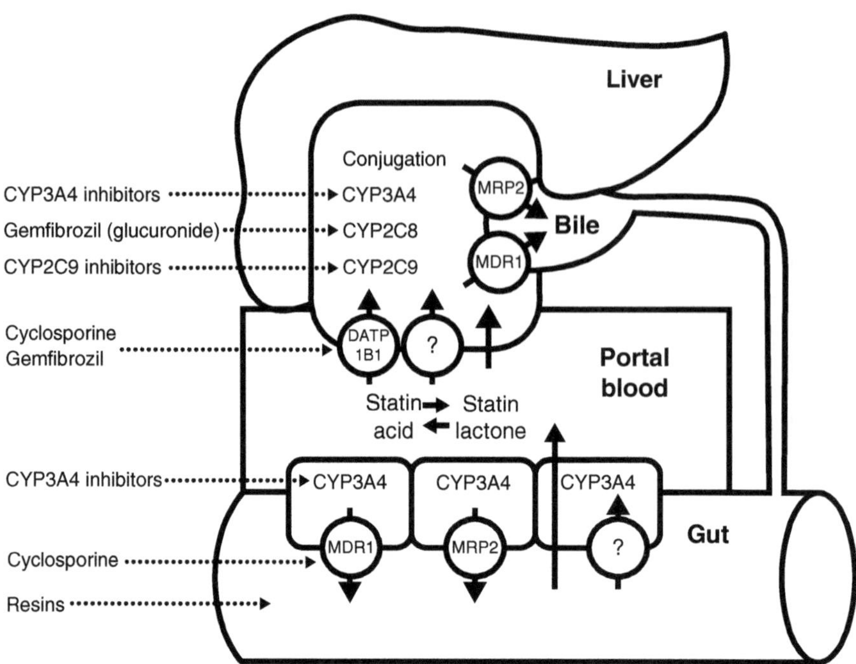

Fig. 8.2 Enzymes involved in the metabolism or transport of the statins and potential drug inhibitors. Reprinted by permission from Macmillan Publishers Ltd: Clinical Pharmacology & Therapeutics, Neuvonen PJ, Niemi M, Backman JT. Drug interactions with lipid-lowering drugs: mechanisms and clinical relevance, 80(6), copyright 2006

The lipophilic statins are primarily metabolized via the hepatic cytochrome P450 (CYP) enzyme system. Atorvastatin, lovastatin, and simvastatin are extensively metabolized via CYP 3A4 and 2C8. Significant metabolism by 3A4 in the gastrointestinal tract prior to absorption contributes to the low bioavailability of these agents [29]. Fluvastatin is chiefly metabolized by CYP 2C9, with minor CYP 3A4 metabolism [24]. Pitavastatin undergoes moderate CYP 2C9 metabolism. The hydrophilic statins, pravastatin and rosuvastatin, are not appreciably metabolized via the CYP enzyme [12].

The statins have been identified as substrates for p-glycoprotein and organic anion-transporting polypeptide (OATP) [30]. Active efflux by multidrug-resistant protein 1 (MDR1) and multidrug-resistant associated protein 2 (MRP2) occurs in the intestines and bile canaliculi, reducing statin absorption and increasing excretion, respectively [31]. OATP assists in the hepatic uptake of most statins; however, the effect is most significant for the hydrophilic statins [32] (Fig. 8.2).

The hydrophilic statins have a lower incidence of myopathy and myalgia. It has been speculated that this may be due to decreased tissue penetration; however, it is more likely a result of non-CYP-dependent metabolism. The ubiquity of CYP metabolism, particularly 3A4, results in a multitude of potential drug–drug and drug–food interactions that can occur with atorvastatin, lovastatin, and simvastatin [33, 34]. Potent 3A4 inhibitors such as cyclosporine, diltiazem, verapamil, protease inhibitors, azole antifungals, grapefruit, and the macrolide antibiotics can increase statin AUC by 5- to 20-fold [34]. Additional interactions via inhibition of MDR1 and OATP likely contribute. The increased risk of myopathy and rhabdomyolysis associated with concomitant administration of gemfibrozil may be due to OATP and CYP 2C8 inhibition [35–38].

Fluvastatin, lovastatin, pravastatin, and simvastatin are rapidly eliminated, with half-lives of ≤ 3 h [29]. As such, evening or bedtime dosing results in a clinically significant increase in efficacy due to greater inhibition of nocturnal steroid synthesis. Rosuvastatin, atorvastatin, and pitavastatin exhibit elimination half-lives of 19, 14, and 11 h, respectively [28]. Active metabolites further extend the duration of action of atorvastatin to approximately 20 h. These agents may be administered at any time of day with no decrease in efficacy [39].

The primary route of excretion for both parent compounds and metabolites is in the feces via the bile. Renal excretion varies by drug and but remains low at 2–20 %. In patients with severe renal impairment, it is recommended to start at the lowest statin dose, with the exception of atorvastatin, which is minimally excreted in the urine (<2 %) and does not require dosage adjustment [40]. Significant increases in AUC and Cmax are seen in patients with mild-moderate hepatic impairment [21]. The statins are contraindicated in patients with active liver disease or unexplained increases in serum transaminases [41, 42].

Gemfibrozil decreases serum triglycerides and very low-density lipoprotein (VLDL) cholesterol by enhancing lipoprotein lipase activities and VLDL catabolism [43]. In addition, gemfibrozil increases high-density lipoprotein (HDL) cholesterol with modest decreases in total and low-density lipoprotein (LDL). Following oral administration, gemfibrozil is completely absorbed, reaching peak plasma concentrations 1–2 h after single-dose administration [44]. Gemfibrozil pharmacokinetics properties are affected by the present of meals; both the rate and extent of absorption of the drug are significantly decreased when given with meals. Average AUC was reduced by 14–44 % when gemfibrozil was given 30 min after meals [43]. Gemfibrozil-like statins metabolize through the CYP IIIA oxidation pathway and can significantly alter metabolism of statins [45]. In addition, gemfibrozil may inhibit OATP2 transport pathway, which further may increase plasma concentration of statins. The co-administration of stains and gemfibrozil caused a 4- to 20-fold increase in plasma concentration of statins [46]. Gemfibrozil may increase the risk of myopathy and rhabdomyolysis when used concomitantly with statins. Therefore, the combination of stains and gemfibrozil should be avoided [47]. Renal impairment has less effect on gemfibrozil elimination compared to fibrates. Finally, gemfibrozil has no effect on serum creatinine compared to fenofibrate [48].

Like other fibrates, fenofibrate is indicated for the treatment of hypercholesterolemia to reduce low-density lipoprotein cholesterol (LDL), total cholesterol (TC), triglycerides (TG), and apolipoprotein B (apo B) and to increase HDL cholesterol in patients with primary hypercholesterolemia or mixed dyslipidemia. Fenofibrate is a prodrug. Following oral administration, fenofibrate hydrolyzes in the tissues and plasma to fenofibric acid. Depending on individual formulation, and absorption rate varies from 60 to 90 %, fenofibrate should be taken with meals to improve bioavailability [49]. Fenofibrate is highly protein bound and greater than 90 % bound to serum albumin [50]. Unlike gemfibrozil, fenofibrate is rapidly hydrolyzed by esterases to fenofibric acid and is primarily conjugated with glucuronic acid. Neither fenofibrate nor fenofibric acid utilize CYP–450 enzymes significantly for elimination [51]. However, dosage adjustment is required in patients with CKD and, if possible, should be avoided in patients with advanced renal impairment. (estimated CLcr < 30 mL/min). Treatment with fenofibrate may cause elevations in serum creatinine as well as in serum transaminases. Abnormal laboratory test results caused by fenofibrate are infrequent and transient. Routine monitoring of serum creatinine is not recommended.

Statins in Chronic Kidney Disease

The subject of dyslipidemia's contribution toward CHD morbidity and mortality in the predialysis advanced CKD population has not been well studied, nor has the efficacy of statins in preventing CHD events been well demonstrated in this population. Risk factors for development of CHD in the general population include elevated levels of total cholesterol and triglycerides as well as low levels of HDL cholesterol. While its pathophysiology is not well understood, dyslipidemia in CKD tends to worsen as eGFR declines [52]. Lipid profiles change along the spectrum of CKD to end-stage renal disease (ESRD) to renal transplant recipients (Table 8.3) [4, 5, 53]. Once a patient reaches ESRD, cardiovascular risk seemingly paradoxically increases with lower levels of cholesterol. The explanation for this is that lower cholesterol in these patients correlates with malnutrition and increased inflammatory markers [5]. It has been shown that in a subset of dialysis patients without evidence of systemic inflammation or malnutrition, elevated cholesterol is an independent risk factor for cardiovascular mortality [6]. Lipid profiles are dynamic along the spectrum of CKD to ESRD and kidney transplant recipients (see Table 8.3).

Table 8.3 Dyslipidemia in CKD patients (relative to the general population)[a]

Predialysis		Nephrotic syndrome	Hemodialysis	Kidney transplant
Total cholesterol	Normal	Increased	Normal or decreased	Increased
HDL	Decreased	Decreased or normal	Decreased	Decreased
LDL	Normal or decreased	Increased (increased $Lp_{(a)}$)	Normal or decreased	Increased
VLDL	Increased	Increased	Increased	Increased
triglycerides	Increased	Increased	Increased	increased

[a]Adapted from [6]

Table 8.4 National kidney foundation guidelines for managing dyslipidemias in adults with CKD[a]

Dyslipidemia	Goal	Initiate	Increase	Alternative
TG ≥500 mg/dL	TG <500 mg/dL	TLC	TCL+fibrate or niacin	Fibrate or niacin
LDL-C 100–129 mg/dL	LDL-C <100 mg/dL	TLC	TCL+low dose statin	Bile acid sequestrant or niacin
LDL-C ≥130 mg/dL	LDL-C <100 mg/dL	TCL+low dose statin	TCL+max dose statin	Bile acid sequestrant or niacin
TG ≥200 mg/dL and non-HDL-C ≥130 mg/dL	Non-HDL-C <130 mg/dL	TLC+low dose statin	TCL+max dose statin	Fibrate or niacin

CKD chronic kidney disease, *HDL-C* high-density lipoprotein cholesterol, *LDL-C* low-density lipoprotein cholesterol, *TG* triglycerides, *TCL* therapeutic lifestyle changes
[a]Adapted from [9]

Table 8.5 Cholesterol targets based on patient risk category

Risk category	LDL goal	Drug therapy should be considered
CHD or CHD risk equivalent	<100 mg/dL(2.60 mmol/L)	≥130 mg/dL (at 100–129 mg/dL, drug optional)
2 or more risk factors	<130 mg/dL (3.35 mmol/L)	≥130 mg/dL for 10-year risk of 10–20 %; 160 mg/dL for 10-year risk of <10 %
0 to 1 risk factor	<160 mg/dL (4.15 mmol/L)	≥190 mg/dL (at 160–189 mg/dL, LDL-lowering drug optional)

Increasing triglycerides seems to correlate with decreasing renal function, but once a patient reaches ESRD greater cardiovascular risk exists in the patients with lower cholesterol levels, presumably as there is coexisting malnutrition and low-grade inflammation [7, 53]. It is unlikely that high cholesterol levels confer a protective effect in ESRD patients, and the mechanism by which inflammation and malnutrition confound the association between total cholesterol and cardiovascular outcomes is unclear [54]. In contrast, the renal transplant recipient typically shows a progressive relationship between lipid levels and CHD events, mirroring the pattern seen in the general population [55, 56]. It is for these reasons that assessment of cardiovascular risk in CKD, ESRD, and renal transplant recipients can be difficult [56]. The NCEP and National Kidney Foundation have established guidelines for cholesterol management based on patient risk factors. Patients at greatest risk include those with preexisting CHD or a CHD risk equivalent and individuals with multiple risk factors (Table 8.4) [3, 57]. One guideline suggests that renal insufficiency be considered a CHD risk equivalent [58]. In addition to the traditional risk factors associated with the development and progression of CHD, the prevalence of hypertension and left ventricular hypertrophy increases as GFR declines [59]. The National Kidney Foundation has published guidelines for managing dyslipidemias in adults with CKD (Table 8.5).

In addition to significant cholesterol-lowering effects, statins may also reduce urinary protein excretion, inflammation, and fibrosis of tubular cells, thereby potentially improving renal function [14, 60, 61]. Blood pressure control and reduction of proteinuria reduce the rate of decline of eGFR as evidenced by the GUARD study [62]. Statin therapy has been shown to reduce proteinuria in rat experimental models, which may have implications on progression of renal disease in humans. Two studies demonstrated that in rats fed high-cholesterol diets the severity of hypercholesterolemia was correlated with proteinuria and the number of glomeruli with lipid deposits [61]. A study by Bianchi et al. suggested that statin therapy may reduce proteinuria in humans [63]. In this randomized trial of patients with proteinuria without evidence of systemic disease known to cause glomerulonephritis, atorvastatin provided a significant reduction in urinary protein excretion and a slower decline in creatinine clearance as compared to patients not on statin therapy [64]. In a separate study of patients with well-controlled hypertension and proteinuria without hyperlipidemia, pravastatin significantly reduced proteinuria compared to placebo [65]. There was no difference in serum creatinine or creatinine clearance between groups, and reduction of proteinuria was independent of co-treatment with an angiotensin receptor blocker (ARB). Total and LDL cholesterol levels are higher in patients with nephrotic-range proteinuria as compared to those patients with lower levels of proteinuria. For these reasons, it would be logical to aggressively treat dyslipidemia early in the CKD patient as the benefits of statin therapy on the spectrum to advanced CKD and ESRD are decreased, if at all present. It should be noted that some statins (particularly rosuvastatin) at high doses have been shown to increase proteinuria; however, this effect is transient and mild, of tubular origin [66], and not associated with negative effects on renal function [66, 67]. The Lipid-lowering and Onset of Renal Disease (LORD) study might help to clarify the benefits of statins on slowing the progression of kidney disease in patients along the continuum of CKD [57].

The Treating to New Targets (TNT) study suggested that atorvastatin reduced progression of renal disease as well as cardiovascular risk [68]. This study showed a slower rate of decline in renal function that was dose related in patients with an eGFR of >60 mL/min. The Pravastatin Pooling Project combined data from a subgroup of patients with eGFR between 30 and 90 mL/min from three randomized trials (CARE, LIPID, WOSCOPS) that were initially conducted on the general population [54]. The study showed an increased risk of myocardial infarction, coronary death, or coronary revascularization in the subgroup with moderate CKD. Among those CKD patients on statin therapy, there was an associated risk reduction of 20 % in the composite outcome over 5 years, similar to the effect seen in patients without CKD.

Statins have been proven to be safe and well tolerated by the majority of patients, but this class of drugs is not entirely free of adverse drug reactions. Patients with CKD are at increased risk of these adverse effects and should be monitored carefully for tolerability and toxicity. Though there is little published data, KDOQI, in accordance with Adult Treatment Panel III, recommend dosage reductions of several of the statins by approximately 50 % in patients with stage IV or V CKD. Dosage recommendations are outlined in Table 8.6 [69].

Table 8.6 Outcome studies of statin in dialysis patients

Study	Type of study	Treatment (n)	Patient population	Primary outcome	Study results
Die Deutsche Diabetes Dialyse Study (**4D**) [77]	Prospective, Randomized, double-blind, placebo control	Placebo Atorvastatin 20 mg $n=1,255$	Age 18–80 years old Type 2 diabetes and receiving hemodialysis for no more than 24 months	Cardiac death, fatal or nonfatal stroke, or nonfatal MI	No significant trend in occurrence of the primary endpoints was noted with atorvastatin (relative risk [RR] 0.92, 95 % confidence interval [CI] 0.77–1.10, $p=0.37$)
Evaluation of the Use of Rosuvastatin in Subjects on Regular Hemodialysis (**AURORA**) [78]	Randomized, double-blind, placebo control	Placebo Rosuvastatin 10 mg $n=2,776$	Age 50–80 years old on long-term hemodialysis	Cardiac death, nonfatal stroke, or nonfatal MI	No significant difference was noted in the primary endpoint with rosuvastatin compared with placebo (hazard ratio [HR] 0.96, 95 % CI 0.84–1.11, $p=0.59$)
The Study of Heart and Renal Protection (**SHARP**) [74]	Randomized, double-blind, placebo control	Placebo	Age ≥40 years old	Major vascular events: nonfatal MI, cardiac death, revascularization, nonfatal or fatal stroke	For the primary endpoint of major vascular events, patients in the active-treatment group experienced a 15.3 % reduction ($p=0.0012$), as compared with placebo
		Simvastatin 20 mg	Chronic kidney disease	Major atherosclerotic events: coronary death, MI, non-hemorrhagic stroke, or revascularization	After a median follow-up of 4.9 years, patients randomized to the ezetimibe/simvastatin combination experienced a 17 % reduction in major atherosclerotic events compared with the placebo group ($p=0.0022$)
		Simvastatin 20 mg/Ezetimibe 10 mg $n=9,000$	Scr ≥ 1.7 mg/dL (men) Scr ≥ 1.5 mg/dL (women) Peritoneal or hemodialysis No history of CVD		But no benefit in dialysis patients

Two recent studies, the Prospective Evaluation of Proteinuria and Renal Function in Diabetic Patients With Progressive Renal Disease (PLANET I $n=325$) and (PLANET II $n=220$) enrolled patients with urinary protein/creatinine ratios of 500–5,000 mg/g, and a fasting LDL of 90 mg/dL or higher. Patients were stable on and had used angiotensin-converting enzyme (ACE) inhibitors or ARBs for at least 3 months before enrollment. Patients were randomized to atorvastatin 80 mg, rosuvastatin 10 mg, and rosuvastatin 40 mg per day. In PLANET I, atorvastatin was associated with a significant reduction in proteinuria by approximately 20 % and no effect on GFR, while rosuvastatin was associated with a decline in GFR by 8 mL/min per year and had no effect on proteinuria [70]. Similar results were noted in the PLANET II study [71]. The incidence of renal adverse reactions was higher with the use of rosuvastatin compared to atorvastatin.

A recent Cochrane Review of statin therapy in non-dialysis CKD patients found that among 26 studies, statins significantly reduced total cholesterol, LDL, and triglyceride levels compared to placebo, though no significant change HDL cholesterol was noted [72, 73]. Overall there was a significant reduction in all-cause and cardiovascular mortality, as well as nonfatal cardiovascular events with statin use in comparison to placebo. There were no significant differences in adverse effects, withdrawal rates, rhabdomyolysis, or abnormal liver function in the CKD patients on statins compared to those on placebo. The renoprotective effects of statins could not be confirmed, as there was no significant difference in the change in creatinine clearance compared to placebo.

The Study of Heart and Renal Protection (SHARP) aimed to assess the effects of lowering LDL on the time to a first major vascular event among patients with moderate to severe kidney disease [74]. The SHARP study was a prospective, randomized, multinational, double-blind placebo-controlled trial comparing the efficacy and safety of ezetimibe/simvastatin daily versus placebo. For the first year, the study randomized 9,270 patients with CKD (3,023 on dialysis) and similar baseline characteristics in a ratio of 4:4:1 to placebo, ezetimibe/simvastatin 10/20 mg, and simvastatin 20 mg. After 1 year, those receiving simvastatin monotherapy were randomly assigned 1:1 to placebo or ezetimibe/simvastatin. The primary efficacy outcome was the occurrence of a major atherosclerotic event, defined as coronary death, myocardial infarction, non-hemorrhagic stroke, or need for revascularization. In addition, this trial was designed to test the secondary hypothesis that cholesterol reduction slows progression to ESRD among predialysis patients. Inclusion criteria consisted of documentation of CKD defined as serum creatinine greater than or equal to 1.7 mg/dL in men, or greater than or equal to 1.5 mg/dL in women or patients whom were receiving dialysis (hemodialysis or peritoneal dialysis), aged greater than or equal to 40 years. Exclusion criteria were definite history of myocardial infarction or coronary revascularization procedure, renal transplantation, past medical history significant for chronic liver disease, or abnormal liver function, clinical evidence of active muscle disease, or previous history of adverse drug reaction to a statin or to ezetimibe.

Patients were assessed at 2 months, 6 months, and every 6 months thereafter. Results of the study showed that in patients with moderate to severe CKD and no history of myocardial infarction or coronary revascularization, treatment with ezetimibe/simvastatin after a median follow-up of 4.9 years resulted in fewer major atherosclerotic events (13.4 % in the placebo arm and 11.3 % in the treatment arm) with a relative risk reduction of 17 % (95 % CI 0.74–0.94; $p=0.0021$). The results are similar whether or not one includes the approximate 10 % of patients initially assigned to simvastatin monotherapy during the first year. In secondary and exploratory analyses, nonfatal myocardial infarction, ischemic stroke, and coronary revascularization contribute substantially to the composite endpoint, although reductions in nonfatal myocardial infarctions or coronary mortality did not reach statistical significance. In the pre-specified subgroup analysis, among the patients not on dialysis at randomization, treatment reduced the relative risk of the primary composite endpoint by 20 % compared with placebo. Among the patients on dialysis at randomization, treatment did not result in a statistically significant reduction in the primary endpoint. The SHARP study was not able to provide evidence for an effect of ezetimibe/simvastatin on reducing the risk for progressing to ESRD; 33.9 % of predialysis patients assigned to the treatment group and 34.6 % assigned to placebo developed ESRD. It was determined that after the fourth year of follow-up 68 % of patients allocated to ezetimibe/simvastatin remained compliant (80 % of doses) or were taking a non-study statin, and 14 % of patients assigned placebo were taking a non-study statin. As a result, the intention-to-treat comparisons exclude the approximate one-third of participants not taking lipid-lowering treatment daily. With regard to safety outcomes, there was no significant increase in the occurrence of any incident cancer (9.4 % vs. 9.5 %), elevated transaminases (0.7 % vs. 0.6 %), hepatitis (0.5 % vs. 0.4 %), myopathy (9 vs. 5 patients), or rhabdomyolysis (4 vs. 1 patient) in the treatment arm compared to placebo, respectively.

The SHARP study provides evidence that lowering LDL cholesterol with ezetimibe/simvastatin in patients with CKD reduces cardiovascular risk. However, the treatment effect appears to be largely driven by the effect in predialysis patients and very small overall reduction. In addition, the re-randomization of the simvastatin monotherapy group to ezetimibe/simvastatin or placebo after 1 year does not allow for direct comparison to determine if the combination therapy is clinically more effective than simvastatin alone in reducing cardiovascular risk. The Effect of Ezetimibe Plus Simvastatin Versus Simvastatin Alone on Atherosclerosis in the Carotid Artery (ENHANCE) study provides some data with regard to ezetimibe/simvastatin combination therapy compared to simvastatin monotherapy [75]. Despite decreases in levels of LDL cholesterol and C-reactive protein (CRP), combined therapy with ezetimibe/simvastatin did not show clinically or statistically significant differences in intima-media thickness as compared with simvastatin alone. It was also reported in the Arterial Biology for the Investigation of the Treatment Effects of Reducing Cholesterol 6–HDL and LDL Treatment Strategies

(ARBITER 6–HALTS) trial that addition of ezetimibe was no more effective than niacin in decreasing the progression of carotid intima-media thickness in patients receiving statin therapy [76].

Finally, two randomized clinical studies and subset analysis of SHARP study have shown no statistically significant effect on the composite primary endpoint of cardiovascular death, nonfatal myocardial infarction, and stroke in patients on hemodialysis [77, 78].

Safety of Lipid-Lowering Agents in Advanced CKD

In general, cumulative data from both primary and secondary prevention studies of statins indicate that the HMG-CoA reductase inhibitors have an excellent safety record and a favorable risk-benefit profile, with a low risk of significant adverse events (<1 % incidence) [79]. However, epidemiological studies indicate the discontinuation rates for lovastatin and simvastatin were 3 % and 6 %, respectively, and there was a much higher incidence of myopathy at high doses (80 mg daily) [80, 81]. In another cohort study, the high-potency statins group was associated with high risk of relative hospitalization rates for acute kidney injury compared to the low-potency statin group within the first 120 days post-exposure to high-potency statins compared with low-potency statins. The effect seems to be strongest in the first 120 days after initiation of statin treatment [67].

Myopathy

Myopathy is the major adverse effect of the statins and is defined as muscle pain or weakness associated without elevation of creatine kinase (CK) levels, while myositis is defined as muscle pain with elevation of CK levels greater than ten times the upper limit of normal. For all statins, the overall risk of rhabdomyolysis is less than 0.5 % in the general population [82]. This risk may be higher in patients with CKD, the elderly, and in patients taking other drugs or food that inhibit CYP 3A4, specifically grapefruit, cyclosporine, azole antifungals, macrolide antibiotics, and fibrates (Table 8.7) [47]. Although the exact pathogenesis of myopathy has not been determined, numbers of mechanisms have been postulated. The etiology of myopathy is most likely related to mitochondrial dysfunction and muscle protein degradation. It has become clear that SLCO1B1 is among the strongest PK predictors of myopathy risk [83]. Rhabdomyolysis and acute renal failure may result if myopathy is not recognized and the drug is continued. For most cases, statins should be discontinued promptly and alternative class of lipid-lowering therapy should be considered.

Table 8.7 Profile of reports of rhabdomyolysis associated with statins[a]

Statin	Frequency of reports/ unique cases	No. of cases associated with potentially interacting drugs (*n*)	
Simvastatin	321/215	Mibefradil (48)	Azole antifungals (4)
		Fibrates (33)	Chlorzoxazone (2)
		Cyclosporine (31)	Nefazodone (2)
		Warfarin (12)	Niacin (2)
		Macrolide antibiotics (10)	Tacrolimus (1)
		Digoxin (9)	Fusidic acid (1)
Cerivastatin	231/192	Fibrates (22)	
		Digoxin (7)	
		Warfarin (6)	
		Macrolide antibiotics (2)	
		Cyclosporine (1)	
		Mibefradil (1)	
Atorvastatin	105/73	Mibefradil (45)	
		Fibrates (10)	
		Macrolide antibiotics (13)	
		Warfarin (7)	
		Cyclosporine (5)	
		Digoxin (5)	
		Azole antifungals (2)	
Pravastatin	98/71	Fibrates (6)	
		Macrolide antibiotics (6)	
		Warfarin (5)	
		Cyclosporine (2)	
		Digoxin (2)	
		Mibefradil (1)	
		Niacin (1)	
Lovastatin	51/40	Cyclosporine (12)	Digoxin (2)
		Macrolide antibiotics (11)	Nefazodone (2)
		Azole antifungals (6)	Niacin (1)
		Fibrates (5)	Warfarin (1)
		Mibefradil (3)	
Fluvastatin	11/10	Fibrates (4)	
		Warfarin (2)	
		Digoxin (1)	
		Mibefradil (1)	

[a]Adapted from [81, 89]

Hepatotoxicity

Previously, hepatocellular necrosis and hepatotoxicity induced by statins were considered a myth [84]. A recent study has concluded that idiosyncratic hepatotoxicity may be associated with the use of statins [41]. Asymptomatic hepatic transaminase elevation (greater than three times the upper limit of normal) may occur in 1–2 % of patients on an HMG-CoA reductase inhibitor and in general is dose related. In most patients, elevation of transaminase enzymes are resolved spontaneously with continued therapy, although discontinuation may be required in some patients.

Conclusion

For more than three decades, statins have been used in clinical practice to treat hyperlipidemia and play an important role in long-term management of various CVDs, including post-ACS, stroke, and peripheral vascular disease. These agents are categorized into two distinctive classes according to their hydrophobicity. Pravastatin and fluvastatin are almost completely absorbed after oral administration and are active as such (no conversion), while oral doses of lovastatin and simvastatin are 5 % absorbed and must be hydrolyzed to their acid form. Pravastatin is a more hydrophilic agent and required active transport into the liver. In addition, pravastatin is metabolized significantly by the CYP family and exhibits more renal elimination compared to other agents. Hydrophilic compounds such as simvastatin and lovastatin are transported by passive diffusion. These agents are metabolized in the liver and are substrate CYP 3A4. After their biotransformation, the drugs' elimination may also be influenced by P-glycoprotein transporter system. For example, both rosuvastatin and fluvastatin are primarily metabolized via CYP 2C9 and are vulnerable to interactions with drugs known to inhibit CYP 3A metabolism. There are other mechanisms that may be responsible for altering statin pharmacokinetics and pharmacodynamics and are mediated by transporter proteins including P-glycoprotein (P-gp) and various organic anion transport polypeptides (OATPs). ABC and other P-glycoprotein (MDR1 gene—multiple drug resistance) are responsible for the biliary efflux of statins. This might explain, in part, some of the potential for drug accumulation, toxicity, and interactions.

With the increasing incidence of chronic renal disease, regular renal function monitoring and dosage adjustment of lipid-lowering agents according to eGFR and pharmacokinetic data are of major importance. Because large studies of the safety of these agents in patients with CKD are lacking, drug–drug interactions and dosage-adjustment recommendations need to be regularly updated following the results of epidemiological studies and long-term follow-up (Tables 8.8 and 8.9) [85]. Generic low-dose statins (simvastatin 20 mg per day, or atorvastatin 10 mg per day) should be considered the drug and dose of choice for most patients with CKD. Pravastatin and fluvastatin are the most suitable agents for transplant patients to achieve target cholesterol levels due to reduced risk of drug interactions [37, 86].

Table 8.8 Dosing adjustment for lipid-lowering agents in chronic kidney disease [87, 88]

Drug class	Medications	Dosing in renal impairment
HMG-CoA reductase inhibitor	Atorvastatin (Lipitor®)	No adjustment is necessary
	Fluvastatin (Lescol®)	Mild-to-moderate renal impairment: no dosage adjustment necessary Severe renal impairment: use with caution (particularly at doses >40 mg/day; has not been studied)
	Lovastatin (Mevacor®)	When ClCr <30 Use IR >20 mg daily with caution Use initial ER 20 mg QHS; (doses >20 mg daily with caution)
	Pitavastatin (Livalo®)	ClCr 15–60 (not receiving HD): initial 1 mg QD; max 2 mg QD ESRD: initial 1 mg QD; max 2 mg QD
	Pravastatin (Pravacho®)	Significant impairment: initial 10 mg/day
	Rosuvastatin (Crestor®)	Mild-to-moderate impairment: no dosage adjustment required ClCr <30: initial 5 mg/day; NTE 10 mg QD
	Simvastatin (Zocor®)	Manufacturer's recommendations Mild-to-moderate renal impairment: no dosage adjustment necessary Severe renal impairment: ClCr <30: initial 5 mg/day with close monitoring Alternative recommendation: no dosage adjustment necessary for any degree of renal impairment
Bile acid sequestrants	Colesevelam (Welchol®)	No dosage adjustment necessary; not absorbed from the GI tract
	Cholestyramine	No dosage adjustment provided in manufacturer's labeling; however, use with caution in renal impairment; may cause hyperchloremic acidosis
	Colestipol	No dosage adjustment necessary; not absorbed from the gastrointestinal tract
Nicotinic acid	Niacor®; Niaspan®	No dosage adjustment recommended; use with caution
Fibric acid derivatives	Gemfibrozil	Mild-to-moderate impairment: use caution; deterioration of renal function has been reported in patients with baseline SCr >2 Severe impairment: contraindicated HD: not removed by HD; supplemental dose is not necessary
	Fenofibrate Antara®; Fenoglide®; Lipofen®; Lofibra®; TriCor®; Triglide®	ClCr ≥50: no dosage adjustment necessary ClCr <50: initiate at 45 mg/day Contraindicated in severe impairment

(continued)

Table 8.8 (continued)

Drug class	Medications	Dosing in renal impairment
Cholesterol absorption inhibitor	Ezetimibe	AUC increased with severe impairment (ClCr <30); no dosing adjustment necessary
Omega-3 fatty acid	Lovaza®	No dosage adjustment provided in manufacturer's labeling (has not been studied)
Nicotinic Acia	Niacor®; Niaspan®	No dosage adjustment recommended; use with caution
Fibric acid derivatives	Gemfibrozil	Mild-to-moderate impairment: use caution; deterioration of renal function has been reported in patients with baseline SCr >2 Severe impairment: contraindicated HD: not removed by HD; supplemental dose is not necessary
	Fenofibrate Antara®; Fenoglide®; Lipofen®; Lofibra®; TriCor®; Triglide®	ClCr ≥50: no dosage adjustment necessary ClCr <50: initiate at 45 mg/day Contraindicated in severe impairment
Cholesterol absorption inhibitor	Ezetimibe	AUC increased with severe impairment (ClCr <30); no dosing adjustment necessary
Omega-3 fatty acid	Lovaza®	No dosage adjustment provided in manufacturer's labeling (has not been studied)

Table 8.9 Common drug interactions of lipid-lowering agents[a]

Atorvastatin	• Avoid combining atorvastatin with telaprevir, tipranavir+ritonavir, gemfibrozil, or cyclosporine • Strong CYP 3A4 inhibitors (e.g., clarithromycin, itraconazole, HIV protease inhibitors [saquinavir+ritonavir, darunavir+ritonavir, fosamprenavir +/– ritonavir]): do not exceed atorvastatin 20 mg daily • Lopinavir+ritonavir: use with caution and use the lowest necessary dose of atorvastatin • Boceprevir: use lowest effective atorvastatin dose, but do not exceed atorvastatin 40 mg daily • Nelfinavir: do not exceed atorvastatin 40 mg daily • In patients taking rifampin and atorvastatin, simultaneous co-administration is recommended • Other fibrates (e.g., fenofibrate) or lipid-lowering doses of niacin (>1 g/day): may increase the risk for skeletal muscle effects. Lower starting and maintenance doses of atorvastatin should be considered when combined with fibrates or niacin. In general, statin–fibrate combinations are not recommended • Cases of myopathy, including rhabdomyolysis, have been reported with co-administration of atorvastatin and colchicine. Caution should be used when prescribing atorvastatin and colchicine

(continued)

Table 8.9 (continued)

Fluvastatin	• Cyclosporine or fluconazole: limit fluvastatin to 20 mg daily • Gemfibrozil: concomitant use with fluvastatin should be avoided • Other fibrates (e.g., fenofibrate) or lipid-lowering doses of niacin (>1 g/day): may increase the risk for skeletal muscle effects. Lower starting and maintenance doses of fluvastatin should be considered when combined with niacin. In general, statin–fibrate combinations are not recommended • Cases of myopathy, including rhabdomyolysis, have been reported with co-administration of fluvastatin and colchicine. Caution should be used when prescribing fluvastatin and colchicine
Lovastatin+[1]	• Lovastatin is *contraindicated* with HCV protease inhibitors (boceprevir or telaprevir), intraconazole, ketoconazole, posaconazole, erythromycin, clarithromycin, telithromycin, HIV protease inhibitors, and nefazodone • Avoid combining lovastatin with gemfibrozil or cyclosporine • Danazol, diltiazem, or verapamil: lovastatin 20 mg daily • Amiodarone: do not exceed lovastatin 40 mg daily • Other fibrates (e.g., fenofibrate) or lipid-lowering doses of niacin (>1 g/day): may increase the risk for skeletal muscle effects. In general, statin–fibrate combinations are not recommended. • Avoid large quantities of grapefruit juice (>1 quart daily) • Cases of myopathy, including rhabdomyolysis, have been reported with co-administration of lovastatin and colchicine. Caution should be used when prescribing lovastatin and colchicine. • Risk of myopathy, including rhabdomyolysis, may be increased by concomitant administration of ranolazine. Dose adjustment of lovastatin may be considered when combined with ranolazine. • Severe renal impairment (CrCl <30 mL.min): doses >20 mg daily should be carefully considered and cautiously implemented.
Pravastatin+	• Cyclosporine: limit pravastatin to 20 mg daily • Clarithromycin: limit pravastatin to 40 mg daily • Boceprevir: concomitant pravastatin and boceprevir increased exposure to pravastatin. Treatment with pravastatin can be initiated at the recommended dose but close clinical monitoring is warranted • Other fibrates (e.g., fenofibrate) or lipid-lowering doses of niacin (>1 g/day): may increase the risk for skeletal muscle effects. In general, statin–fibrate combinations are not recommended
Simvastatin+[2]	• Simvastatin is *contraindicated* with: itraconazole, ketoconazole, posaconazole, erythromycin, clarithromycin, telithromycin, HIV protease inhibitors, nefazodone, gemfibrozil, cyclosporine, danazol, and HCV protease inhibitors [boceprevir and telaprevir] • Verapamil or diltiazem: do not exceed simvastatin 10 mg daily • Amiodarone, amlodipine, or ranolazine: do not exceed simvastatin 20 mg daily • Other fibrates (e.g., fenofibrate) or lipid-lowering doses of niacin (>1 g/day): may increase the risk for skeletal muscle effects. In general, statin–fibrate combinations are not recommended • Cases of myopathy, including rhabdomyolysis, have been reported with co-administration of simvastatin and colchicine. Caution should be used when prescribing simvastatin and colchicine • Avoid large quantities of grapefruit juice (>1 quart daily) • Severe renal impairment (CrCl <30 mL/min): initiate dosing at 5 mg daily and be closely monitored

(continued)

Table 8.9 (continued)

Rosuvastatin	• Cyclosporine: limit rosuvastatin to 5 mg daily • Gemfibrozil: combination should be avoided. If used together, limit rosuvastatin to 10 mg daily • Other fibrates (e.g., fenofibrate) and niacin >1 g/day may increase risk of skeletal muscle effects. In general, statin–fibrate combinations are not recommended • Lopinavir/ritonavir, atazanavir/ritonavir: limit rosuvastatin to 10 mg daily • Patients with severe renal impairment (CrCl <30 mL/min), not receiving dialysis, should be started on rosuvastatin 5 mg daily and limited to 10 mg daily • Initial dose is rosuvastatin 5 mg daily in Asian patients • The 40 mg dose of rosuvastatin can be considered only after confirmation of compliance with the lipid-lowering regimen; after a careful assessment of the benefits and risks in an individual patient; and only if the patient has not met their LDL-C goal on 20 mg daily. Factors that can increase the risk for serious adverse events (myopathy and rhabdomyolysis) should be considered in the risk assessment. These factors are noted in the footnote below. If unexplained, persistent proteinuria is noted in a patient receiving rosuvastatin 40 mg daily during routine urinalysis testing, consider reducing the dose of rosuvastatin
Pitavastatin	• Pitavastatin is *contraindicated* with cyclosporine • Erythromycin: limit pitavastatin to 1 mg daily • Rifampin: initiate pitavastatin 1 mg daily (initial dose), maximum dose 2 mg daily • Use with fibrate products or lipid-lowering doses of niacin (>1 g/day) may increase the risk for adverse skeletal muscle events; pitavastatin–fibrate combination use is not recommended • Use with niacin may increase the risk for skeletal muscle adverse events • Moderate to severe renal impairment (CrCl 30–59 mL/min [moderate], CrCl <30 mL/min [severe]): pitavasatin 1 mg daily (initial dose), maximum dose 2 mg daily

[a]Adapted from [85]

References

1. Kochanek KD, Xu JQ, Murphy SL, Miniño AM, Kung HC. Deaths: final data for 2009 [PDF-2M]. Nat Vital Stat Rep. 2011;60(3):2013.
2. Downs JR, Clearfield M, Weis S, Whitney E, Shapiro DR, Beere PA, et al. Primary prevention of acute coronary events with lovastatin in men and women with average cholesterol levels: results of AFCAPS/TexCAPS. Air Force/Texas Coronary Atherosclerosis Prevention Study. JAMA. 1998;279(20):1615–22.
3. Third Report of the National Cholesterol Education Program (NCEP). Expert panel on detection, evaluation, and treatment of high blood cholesterol in adults (adult treatment panel III) final report. Circulation. 2002;106(25):3143–421.
4. Attman PO, Alaupovic P, Tavella M, Knight-Gibson C. Abnormal lipid and apolipoprotein composition of major lipoprotein density classes in patients with chronic renal failure. Nephrol Dial Transplant. 1996;11(1):63–9.
5. Coresh J, Longenecker JC, Miller III ER, Young HJ, Klag MJ. Epidemiology of cardiovascular risk factors in chronic renal disease. J Am Soc Nephrol. 1998;9(12 Suppl):S24–30.

6. Fellstrom B, Holdaas H, Jardine AG, Svensson MK, Gottlow M, Schmieder RE, et al. Cardiovascular disease in patients with renal disease: the role of statins. Curr Med Res Opin. 2009;25(1):271–85.
7. Jardine AG, Fellstrom B, Logan JO, Cole E, Nyberg G, Gronhagen-Riska C, et al. Cardiovascular risk and renal transplantation: post hoc analyses of the Assessment of Lescol in Renal Transplantation (ALERT) Study. Am J Kidney Dis. 2005;46(3):529–36.
8. U.S renal data system, USRDS 2006 annual data report: Atlas of end-stage Renal disease in the united states, national institutes of health, national institute of diabetes and digestive and kidney diseases, Bethesda, MD; 2008.2009. 2010.
9. Kidney Disease Outcomes Quality Initiative (K/DOQI) Group. K/DOQI clinical practice guidelines for management of dyslipidemias in patients with kidney disease. Am J Kidney Dis. 2003;41(4 Suppl 3):S1–91.
10. Brown AG, Smale TC, King TJ, Hasenkamp R, Thompson RH. Crystal and molecular structure of compactin, a new antifungal metabolite from Penicillium brevicompactum. J Chem Soc Perkin 1. 1976;11:1165–70.
11. Corsini A, Bellosta S, Baetta R, Fumagalli R, Paoletti R, Bernini F. New insights into the pharmacodynamic and pharmacokinetic properties of statins. Pharmacol Ther. 1999;84(3):413–28.
12. Saito Y. Pitavastatin: an overview. Atheroscler Suppl. 2011;12(3):271–6.
13. Teresi RE, Planchon SM, Waite KA, Eng C. Regulation of the PTEN promoter by statins and SREBP. Hum Mol Genet. 2008;17(7):919–28.
14. Blum A, Shamburek R. The pleiotropic effects of statins on endothelial function, vascular inflammation, immunomodulation and thrombogenesis. Atherosclerosis. 2009;203(2):325–30.
15. Maron DJ, Fazio S, Linton MF. Current perspectives on statins. Circulation. 2000;101(2): 207–13.
16. Bianco AM, Zanin V, Marcuzzi A, Crovella S. Clarification of the pleiotropic effects of statins on mevalonate pathway and the feedback regulation of isoprenoids requires more comprehensive investigation. Cell Biochem Funct. 2012;30(2):176.
17. Laufs U. Beyond lipid-lowering: effects of statins on endothelial nitric oxide. Eur J Clin Pharmacol. 2003;58(11):719–31.
18. Callahan III AS. Vascular pleiotropy of statins: clinical evidence and biochemical mechanisms. Curr Atheroscler Rep. 2003;5(1):33–7.
19. Istvan ES. Structural mechanism for statin inhibition of 3-hydroxy-3-methylglutaryl coenzyme A reductase. Am Heart J. 2002;144(6 Suppl):S27–32.
20. Lennernas H, Fager G. Pharmacodynamics and pharmacokinetics of the HMG-CoA reductase inhibitors. Similarities and differences. Clin Pharmacokinet. 1997;32(5):403–25.
21. Simonson SG, Martin PD, Mitchell P, Schneck DW, Lasseter KC, Warwick MJ. Pharmacokinetics and pharmacodynamics of rosuvastatin in subjects with hepatic impairment. Eur J Clin Pharmacol. 2003;58(10):669–75.
22. Martin PD, Mitchell PD, Schneck DW. Pharmacodynamic effects and pharmacokinetics of a new HMG-CoA reductase inhibitor, rosuvastatin, after morning or evening administration in healthy volunteers. Br J Clin Pharmacol. 2002;54(5):472–7.
23. Pan HY, DeVault AR, Wang-Iverson D, Ivashkiv E, Swanson BN, Sugerman AA. Comparative pharmacokinetics and pharmacodynamics of pravastatin and lovastatin. J Clin Pharmacol. 1990;30(12):1128–35.
24. Tse FL, Jaffe JM, Troendle A. Pharmacokinetics of fluvastatin after single and multiple doses in normal volunteers. J Clin Pharmacol. 1992;32(7):630–8.
25. Radulovic LL, Cilla DD, Posvar EL, Sedman AJ, Whitfield LR. Effect of food on the bioavailability of atorvastatin, an HMG-CoA reductase inhibitor. J Clin Pharmacol. 1995;35(10): 990–4.
26. Bellosta S, Paoletti R, Corsini A. Safety of statins: focus on clinical pharmacokinetics and drug interactions. Circulation. 2004;109(23 Suppl 1):III50–7.
27. Garcia MJ, Reinoso RF, Sanchez NA, Prous JR. Clinical pharmacokinetics of statins. Methods Find Exp Clin Pharmacol. 2003;25(6):457–81.

28. Neuvonen PJ, Backman JT, Niemi M. Pharmacokinetic comparison of the potential over-the-counter statins simvastatin, lovastatin, fluvastatin and pravastatin. Clin Pharmacokinet. 2008; 47(7):463–74.
29. Shitara Y, Sugiyama Y. Pharmacokinetic and pharmacodynamic alterations of 3-hydroxy-3-methylglutaryl coenzyme A (HMG-CoA) reductase inhibitors: drug-drug interactions and interindividual differences in transporter and metabolic enzyme functions. Pharmacol Ther. 2006;112(1):71–105.
30. Hua WJ, Hua WX, Fang HJ. The role of OATP1B1 and BCRP in pharmacokinetics and DDI of novel statins. Cardiovasc Ther. 2012;30(5):e234–41.
31. Ma TK, Lam YY, Tan VP, Kiernan TJ, Yan BP. Impact of genetic and acquired alteration in cytochrome P450 system on pharmacologic and clinical response to clopidogrel. Pharmacol Ther. 2010;125(2):249–59.
32. Tomita Y, Maeda K, Sugiyama Y. Clin Pharmacol Ther. 2013;94(1):37–51.
33. Yang SH, Choi JS, Choi DH. Effects of HMG-CoA reductase inhibitors on the pharmacokinetics of losartan and its main metabolite EXP-3174 in rats: possible role of CYP3A4 and P-gp inhibition by HMG-CoA reductase inhibitors. Pharmacology. 2011;88(1–2):1–9.
34. Backes JM, Howard PA, Ruisinger JF, Moriarty PM. Does simvastatin cause more myotoxicity compared with other statins? Ann Pharmacother. 2009;43(12):2012–20.
35. Feng Q, Wilke RA, Baye TM. Individualized risk for statin-induced myopathy: current knowledge, emerging challenges and potential solutions. Pharmacogenomics. 2012;13(5):579–94.
36. Voora D, Ginsburg GS. Clinical application of cardiovascular pharmacogenetics. J Am Coll Cardiol. 2012;60(1):9–20.
37. Kajinami K, Masuya H, Hoshiba Y, Takeda K, Sato R, Okabayashi M, et al. Statin response and pharmacokinetics variants. Expert Opin Pharmacother. 2005;6(8):1291–7.
38. Gallelli L, Ferraro M, Spagnuolo V, Rende P, Mauro GF, De SG. Rosuvastatin-induced rhabdomyolysis probably via CYP2C9 saturation. Drug Metabol Drug Interact. 2009;24(1):83–7.
39. Cilla Jr DD, Gibson DM, Whitfield LR, Sedman AJ. Pharmacodynamic effects and pharmacokinetics of atorvastatin after administration to normocholesterolemic subjects in the morning and evening. J Clin Pharmacol. 1996;36(7):604–9.
40. Poli A. Atorvastatin: pharmacological characteristics and lipid-lowering effects. Drugs. 2007;67 Suppl 1:3–15.
41. Bjornsson E, Jacobsen EI, Kalaitzakis E. Hepatotoxicity associated with statins: reports of idiosyncratic liver injury post-marketing. J Hepatol. 2012;56(2):374–80.
42. Calderon RM, Cubeddu LX, Goldberg RB, Schiff ER. Statins in the treatment of dyslipidemia in the presence of elevated liver aminotransferase levels: a therapeutic dilemma. Mayo Clin Proc. 2010;85(4):349–56.
43. Todd PA, Gemfibrozil WA. A review of its pharmacodynamic and pharmacokinetic properties, and therapeutic use in dyslipidaemia. Drugs. 1988;36(3):314–39.
44. Benko S, Drabant S, Grezal G, Urmos I, Csorgo M, Klebovich I. Pharmacokinetic and bioequivalence study of two gemfibrozil preparations. Arzneimittelforschung. 1997;47(8):913–6.
45. Jacobson TA. Myopathy with statin-fibrate combination therapy: clinical considerations. Nat Rev Endocrinol. 2009;5(9):507–18.
46. Shitara Y, Hirano M, Sato H, Sugiyama Y. Gemfibrozil and its glucuronide inhibit the organic anion transporting polypeptide 2 (OATP2/OATP1B1:SLC21A6)-mediated hepatic uptake and CYP2C8-mediated metabolism of cerivastatin: analysis of the mechanism of the clinically relevant drug-drug interaction between cerivastatin and gemfibrozil. J Pharmacol Exp Ther. 2004;311(1):228–36.
47. Bellosta S, Corsini A. Statin drug interactions and related adverse reactions. Expert Opin Drug Saf. 2012;11(6):933–46.
48. McQuade CR, Griego J, Anderson J, Pai AB. Elevated serum creatinine levels associated with fenofibrate therapy. Am J Health Syst Pharm. 2008;65(2):138–41.
49. Balfour JA, McTavish D, Heel RC. Fenofibrate. A review of its pharmacodynamic and pharmacokinetic properties and therapeutic use in dyslipidaemia. Drugs. 1990;40(2):260–90.

50. Brown WV. Potential use of fenofibrate and other fibric acid derivatives in the clinic. Am J Med. 1987;83(5B):85–9.
51. Caldwell J. The biochemical pharmacology of fenofibrate. Cardiology. 1989;76 Suppl 1:33–41.
52. Harper CR, Jacobson TA. Managing dyslipidemia in chronic kidney disease. J Am Coll Cardiol. 2008;51(25):2375–84.
53. Liu Y, Coresh J, Eustace JA, Longenecker JC, Jaar B, Fink NE, et al. Association between cholesterol level and mortality in dialysis patients: role of inflammation and malnutrition. JAMA. 2004;291(4):451–9.
54. Tonelli M, Isles C, Curhan GC, Tonkin A, Pfeffer MA, Shepherd J, et al. Effect of pravastatin on cardiovascular events in people with chronic kidney disease. Circulation. 2004;110(12): 1557–63.
55. Akioka K, Takahara S, Ichikawa S, Yoshimura N, Akiyama T, Ohshima S. Factors predicting long-term graft survival after kidney transplantation: multicenter study in Japan. World J Surg. 2005;29(2):249–56.
56. Kimak E, Ksiazek A, Baranowicz-Gaszczyk I, Solski J. Disturbed lipids, lipoproteins and triglyceride-rich lipoproteins as well as fasting and nonfasting non-high-density lipoprotein cholesterol in post-renal transplant patients. Ren Fail. 2007;29(6):705–12.
57. Fassett RG, Ball MJ, Robertson IK, Geraghty DP, Coombes JS. The Lipid-lowering and Onset of Renal Disease (LORD) Trial: a randomized double blind placebo controlled trial assessing the effect of atorvastatin on the progression of kidney disease. BMC Nephrol. 2008;9:4.
58. Lewis D, Haynes R, Landray MJ. Lipids in chronic kidney disease. J Ren Care. 2010;36 Suppl 1:27–33.
59. Tomilina NA, Storozhakov GI, Gendlin GE, Badaeva SV, Zhidkova DA, Kim IG, et al. [Risk factors and pathogenetic mechanisms of left ventricular hypertrophy in progressive chronic kidney disease and after transplantation of the kidney]. Ter Arkh. 2007;79(6):34–40.
60. Muntner P, He J, Astor BC, Folsom AR, Coresh J. Traditional and nontraditional risk factors predict coronary heart disease in chronic kidney disease: results from the atherosclerosis risk in communities study. J Am Soc Nephrol. 2005;16(2):529–38.
61. Rayner HC, Ross-Gilbertson VL, Walls J. The role of lipids in the pathogenesis of glomerulosclerosis in the rat following subtotal nephrectomy. Eur J Clin Invest. 1990;20(1):97–104.
62. Bakris GL, Toto RD, McCullough PA, Rocha R, Purkayastha D, Davis P. Effects of different ACE inhibitor combinations on albuminuria: results of the GUARD study. Kidney Int. 2008;73(11):1303–9.
63. Bianchi S, Bigazzi R, Caiazza A, Campese VM. A controlled, prospective study of the effects of atorvastatin on proteinuria and progression of kidney disease. Am J Kidney Dis. 2003; 41(3):565–70.
64. Olyaei A, Greer E, Delos SR, Rueda J. The efficacy and safety of the 3-hydroxy-3-methylglutaryl-CoA reductase inhibitors in chronic kidney disease, dialysis, and transplant patients. Clin J Am Soc Nephrol. 2011;6(3):664–78.
65. Lee TM, Su SF, Tsai CH. Effect of pravastatin on proteinuria in patients with well-controlled hypertension. Hypertension. 2002;40(1):67–73.
66. Buyukhatipoglu H, Sezen Y, Guntekin U, Kirhan I, Dag OF. Acute renal failure with the combined use of rosuvastatin and fenofibrate. Ren Fail. 2010;32(5):633–5.
67. Dormuth CR, Hemmelgarn BR, Paterson JM, James MT, Teare GF, Raymond CB, et al. Use of high potency statins and rates of admission for acute kidney injury: multicenter, retrospective observational analysis of administrative databases. BMJ. 2013;346:f880.
68. Shepherd J, Kastelein JJ, Bittner V, Deedwania P, Breazna A, Dobson S, et al. Intensive lipid-lowering with atorvastatin in patients with coronary heart disease and chronic kidney disease: the TNT (Treating to New Targets) study. J Am Coll Cardiol. 2008;51(15):1448–54.
69. Munar MY, Singh H. Drug dosing adjustments in patients with chronic kidney disease. Am Fam Physician. 2007;75(10):1487–96.

70. Prospective Evaluation of Proteinuria and Renal Function in Diabetic Patients With Progressive Renal Disease. XLVII European Renal Association-European Dialysis and Transplant Association (ERA-EDTA) Congress, June 25–28, 2010, Munich, Germany; 2010.
71. de Zeeuw D. Prospective evaluation of proteinuria and renal function in nondiabetic patients with progressive renal disease. 2010.
72. Navaneethan SD, Pansini F, Perkovic V, Manno C, Pellegrini F, Johnson DW, et al. HMG CoA reductase inhibitors (statins) for people with chronic kidney disease not requiring dialysis. Cochrane Database Syst Rev. 2009;(2):CD007784.
73. Navaneethan SD, Hegbrant J, Strippoli GF. Role of statins in preventing adverse cardiovascular outcomes in patients with chronic kidney disease. Curr Opin Nephrol Hypertens. 2011;20(2):146–52.
74. Baigent C, Landray MJ, Reith C, Emberson J, Wheeler DC, Tomson C, et al. The effects of lowering LDL cholesterol with simvastatin plus ezetimibe in patients with chronic kidney disease (Study of Heart and Renal Protection): a randomised placebo-controlled trial. Lancet. 2011;377(9784):2181–92.
75. Kastelein JJ, Akdim F, Stroes ES, Zwinderman AH, Bots ML, Stalenhoef AF, et al. Simvastatin with or without ezetimibe in familial hypercholesterolemia. N Engl J Med. 2008; 358(14):1431–43.
76. Villines TC, Stanek EJ, Devine PJ, Turco M, Miller M, Weissman NJ, et al. The ARBITER 6-HALTS Trial (Arterial Biology for the Investigation of the Treatment Effects of Reducing Cholesterol 6-HDL and LDL Treatment Strategies in Atherosclerosis): final results and the impact of medication adherence, dose, and treatment duration. J Am Coll Cardiol. 2010; 55(24):2721–6.
77. Wanner C, Krane V, Marz W, Olschewski M, Mann JF, Ruf G, et al. Atorvastatin in patients with type 2 diabetes mellitus undergoing hemodialysis. N Engl J Med. 2005;353(3):238–48.
78. Fellstrom BC, Jardine AG, Schmieder RE, Holdaas H, Bannister K, Beutler J, et al. Rosuvastatin and cardiovascular events in patients undergoing hemodialysis. N Engl J Med. 2009;14:1395–407.
79. Brown AS, Bakker-Arkema RG, Yellen L, Henley Jr RW, Guthrie R, Campbell CF, et al. Treating patients with documented atherosclerosis to National Cholesterol Education Program-recommended low-density-lipoprotein cholesterol goals with atorvastatin, fluvastatin, lovastatin and simvastatin. J Am Coll Cardiol. 1998;32(3):665–72.
80. FDA. FDA: Limit Use of 80 mg Simvastatin. This article appears on FDA's Consumer Updates page4, which features the latest on all FDA-regulated products June 8, 2011; 2011.
81. Omar MA, Wilson JP. FDA adverse event reports on statin-associated rhabdomyolysis. Ann Pharmacother. 2002;36(2):288–95.
82. McKenney JM, Davidson MH, Jacobson TA, Guyton JR. Final conclusions and recommendations of the National Lipid Association Statin Safety Assessment Task Force. Am J Cardiol. 2006;97(8A):89C–94C.
83. Strain JD, Farver DK, Clem JR. A review on the rationale and clinical use of concomitant rosuvastatin and fenofibrate/fenofibric acid therapy. Clin Pharmacol. 2010;2:95–104.
84. Bader T. The myth of statin-induced hepatotoxicity. Am J Gastroenterol. 2010;105(5):978–80.
85. http://www.pbm.va.gov or http://vaww.pbm.va.gov. (Pravastatin, Rosuvastatin, Fluvastatin, Fluvastatin XL, Pitavastatin) VHA Pharmacy Benefits Management (PBM) Services, Medical Advisory Panel (MAP) and VISN Pharmacist Executives (VPEs). 2013.
86. Jardine AG, Holdaas H, Fellstrom B, Cole E, Nyberg G, Gronhagen-Riska C, et al. Fluvastatin prevents cardiac death and myocardial infarction in renal transplant recipients: post-hoc subgroup analyses of the ALERT Study. Am J Transplant. 2004;4(6):988–95.
87. Schachter M. Chemical, pharmacokinetic and pharmacodynamic properties of statins: an update. Fundam Clin Pharmacol. 2005;19(1):117–25.
88. Neuvonen PJ, Niemi M, Backman JT. Drug interactions with lipid-lowering drugs: mechanisms and clinical relevance. Clin Pharmacol Ther. 2006;80(6):565–81.
89. Omar MA, Wilson JP, Cox TS. Rhabdomyolysis and HMG-CoA reductase inhibitors. Ann Pharmacother. 2001;35(9):1096–107.

Chapter 9
Non-statin Therapies for CKD with Dyslipidemia

Istvan Mucsi

Introduction

Disorders of lipid metabolism and altered serum lipid and lipoprotein profile (dyslipidemia) are very common in patients with various stages of chronic kidney disease (CKD). Patients not on renal replacement therapy (RRT) and also individuals receiving various RRTs (including peritoneal dialysis [PD], hemodialysis [HD] or kidney transplantation [KTx]) usually have elevated TG, reduced HDL-C levels, with variable changes in LDL-C. It is likely that dyslipidemia contributes to the high risk of cardiovascular disease (CVD) in patients with CKD [1]. In fact, CKD is considered a coronary heart disease (CHD) risk equivalent, and it is recommended that patients with CKD be considered at the "highest level" of CHD risk for treatment decisions [2, 3]. These treatment considerations are usually based on measured serum lipid levels and also pre-specified target ranges. These quantitative parameters, however, have somewhat limited value in patients with CKD, since the multitude of coexistent traditional and novel CV risk factors, the presence of protein-energy wasting, various modifications of lipoprotein moieties may both quantitatively and qualitatively alter the lipoprotein particles and the pathophysiology of dyslipidemia [4–8]. These CKD-specific factors and modifications likely modify the pathophysiological significance and disease associations of lipoproteins substantially [4, 5, 8]. In addition these disease-specific characteristics and processes may, at least in part, explain the reverse epidemiology of dyslipidemia described in patients with various stages of CKD, and also may explain, to some extent, the sometimes surprising results of recent negative clinical trials. Therefore, it would be very important that treatment decisions concerning lipid lowering could be based on data specifically obtained in appropriate, well-designed RCTs that include patients with CKD. Since disease

I. Mucsi, M.D., Ph.D. (✉)
Department of Medicine, Division of Nephrology, McGill University Health Centre,
Royal Victoria Hospital, 687 Pine Avenue West, Room R2.37, Montreal, QC, Canada, H3A 1A1
e-mail: istvan.mucsi@mcgill.ca

A. Covic et al. (eds.), *Dyslipidemias in Kidney Disease*, DOI 10.1007/978-1-4939-0515-7_9,

associations are also likely to be significantly modified by the specific modality of RRT utilized, treatment recommendations should ideally be based on data obtained in studies enrolling individuals in the specific RRT modality.

The National Kidney Foundation–Kidney Disease Outcomes Quality Initiative (KDOQI) developed clinical practice guidelines that recommend aggressive therapy of dyslipidemia in patients who have kidney disease [2, 9]. The recommendations of the KDOQI guidelines are similar to the ones of the National Cholesterol Education Program Adult Treatment Panel (NCEP ATP) III [2, 10]. Due to the lack of published RCTs in patients with CKD, those treatment guidelines had to rely on evidence relevant to the general population with their results extrapolated to patients with CKD. Specifically, the guidelines suggest treating patients with CKD according to their levels of CHD risk and LDL-C, as recommended by the NCEP ATP III guideline [10].

The results of several treatment trials, mainly focusing on the clinical effectiveness of statins, have been published since the publication of the KDOQI guidelines. Evidence from those trials and from subsequent systematic reviews and meta-analyses [11] suggest that statin therapy is beneficial in individuals with CKD, both to reduce increased LDL-C and TC levels, reduce TG levels, and also to improve clinical outcomes. A recent meta-analysis also supports the clinical effectiveness of fibrates in this patient population [12].

No CKD-specific guidelines have been published since the KDOQI guidelines; the European Renal Best Practice website [13] refers to the KDOQI guidelines and also to the recent recommendations issued by the Canadian Cardiovascular Society [14]. This latter and perhaps most recent guideline considers individuals with CKD as "high" cardiovascular risk patients and recommends following screening and treatment target strategies accordingly. The KDIGO clinical practice guidelines are expected to be published in 2013 to support the management of dyslipidemia of individuals with CKD utilizing the best and most current available evidence. However, considering the paucity of published studies concerning lipid-lowering agents other than statins in individuals with CKD, it is expected that only limited specific evidence will support the use of those lipid-lowering regimens in patients with CKD [1].

In the absence of high-grade evidence, clinicians will still need to make decisions, and those decisions concerning non-statin lipid-lowering treatments will need to be based on available lower-grade evidence and on clinical judgment, also considering patient views and preferences. This mainly applies to patients receiving maintenance dialysis and to kidney transplant recipients, for whom the available evidence to support the use of various lipid-lowering regimens is very limited.

With all the above considerations in mind, we will review data from the general population concerning the therapeutic interventions. We will add CKD-specific information when available. We will focus on treatment interventions (others than statins) that are specifically targeting lipid disorders, namely therapeutic lifestyle changes (TLC), fibrates, nicotinic acid (NA), bile acid sequestrants, omega-3 fatty acids (fish oil), and inhibitors of cholesteryl ester transfer protein (CETPi). Other, non-specific interventions (optimal treatment of diabetes, reducing proteinuria with the use of ACEI, optimizing medication use) will not be covered here.

Therapeutic Lifestyle Changes

The available guidelines all support the use of TLCs as the first step to reduce CV risk and also to improve dyslipidemias [2, 9, 10]. In fact, TLCs may be the only intervention needed for a significant proportion of cooperating patients. TLCs include dietary changes, smoking cessation, regular exercise, weight loss–weight management, and modification of alcohol consumption. Both observational data and intervention trials (mainly dietary interventions) have confirmed that TLCs will effectively reduce serum lipid levels and also substantially reduce CV risk. The magnitude of the effect of TLCs on clinical outcome likely exceeds that of pharmacotherapy [15–17]. Changing lifestyle, modifying dietary habits and activity pattern, however, is quite difficult and requires a concerted multidisciplinary approach [18–21].

Polyunsaturated Fatty Acids

A large body of evidence links nutritional factors to serum lipid levels in the general population [10, 22]. The effects of dietary cholesterol intake on cholesterol absorption and serum cholesterol levels show marked inter-individual variability [23, 24]. Perhaps the strongest effect on serum TC and LDL-C levels is attributed to dietary saturated fatty acids (SFAs) [25]. Trans fatty acids (found in diary products, red meat and "partially hydrogenated fatty acids") increase LDL-C similar to SFAs [26]. These factors have only limited effect on HDL-C [25]. Replacing SFAs by monounsaturated fatty acids (MUFAs), omega-6 polyunsaturated fatty acids (PUFAs), or by carbohydrate will reduce LDL-C [25]. MUFAs will also improve insulin sensitivity and reduce TG [27].

Omega-3 fatty acids (eicosapentaenoic acid [EPA] and docosahexaenoic acid [DHA]) are components of fish oil and the Mediterranean diet, and have been shown to lower TG by about 30 %, but not LDL-C. Omega-3 fatty acids at pharmacological doses (2 g/day or more) affect serum lipids and lipoproteins, in particular VLDL concentration. The underlying mechanism may involve interactions with PPARs and reduced secretion of apoB [25, 27]. The Food and Drug Administration (FDA) has approved the use of omega-3 fatty acids (prescription products) as an adjunct to the diet if TG exceed 5.6 mmol/L, but more data on clinical outcomes are needed to justify the use of prescription omega-3 fatty acids [28]. A recent Japanese study in patients with hypercholesterolemia reported a 19 % reduction in CV outcomes [29], but the data remain inconclusive and the clinical efficacy of fish oil may be related to non-lipid effects [30]. The recommended dose of total EPA and DHA to lower TG is between 2 and 4 g/day. The administration of omega-3 fatty acids appears to be safe. They also exert antithrombotic effects that need to be considered when they are co-administered with aspirin/clopidogrel.

Dietary Carbohydrate and Alcohol

Dietary carbohydrate is "cholesterol neutral," while dietary fiber (legumes, fruit, vegetables, and whole meal cereals) has a direct hypocholesterolemic effect [31]. High carbohydrate diet, on the other hand, especially foods with a high glycemic index/low fiber content, will significantly increase TG and reduce HDL-C, whereas fiber-rich, low glycemic index foods will have much less such effect on TG and HDL-C levels [25, 32].

Alcohol consumption (even small amounts) may substantially increase TG levels, especially in individuals with high fasting TG concentrations [33]. On the other hand, moderate amount of alcohol consumption is associated with increased HDL-C compared to non-drinkers [34].

Weight Loss

Although overweight and obesity is associated with dyslipidemia, the effect of weight reduction on TC and LDL-C is modest. Similarly, small cholesterol-lowering effect was shown for regular exercise [35, 36]. Weight reduction improves insulin sensitivity and decreases TG levels and the effect is maintained as long as weight is not regained [36]. Weight reduction and physical exercise also have a beneficial influence on HDL-C levels [37].

TLC in Patients with CKD

In CKD, current data regarding the relationship between dietary fat and CVD are unclear [38]. Similarly, there is a lack of data on which suggestions concerning the optimal composition of macronutrients in these patients could be based. Consequently, CKD patients are advised to follow a diet with nutrient composition similar to the general population [39–41]. However, it would appear advisable to maintain a high energy intake, to use sources of unsaturated fat rather than saturated or trans fats, and to maintain lower dietary intake of cholesterol [38].

Polyunsaturated Fatty Acids

Observational studies reported an inverse association between omega-3 PUFA consumption and mortality in maintenance dialysis patients [42, 43]; however, it was not possible to exclude confounding effects (e.g., socioeconomic status, overall nutritional intake, etc.) [44]. Data from small, randomized clinical trials suggest that the triglyceride-lowering effect of omega-3 PUFA extends to individuals with advanced CKD and end-stage renal disease (ESKD) [45, 46]. One clinical trial reported the effects of omega-3 PUFA supplementation 1.7 g daily on secondary

CV events over a 2-year period in 206 chronic hemodialysis patients [47]. Omega-3 PUFA did not reduce the composite endpoint of CV events and death, although the rate of myocardial infarction was reduced.

Although the 2005 NKF-K/DOQI Clinical Practice Guidelines for Cardiovascular Disease in Dialysis Patients recommends further research on the use of omega-3 PUFA in CKD [48], no intake guidelines have thus far been established. Based on the above, however, it is not unreasonable to suggest that the current AHA intake guidelines [49] be applied to patients with CKD. These guidelines suggest to consume about 1 g EPA+DHA daily, preferably from fatty fish. Fish oil in capsule form can also be considered [49].

Aerobic Exercise

Several small studies looked at the effects of aerobic exercise training on blood lipids in patients with CKD [19, 50–53]. Most of these studies were not able to demonstrate significant improvement of dyslipidemia with exercise training, although insufficient statistical power may have played a role [50]. However, given the beneficial effects of exercise training on CV risk, physical functioning, and quality of life, regular, moderate intensity aerobic exercise is recommended to patients with CKD.

Weight Loss

Very little is known about the effect of weight loss on dyslipidemia in overweight or obese individuals with CKD. This question is also complicated by the "reverse epidemiology" of obesity observed in individuals with CKD and on dialysis and the problems surrounding the best method to estimate or measure clinically significant adiposity [4, 54–56]. However, the few trials evaluating weight loss in CKD [57, 58] have shown a favorable outcome. It has also been suggested by studies that weight loss in overweight patients or obese patients with CKD may reduce albuminuria and improve renal outcomes [59]. Given the concerns about protein-energy wasting in this patient population, it is important that weight loss attempts be monitored by the managing team, including dieticians and also preferably done as part of a complex, multi-faceted risk management program.

Recommendations for TLCs [2, 10, 60]

Individuals with excessive weight (BMI>25 kg/m^2) and/or abdominal adiposity (waist circumference >94 cm for males, >80 cm for females if Caucasians) should reduce caloric intake and increase energy expenditure, creating a daily deficit of 300–500 kcal/day. This should be achieved by following structured lifestyle education programs and engaging in regular physical exercise.

The recommended total fat intake is between 25 and 35 % of calories for adults depending upon individual preferences and characteristics. The type of fat intake should predominantly come from sources of MUFAs and both omega-6 and omega-3 PUFAs. Available data are insufficient to define an optimal omega-3/omega-6 fatty acid ratio. To achieve optimal lipid levels, saturated fat intake should be less than 10 % of the total caloric intake. Trans fat consumption should be minimal, below 1 % of energy consumed. Cholesterol intake should not exceed 300 mg/day.

Carbohydrate intake may range between 45 and 55 % of total energy. Consumption of vegetables and other foods rich in dietary fiber with a low glycemic index (legumes, fruits, nuts, and wholegrain cereals) should be an important part of everyday diet. Intake of sugars should not exceed 10 % of total energy intake.

Moderate alcohol consumption (up to 20–30 g/day for men and 10–20 g/day for women) is acceptable, provided that TG levels are not elevated. Smoking cessation should be strongly encouraged for, among other reasons, its clear benefits on HDL-C.

Pharmacotherapy to Lower TC and LDL-C

Available high-grade evidence from RCTs and systematic reviews support the effectiveness of using statins to reduce LDL-C and to reduce CVD event rate proportional to the achieved reduction in LDL-C [61]. Recent analyses indicate that this association between LDL-C and CVD risk persists throughout even very low LDL-C concentrations, lending further support to intensive statin therapy [62, 63]. However, a review of recent RCTs revealed a substantial CVD event rate in those treated to achieve even the most stringent LDL-C targets [64–66]. Recognition of this sizable residual risk has intensified efforts to identify alternative therapeutic interventions. These therapeutic alternatives are also necessary for those patients who cannot take statins or do not tolerate large enough dose. Below we will review the available pharmacotherapeutic alternatives, emphasizing that these medications should only be considered after TLCs and statins have been utilized or in addition to those interventions.

Cholesterol Absorption Inhibitors

Ezetimibe inhibits intestinal cholesterol absorption, likely interacting with the NPC1L1 protein of the intestinal brush border. This will result in reduced amount of lipoprotein cholesterol reaching the liver and a consequent up-regulation of the LDLR, which in turn leads to increased clearance of LDL from the blood.

Ezetimibe monotherapy reduces LDL-C in hypercholesterolemic patients by 15–22 %. Combined therapy with ezetimibe and a statin provides an incremental reduction in LDL-C levels of 15–20 % [67–69].

Ezetimibe is rapidly absorbed and metabolized to the pharmacologically active ezetimibe glucuronide. It can be taken in the morning or evening without regard to food intake. There are no clinically significant effects of age, sex, or race on ezetimibe pharmacokinetics, and no dosage adjustment is necessary in patients with mild hepatic impairment or mild to severe renal insufficiency. Ezetimibe can be co-administered with any dose of any statin. No major side effects have been reported. Occasionally, moderate elevations of liver enzymes, and muscle pain can be encountered.

The safety and effectiveness of ezetimibe in patients with CKD has been demonstrated in the Study of Heart and Renal Protection (SHARP) (see above) [69]. Unfortunately, we do not have data about the efficacy and effectiveness of ezetimibe alone or combined with lipid lowering agents other than statins in patients with CKD.

Bile Acid Sequestrants

Bile acid sequestrants (cholestyramine, colestipol, and colesevelam) are bile acid-binding exchange resins that reduce serum LDL-C concentration by about 20 % [70]. No clinically significant effect on TG or HDL-C levels was reported.

These compounds are not absorbed or altered by digestive enzymes. Bile acids are synthesized in the liver from cholesterol and are excreted into the intestinal lumen with the bile. Most of the bile acid is reabsorbed in the terminal ileum and is returned to the liver. Bile acid sequestrants bind the bile acids in the gut, preventing their entry into the circulation. The resulting increase in cholesterol catabolism leads to a compensatory increase in hepatic LDLR activity, which promotes clearing LDL-C from the circulation and thus reducing LDL-C levels.

Gastrointestinal adverse effects (most commonly flatulence, constipation, dyspepsia, and nausea) are relatively frequent with these drugs. To reduce these side effects, the dose should be increased gradually and ample amounts of fluid should be ingested with the drug. Reduced absorption of fat-soluble vitamins has been reported. Bile acid sequestrants have important drug interactions with many commonly prescribed drugs and should therefore be administered either 4 h before or 1 h after other drugs [71].

No dose adjustments are needed when these medications are used in individuals with impaired kidney function since these drugs are not absorbed [72]. Bile acid sequestrants do interfere with cyclosporine absorption in kidney transplant recipients, however, and may also increase triglyceride levels. There are little data on the safety and cardiac outcomes of these agents in the CKD population. A recent, small study using colesevelam 1.5 g before meals for 6 months reported a significant 20 % reduction in non–HDL-C and a 63 % reduction in median CRP [73].

Sevelamer is a cationic polymer that binds phosphates via ion exchange. It also has been found to reduce TC by about 20 % and LDL-C by 30–40 % by binding bile acids in the intestine [74]. An open-label study involving 192 patients treated by hemodialysis who used sevelamer for 46 weeks showed a 36 % reduction in LDL cholesterol level and an 18 % increase in HDL cholesterol level [75]. In the Treat to Goal Study, patients receiving sevelamer had significantly lower rates of coronary artery calcification and a reduction in LDL-C [76]. The clinical relevance of this effect of sevelamer, however, in improving CV outcomes in patients with CKD has not been clearly documented.

Nicotinic Acid (See Also Under TG and HDL)

Nicotinic acid reduces both LDL-C by 15–18 % and TG by 20–40 % at the maximum recommended dose (2 g/day). It also lowers Lp(a) levels by up to 30 %, which is a unique effect. It also increases HDL-C by about 25 %. Nicotinic acid may be used in combination with statins [77].

Combination Therapy to Reduce TC and LDL-C

Although in the majority of cases therapeutic targets can be reached using TLC and statin monotherapy, patients who do not tolerate high doses of statins may benefit from combination therapy.

Adding bile acid sequestrant to statins results in an additional 15–20 % reduction of LDL-C. This combination reportedly reduced atherosclerotic coronary changes [78, 79], but no studies with hard clinical endpoints have been published so far using this combination.

Similarly, adding ezetimibe to statins results in an additional 15–20 % reduction of LDL-C [80]. This combination has been shown to significantly reduce clinically meaningful outcome measure both in the general population [67] and in patients with various stages of CKD in the SHARP study [69].

Co-administration of ezetimibe and bile acid sequestrants also has an additive effect in reducing LDL-C levels without any additional adverse effects. Similarly, adding ezetimibe to nicotinic acid further reduces LDL-C and does not affect nicotinic acid-induced HDL-C increase. Triple therapy (bile acid sequestrant, statin, and ezetimibe or nicotinic acid) will further reduce LDL-C, but the clinical significance of these combinations has not been tested.

Pharmacotherapy to Reduce Hypertriglyceridemia

Although much of the available evidence points to the importance of cholesterol in determining CV risk, high TG levels may also contribute [81]. Hypertriglyceridemia (HTG) is also a significant risk factor for pancreatitis, even at moderately elevated (5 and 10 mmol/L) levels. In spite of the uncertainties surrounding the role of TG as a CV risk factor, current guidelines suggest to maintain a level of fasting TG 1.7 mmol/L or less [2, 10, 60].

After considering and addressing potential correctable underlying causes for HTG, the first step in the management of the condition is to strongly emphasize TLC to reduce TG levels. Pharmacotherapy to lower TG should only be considered in subjects with TG >2.3 mmol/L in whom lifestyle measures are not sufficient to reach the suggested target, and if the subject is at high CV risk. Statins, fibrates, nicotinic acid, and omega-3 PUFAs have all showed efficacy to reduce TG levels. As statins were shown to reduce mortality as well as most CVD outcome parameters, these drugs are the first choice to reduce both total CVD risk and moderately elevated TG levels.

Fibrates

Fibrates are agonists of peroxisome proliferator-activated receptor-alpha (PPAR-alpha), and regulate lipid and lipoprotein metabolism through a complex network of signaling mechanisms eventually modulating gene expression. Fibrates effectively reduced both fasting and post-prandial TG levels and also triglyceride-rich lipoprotein (TRL) remnant particles in prospective clinical trials [82–85]. In these studies, fibrates have consistently reduced the rates of non-fatal MI by the fibrates studied (although often only in post-hoc analyses). The observed effect was the most obvious in subjects with elevated TG/low HDL-C levels. However, the data on other outcome measures have remained equivocal. Recent meta-analyses confirmed that fibrate therapy reduced major CVD events by 13 % (95 % confidence interval [CI] 7–19) in the general population [86] and both MACE and CV death, but not all-cause mortality in patients with CKD [12].

Fibrates are generally well tolerated, the side effects are usually mild and do not prompt discontinuation of the medication. These side effects include gastrointestinal disturbance, skin rash, myopathy and CK elevation, increased liver enzymes, and cholelithiasis [87]. In addition, small increases in the incidence of pancreatitis, pulmonary embolism, and deep vein thrombosis were reported in those taking fibrates [85].

The risk of myopathy varies if fibrates and statins were used in combination. Gemfibrozil inhibits the metabolism of statins via the glucuronidation pathway that leads to highly increased plasma concentrations of statins. As fenofibrate does not share the same pharmacokinetic pathways, the risk of myopathy is much less with the combination therapy including fenofibrate and statins [87].

Fibrates have been reported to raise serum creatinine concentration in both short-term and long-term studies. Whether or not the increase of serum creatinine reflects kidney dysfunction is a matter of ongoing debate. Monitoring serum creatinine in patients taking fibrates, particularly in people with type 2 diabetes, is necessary.

Fibrates also increase serum homocysteine level. This may blunt the increases in both HDL-C and apo A1, and may contribute to the smaller than estimated CV benefits of these medications [88]. High homocysteine levels also promote thrombosis, and this may explain the increased incidence of thromboembolic events associated with fibrates.

Fibrates are effective in improving lipid profiles and reducing the risk of cardiovascular events with evidence showing greater efficacy of fibrates in people with baseline HTG [86, 89]. The higher levels of triglycerides and the lower HDL levels in the CKD population therefore provide a strong rationale for expecting greater magnitudes of benefit in CKD. However, in recent trials, co-administration of fenofibrate and niacin with simvastatin did not reduce CVD events more than simvastatin alone in patients with type II diabetes and established atherosclerotic disease, respectively [90–92].

A meta-analysis of studies assessing the effects of fibrates on cardiovascular events in the broader population has reported overall benefit, with consistent evidence of greater effects for subgroups with elevated triglyceride and/or decreased HDL levels [86].

Gemfibrozil was associated with 20 % reduction in cardiovascular events in patients who had mild to moderate renal insufficiency (GFR 30–75 mL/min/1.73 m^2 bsa) in the VA-HIT (Veterans Affairs Cooperative HDL Cholesterol Intervention Trial) [93]. Fenofibrate reduced total cardiovascular events in diabetic patients with mild to moderate renal insufficiency in the FIELD (Fenofibrate Intervention and Event Lowering in Diabetes) trial [94]. A recently published systematic review of eight randomized controlled trials published in ten articles, including a total of 16,869 patients analyzed the effects of fibrates on various CV and renal outcomes in patients with CKD [12]. In addition to the results described below this chapter also highlights the lack of data in patients with advanced kidney disease (eGFR <30 mL/min/1.73 m^2). Analysis of the available data suggested that fibrate therapy reduces the risk of cardiovascular events in patients with CKD including protection against cardiovascular death [12]. The effects in people with CKD appeared at least as large as the effects in people with normal kidney function. No significant effect was seen in the risk of stroke or all-cause mortality. Fibrates also reduced the progression of albuminuria. Another systematic review and meta-analysis of available data in patients with diabetes and albuminuria demonstrated that fenofibrate treatment increased regression from micro- to normoalbuminuria and from macro- to micro-albuminuria compared to placebo [95]. In these systematic analyses, fibrates did not seem to alter the risk of ESKD.

The risk of myopathy may also be increased in patients with CKD, although in patients treated with continuous ambulatory peritoneal dialysis, gemfibrozil led to significant reductions in triglyceride levels without myositis or liver toxicity [96, 97]. The dose used in these studies was less than that used in the general population (600 mg/day or 600 mg every other day). Several case reports have documented rhabdomyolysis associated with use of fibrates in ESKD and hypothyroidism, however [98]. Recent guidelines discourage the use of fibrates in patients who have a GFR of less than 15 mL/min/1.73 m^2 [2].

Both uncertainty about efficacy and longer-term renal outcomes, and concerns about safety related to increases in serum creatinine [99–103], associations with increased hospitalization [104] have limited the utilization of fibrates in CKD. The National Kidney Foundation and the National Lipid Association have both recommended cautious use of fibrates in patients with CKD based on this perceived risk [2].

There have been conflicting reports regarding the impact of fibrate therapy on kidney function [105, 106]. The systematic review by Jun et al. has confirmed that fibrate therapy is associated with an acute reduction in eGFR [12]. A recent post hoc analysis of the FIELD study, however, suggested that this is likely to be reversible; in fact, plasma creatinine levels in a cohort of 661 "substudy washout participants" were significantly lower in participants who had received fenofibrate compared to placebo 8 weeks after withdrawal from study treatment, even suggesting longer-term renoprotective effects [105]. Acute increase in serum creatinine was also reversible in the ACCORD study, as well [107].

The increase in serum creatinine with fibrate therapy may be explained by the interference of the drugs with the generation of vasodilatory prostaglandins due to the activation of peroxisome proliferator-activated receptors [108]. This would cause a change in renal blood flow and consequently increased serum creatinine and reduced eGFR. Hottelart and colleagues reported that serum creatinine was elevated with fenofibrate but mGFR as assessed by inulin clearances was unchanged [102]. These observations support the view that the drug-induced elevation in serum creatinine does not reflect true deterioration of renal function, and Jun et al. have concluded their meta-analysis that the available data support the overall safety and potential benefits of this class of agents [12]. However, a large outcome trial conducted specifically in this population is required to more clearly dissolve concerns regarding the safety of fibrates in CKD.

The results of the systematic review and the observations described above suggest that fibrate therapy does not lead to adverse effects on major clinical renal outcomes, and even suggest the possibility of long-term renal benefit. This should provide strong rationale for an outcome trial specifically conducted in people with CKD.

Nicotinic Acid

Nicotinic acid (NA) is a broad-spectrum lipid-regulating agent which inhibits diacylglycerol acyltransferase-2 (DGAT-2) in the liver that results in the reduced secretion of VLDL particles from the liver, and consequent reductions of both IDL and LDL particles [109]. Nicotinic acid stimulates apo A1 production and also regulates the activity of hormone-sensitive lipase in the adipose tissue [109].

Nicotinic acid exerts pleiotropic actions which are reflected in multiple beneficial changes in serum lipid and lipoprotein levels [109]. In addition to the mentioned effects of LDL-C and HDL-C, i.e., reductions in apoB and increases in apoA1-containing lipoproteins, NA at the daily dose of 2 g or more reduces TG by 20–40 % [109].

Only a few prospective trials have looked at the effect of NA on clinical outcomes, mainly surrogate angiographic outcomes [110–113]. The favorable effect of NA on various vascular parameters reported in these prospective randomized trials have been challenged by the recently published results of the AIM-HIGH (Atherothrombosis Intervention in Metabolic Syndrome with Low HDL/High Triglycerides: Impact on Global Health Outcomes trial) [91], which was designed to evaluate the addition of extended-release NA to intensive statin therapy in patients with established CVD and atherogenic dyslipidemia (characterized by low HDL-C, elevated triglycerides, and small, dense LDL-C), compared with statin use alone. After 2 years of NA treatment HDL cholesterol level had increased by 25.0 % in the NA group, whereas it had increased by about 10 % in the placebo group. TG levels had decreased by 29 % in the NA group and by 8 % in the placebo group. The LDL cholesterol level had further decreased by 12 % in the NA group and by 5 % in the placebo group (all significant differences between the active and placebo arm). These lipid findings persisted through 3 years of follow-up [91]. The study, however, was stopped prematurely after an interim analysis revealed futility with respect to the primary clinical endpoint and a trend toward increased stroke incidence in NA-treated subjects. A subsequent systematic review, meta-analysis, and meta-regression analyzed data from 11 trials (including the AIM-HIGH study) including 9,959 subjects. This analysis reported that NA use was associated with a significant reduction in the composite endpoints of any CV event (OR: 0.66; 95 % confidence interval [CI]: 0.49–0.89) and also MACE (OR: 0.75; 95 % CI: 0.59–0.96) [114]. No significant association was observed between NA and the incidence of stroke. The results of the HPS2-THRIVE (Treatment of HDL to Reduce the Incidence of Vascular Events) trial have been announced in a recent press release [115] after the publication of the systematic review mentioned above. In this trial a NA/laropiprant (ERN/LRPT) combination has been used (laropiprant, a selective antagonist of prostaglandin D2 is added to NA to prevent flushing). This trial, which enrolled 25,000 individuals with high CV risk has concluded that adding ER niacin/laropiprant to current standard treatment did not produce worthwhile reductions in the risk of heart attack, stroke, and revascularization procedures, but it did cause additional side effects [116]. These two large studies, both concluding that NA did not result in meaningful clinical CV benefit, raise very substantial questions about the utility of this medication.

In clinical practice, skin reactions (flushing) associated with itching and tingling are the most frequent and troublesome side effect of NA and its derivatives, often preventing titration of the dose to maximal efficacy and also leading to discontinuation, even when using aspirin as a modulator of flushing. In various studies, at least 20–25 % of individuals will not tolerate the drug [91, 116], mainly due to flushing. Recently, specific NA receptors in adipocytes and in skin macrophages were discovered and are thought to be the link to this robust side effect of NA. The mediator is prostaglandin D2, which can be blocked by laropiprant, a selective antagonist of prostaglandin D2 action at the receptor level [117].

Hyperuricemia, acanthosis nigricans, and elevation of liver enzymes have also been reported, although less commonly, in users of ER nicotinic acid. NA may also interfere with glycemic control by increasing blood glucose and this is obviously of concern for patients with diabetes [77, 109, 118]. In clinical practice, glucose-lowering medications need to be titrated to overcome this unfavorable effect.

A recent review of the U.S. FDA's Adverse Event Reporting System found that prescription NA was associated with a lower rate of serious adverse events (defined as resulting in hospitalization or death), hepatotoxicity, and rhabdomyolysis compared with that of several other commonly used lipid-lowering drugs including statins and fibrates [118]. Some studies reported that the safety profile of NA–statin combination therapy was comparable to that of either drug alone [118, 119]. The recently published results of the HPS2-THRIVE trial, however, suggested that the risk of myopathy was increased by adding ERN/LRPT to simvastatin 40 mg daily (with or without ezetimibe), particularly in Chinese patients who seem to be at higher risk of this complication [116].

The National Kidney Foundation guidelines recommend nicotinic acid as an alternative second agent for LDL cholesterol reduction in combination with a statin [2]. There are limited data on the efficacy and safety of nicotinic acid in CKD, but the recently announced negative results of the AIM-HIGH [91] and the HPS2-THRIVE [116] trials raise serious concerns about the effectiveness of NA to improve clinical outcomes. Pharmacokinetic studies indicate that about one-third of the drug is excreted via the kidneys. The NKF guidelines suggest a 50 % dose reduction for patients with GFR <15 mL/min/1.73 m^2; no dosing changes are recommended in patients with better renal function [2].

Combination Pharmacotherapy to Reduce HTG

Clinical trials have shown that the combination of a statin and a fibrate results in a significantly stronger reduction in LDL-C and TG as well as a greater elevation of HDL-C than monotherapy with either [120].

Furthermore, while in patients with type 2 diabetes combination therapy of fenofibrate with simvastatin did not reduce the rates of CVD as compared with simvastatin alone in the Action to Control Cardiovascular Risk in Diabetes (ACCORD) trial [90], a subgroup analysis of patients who had both TG levels in the higher third (≥2.3 mmol/L) and an HDL-C level below the lower third (≤0.88 mmol/L) suggested an apparent benefit from the combination therapy. These results are similar to those from post hoc analyses of several other prospective randomized trials, suggesting that the addition of fenofibrate to a statin may benefit certain patients with type 2 diabetes with a high TG/low HDL-C dyslipidemic pattern.

Since both fibrate and statin monotherapy are associated with an increased risk of myopathy, the risk could be increased when these drugs are taken together, particularly if the doses of statin are very high. This risk is substantially increased if gemfibrozil is used in combination with statins. In summary, fibrates, particularly fenofibrate due to its lower myopathic potential, can be prescribed concomitantly with statins to improve achievement of lipid goals in patients with atherogenic combined dyslipidemia [6, 60].

The combination of ER nicotinic acid with moderate doses of a statin provided a significantly better increase in HDL-C and decrease in TG than either a high dose of a statin or the combination of a statin and ezetimibe [121]. The combination of statins and NA does not seem to be associated with increased incidence of adverse events, including flushing. Triple combination therapy with NA, simvastatin, and ezetimibe showed a greater reduction of LDL-C and a greater increase in HDL-C than with either drug alone or with statin/ezetimibe treatment [122].

The combination of omega-3 fatty acids and simvastatin more efficiently reduced TG concentrations when compared with statin alone [123]. Adding omega-3 fatty acids to pravastatin and fenofibrate in a triple combination further decreased TG concentrations and homocysteine as well in patients with diabetes and dyslipidemia. Inconclusive data suggest that combination of omega-3 fatty acids and low dose statin, compared with statin therapy alone, reduced CV events [29]. These effects, however, may be mediated by mechanisms other than LDL-C lowering.

Pharmacotherapy to Increase HDL-C

Several observational studies established low levels of HDL-C, a strong, independent predictor of elevated CV risk [124–127], especially if HDL-C is below 1.17 mmol/L [128]. Importantly, low plasma HDL-C is usually seen in patients with CKD, as well as in type 2 diabetes or hepatic insufficiency [92]. These conditions are also associated with moderate or marked HTG. Based on these observations, it has been postulated that interventions that increase HDL-C may lead to improved clinical outcomes, reduced CV events.

There are only a few therapeutic options to increase low HDL-C levels. TLC, including weight reduction, exercise, smoking cessation, and moderate alcohol consumption, will increase HDL-C levels by about 5–10 % [129, 130].

Statins produce a modest, 5–10 % elevation in HDL-C [123], and it is unclear if this contributes to the beneficial effects of statins on CV outcomes.

Although fibrates increased HDL-C by 10–15 % in short-term trials [131], the long-term effects of fibrates on HDL-C is more modest.

Nicotinic Acid

NA is recognized as a potent modulator of HDL-C currently available [114]. It increases HDL-C by both reducing HDL catabolism and increasing apo A1 synthesis by the liver [77]. A current meta-regression analysis of available data from intervention trials, however, failed to demonstrate an association between on-treatment differences in HDL-C concentration and NA-mediated improvement of outcomes [114]. It is possible that the clinical efficacy of NA may result from its effects on lipids, but that these are not captured in the standard lipid measurements reported in clinical trials. For example, NA reduces lipoprotein (a) and exerts presumably favorable effects on both HDL-C and LDL-C particle size distribution, not reflected by typical lipoprotein analysis [132]. It is also possible that the clinical benefits of NA are independent from its effects on serum lipids. Furthermore, the recently announced negative results of the AIM-HIGH and the HPS2-THRIVE trials raise serious concerns about the effectiveness of NA to improve clinical outcomes [91, 116].

Cholesteryl Ester Transfer Protein Inhibitors

To date, the most efficacious approach to increase low HDL-C levels has been the direct inhibition of cholesteryl ester transfer protein (CETP) by small molecule inhibitors, which may induce an increase in HDL-C by ≥100 % on a dose-dependent basis [133–136]. Among three CETP inhibitors developed originally (torcetrapib, dalcetrapib, and anacetrapib), torcetrapib was withdrawn following an excess of mortality in the torcetrapib arm of the Investigation of Lipid Levels Management to Understand its Impact in Atherosclerotic Events (ILLUMINATE) trial [137]. It appears that the deleterious effects of torcetrapib arose primarily from off-target toxicity. The dal-OUTCOMES trial aimed to evaluate the efficacy of dalcetrapib as an adjunct to existing standard of care in secondary prevention of CVD was recently halted due to a lack of clinically meaningful benefit despite increasing HDL-C by more than 25 % during phase II clinical trials [138]. A large phase III trial with anacetrapib (REVEAL) in patients with a history of CV disease was started in 2011 to enroll 30,000 individuals to be completed in 2017. In the meanwhile, however, available evidence does not support the clinical effectiveness of increasing HDL-C to reduce CV disease.

At the present time, the available evidence does not seem to support the viability of HDL-C as both a therapeutic target and surrogate marker of CVD risk. Mendelian randomization analyses failed to establish a relationship between genetic polymorphisms associated with HDL-C levels and CHD event incidence [139]. Furthermore, the negative results of the large NA trials and the negative CETP inhibitor trials may suggest that the augmentation of serum HDL-C as a therapeutic target may be misdirected [114].

Summary and Recommendations for Non-statin Pharmacotherapy to Improve Dyslipidemia in Patients with CKD

The first step in managing dyslipidemia in patients with CKD (any stages) has to be a consistent multidisciplinary effort to implement TLCs with the following cornerstones: smoking cessation; appropriate weight management using dietary changes and regular exercise programs; education and support to implement beneficial dietary changes (reduce saturated fat and increase MUFA); and both omega-6 and omega-3 PUFA intake. See Table 9.1 for a summary of non-statin lipid-lowering therapies.

Table 9.1 Summary of non-statin lipid-lowering therapies

Group	Drug name/intervention	Main therapeutic effects	Potential side effects	CKD-specific data	Dose adjustment in CKD	Comment
Therapeutic lifestyle changes (TLC)	Diet: reduced saturated fatty acids, reduced trans-fatty acids	Reduced LDL-C; increase in HDL-C				
	Diet: omega-3-PUFA	Reduction of LDL-C		[42–47]		
	Diet: omega-6-PUFA	Reduction of TG				
	Diet: fiber	Reduction of LDL-C				
	Exercise	Small reduction of LDL-C and TG; increase of HDL-C		[19, 50–53]		
	Weight loss	Small reduction of LDL-C; reduction of TG; increase of HDL-C		[57–59]		
	Smoking cessation	Increase of HDL-C				
Cholesterol absorption inhibitors	Ezetimibe	Reduction of LDL-C	Occasional elevations of liver enzymes, and muscle pain	[69]	No	Primarily recommended in combination with statins or other lipid lowering agents
Bile acid sequestrants	Cholestyramine, colestipol and colesevelam	Reduced LDL-C	GI side effects Reduced absorption of fat-soluble vitamins drug interactions	[72, 73]	No	Administer 4 h before or 1 h after other drugs
	Sevelamer	Reduced LDL-C Modest increase in HDL-C		[74–76]		

Other	Nicotinic acid	Modest reduction of LDL-C	Flushing associated with itching and tingling		Reduce dose by 50 % in patients with eGFR <15 mL/min/1.73 m^2	Usually used in combination with statins
		Reduction of TG	Hyperuricemia, acanthosis nigricans and elevation of liver enzymes			NA was not associated with improved CV outcomes in recent trials—clinical utility may be questionable
		Increase of HDL-C	Increased blood glucose			
Fibrates	Gemfibrozil, fenofibrate	Reduced TG	Gastrointestinal disturbance, skin rash, myopathy and CK elevation, increased liver enzymes, and cholelithiasis small increases in the incidence of pancreatitis, pulmonary embolism and deep vein thrombosis	[12, 93–95]	Should be used with caution in mild–moderate CKD; their use is contraindicated in severe renal failure (eGFR <20–30 mL/min/1.73 m^2)	Increase in serum creatinine—may not reflect kidney dysfunction
Cholesteryl ester transfer protein inhibitors	Torcetrapib, dalcetrapib, anacetrapib	Increase in HDL-C				Torcetrapib was withdrawn following an excess of mortality in the ILLUMINATE study The dal-OUTCOMES trial (dalcetrapib) was halted due to futility A large phase III trial with anacetrapib (REVEAL) to be completed in 2017

PUFA poly-unsaturated fatty acids, *CKD* chronic kidney disease, *LDL-C* low-density lipoprotein cholesterol, *HDL-C* high-density lipoprotein cholesterol, *TG* triglyceride

CKD 1–4 (eGFR Above 15 mL/min/1.73 m^2) and CKD Tx

In patients in whom pharmacotherapy is indicated statin therapy needs to be initiated (see above).

If additional pharmacotherapy is needed to achieve target levels ezetimibe (10 mg/day) should be added.

In patients who do not tolerate statins, the use of fibrates (gemfibrozil 600 mg daily; fenofibrate 48 mg daily) should be considered in patients with CKD 1–4 and CKD Tx, given the available evidence supporting the efficacy and clinical effectiveness of fibrates to reduce lipid levels and to improve at least some relevant CV and renal outcomes.

If gemfibrozil is used, it should be combined with fluvastatin to avoid the increased risk of myopathy. Fenofibrate could be combined with any statins without increasing the risk of myopathy but needs appropriate dose reduction.

Ezetimibe can be combined with fibrates or statins + fibrates, as well, if necessary.

Bile acid sequestrants, fish oil or nicotinic acid might also be considered in addition to the combinations above; however, no very substantial concerns exist about the clinical effectiveness of these drugs.

CKD 5 (eGFR <15 mL/min/1.73 m^2 and Patients on PD or HD)

Ezetimibe (10 mg/day) can be added to statins if needed.

If target is not reached, fish oil, bile acid sequestrants, or nicotinic acid could be considered (see previous section).

Fibrates are contraindicated in patients on dialysis.

References

1. Kasiske BL, Wheeler DC. The management of dyslipidemia in CKD: new analyses of an expanding dataset. Am J Kidney Dis. 2013;61(3):371–4. Epub 2012/12/25.
2. Kidney Disease Outcomes Quality Initiative (K/DOQI) Group (2003) K/DOQI clinical practice guidelines for management of dyslipidemias in patients with kidney disease. Am J Kidney Dis. 41(4 Suppl 3):I-IV, S1–91. . Epub 2003/04/03.
3. Matsushita K, van der Velde M, Astor BC, Woodward M, Levey AS, de Jong PE, et al. Association of estimated glomerular filtration rate and albuminuria with all-cause and cardiovascular mortality in general population cohorts: a collaborative meta-analysis. Lancet. 2010;375(9731):2073–81. Epub 2010/05/21.
4. Kovesdy CP, Anderson JE, Kalantar-Zadeh K. Inverse association between lipid levels and mortality in men with chronic kidney disease who are not yet on dialysis: effects of case mix and the malnutrition-inflammation-cachexia syndrome. J Am Soc Nephrol. 2007;18(1): 304–11. Epub 2006/12/15.

5. Noori N, Caulfield MP, Salameh WA, Reitz RE, Nicholas SB, Molnar MZ, et al. Novel lipoprotein subfraction and size measurements in prediction of mortality in maintenance hemodialysis patients. Clin J Am Soc Nephrol. 2011;6(12):2861–70. Epub 2011/10/29.
6. Harper CR, Jacobson TA. Managing dyslipidemia in chronic kidney disease. J Am Coll Cardiol. 2008;51(25):2375–84. Epub 2008/06/21.
7. Khoueiry G, Abdallah M, Saiful F, Abi Rafeh N, Raza M, Bhat T, et al. High-density lipoprotein in uremic patients: metabolism, impairment, and therapy. International urology and nephrology. 2014;46(1):27–39. Epub 2013/02/28.
8. Speer T, Rohrer L, Blyszczuk P, Shroff R, Kuschnerus K, Krankel N, et al. Abnormal high-density lipoprotein induces endothelial dysfunction via activation of toll-like receptor-2. Immunity. 2013;38(4):754–68. Epub 2013/03/13.
9. Kasiske B, Cosio FG, Beto J, Bolton K, Chavers BM, Grimm Jr R, et al. Clinical practice guidelines for managing dyslipidemias in kidney transplant patients: a report from the Managing Dyslipidemias in Chronic Kidney Disease Work Group of the National Kidney Foundation Kidney Disease Outcomes Quality Initiative. Am J Transplant. 2004;4 Suppl 7:13–53. Epub 2004/03/19.
10. Third Report of the National Cholesterol Education Program (NCEP). Expert panel on detection, evaluation, and treatment of high blood cholesterol in adults (adult treatment panel III) final report. Circulation. 2002;106(25):3143–421. Epub 2002/12/18.
11. Upadhyay A, Earley A, Lamont JL, Haynes S, Wanner C, Balk EM. Lipid-lowering therapy in persons with chronic kidney disease: a systematic review and meta-analysis. Ann Intern Med. 2012;157(4):251–62. Epub 2012/08/23.
12. Jun M, Zhu B, Tonelli M, Jardine MJ, Patel A, Neal B, et al. Effects of fibrates in kidney disease: a systematic review and meta-analysis. J Am Coll Cardiol. 2012;60(20):2061–71. Epub 2012/10/23.
13. [cited 2013 September 14]. http://www.european-renal-best-practice.org/content/guidelines-topic-ckd-hyperlipidaemia.
14. Anderson TJ, Gregoire J, Hegele RA, Couture P, Mancini GB, McPherson R, et al. 2012 update of the Canadian Cardiovascular Society guidelines for the diagnosis and treatment of dyslipidemia for the prevention of cardiovascular disease in the adult. Can J Cardiol. 2013;29(2):151–67. Epub 2013/01/29.
15. de Lorgeril M, Salen P, Martin JL, Monjaud I, Delaye J, Mamelle N. Mediterranean diet, traditional risk factors, and the rate of cardiovascular complications after myocardial infarction: final report of the Lyon Diet Heart Study. Circulation. 1999;99(6):779–85. Epub 1999/02/17.
16. Trichopoulou A, Costacou T, Bamia C, Trichopoulos D. Adherence to a Mediterranean diet and survival in a Greek population. N Engl J Med. 2003;348(26):2599–608. Epub 2003/06/27.
17. Pereira MA, O'Reilly E, Augustsson K, Fraser GE, Goldbourt U, Heitmann BL, et al. Dietary fiber and risk of coronary heart disease: a pooled analysis of cohort studies. Arch Intern Med. 2004;164(4):370–6. Epub 2004/02/26.
18. Gaede P, Vedel P, Larsen N, Jensen GV, Parving HH, Pedersen O. Multifactorial intervention and cardiovascular disease in patients with type 2 diabetes. N Engl J Med. 2003;348(5):383–93. Epub 2003/01/31.
19. Greenwood SA, Lindup H, Taylor K, Koufaki P, Rush R, Macdougall IC, et al. Evaluation of a pragmatic exercise rehabilitation programme in chronic kidney disease. Nephrol Dial Transplant. 2012;27 Suppl 3:iii126–34. Epub 2012/07/13.
20. MacLaughlin HL, Sarafidis PA, Greenwood SA, Campbell KL, Hall WL, Macdougall IC. Compliance with a structured weight loss program is associated with reduced systolic blood pressure in obese patients with chronic kidney disease. Am J Hypertens. 2012;25(9):1024–9. Epub 2012/06/22.
21. van Zuilen AD, Bots ML, Dulger A, van der Tweel I, van Buren M, Ten Dam MA, et al. Multifactorial intervention with nurse practitioners does not change cardiovascular outcomes in patients with chronic kidney disease. Kidney Int. 2012;82(6):710–7. Epub 2012/06/29.

22. Mente A, de Koning L, Shannon HS, Anand SS. A systematic review of the evidence supporting a causal link between dietary factors and coronary heart disease. Arch Intern Med. 2009;169(7): 659–69. Epub 2009/04/15.
23. Keys A. Serum cholesterol response to dietary cholesterol. Am J Clin Nutr. 1984;40(2):351–9. Epub 1984/08/01.
24. Ordovas JM. Genetic influences on blood lipids and cardiovascular disease risk: tools for primary prevention. Am J Clin Nutr. 2009;89(5):1509S–17. Epub 2009/04/03.
25. Mensink RP, Zock PL, Kester AD, Katan MB. Effects of dietary fatty acids and carbohydrates on the ratio of serum total to HDL cholesterol and on serum lipids and apolipoproteins: a meta-analysis of 60 controlled trials. Am J Clin Nutr. 2003;77(5):1146–55. Epub 2003/04/30.
26. Mozaffarian D, Aro A, Willett WC. Health effects of trans-fatty acids: experimental and observational evidence. Eur J Clin Nutr. 2009;63 Suppl 2:S5–21. Epub 2009/05/09.
27. Mattar M, Obeid O. Fish oil and the management of hypertriglyceridemia. Nutr Health. 2009;20(1):41–9. Epub 2009/03/31.
28. Balk EM, Lichtenstein AH, Chung M, Kupelnick B, Chew P, Lau J. Effects of omega-3 fatty acids on serum markers of cardiovascular disease risk: a systematic review. Atherosclerosis. 2006;189(1):19–30. Epub 2006/03/15.
29. Yokoyama M, Origasa H, Matsuzaki M, Matsuzawa Y, Saito Y, Ishikawa Y, et al. Effects of eicosapentaenoic acid on major coronary events in hypercholesterolaemic patients (JELIS): a randomised open-label, blinded endpoint analysis. Lancet. 2007;369(9567):1090–8. Epub 2007/04/03.
30. Marchioli R, Barzi F, Bomba E, Chieffo C, Di Gregorio D, Di Mascio R, et al. Early protection against sudden death by n-3 polyunsaturated fatty acids after myocardial infarction: time-course analysis of the results of the Gruppo Italiano per lo Studio della Sopravvivenza nell'Infarto Miocardico (GISSI)-Prevenzione. Circulation. 2002;105(16):1897–903. Epub 2002/05/09.
31. Brown L, Rosner B, Willett WW, Sacks FM. Cholesterol-lowering effects of dietary fiber: a meta-analysis. Am J Clin Nutr. 1999;69(1):30–42. Epub 1999/01/30.
32. Kelly S, Frost G, Whittaker V, Summerbell C. Low glycaemic index diets for coronary heart disease. Cochrane Database Syst Rev. 2004;4, CD004467. Epub 2004/10/21.
33. Rimm EB, Williams P, Fosher K, Criqui M, Stampfer MJ. Moderate alcohol intake and lower risk of coronary heart disease: meta-analysis of effects on lipids and haemostatic factors. BMJ. 1999;319(7224):1523–8. Epub 1999/12/11.
34. Mooradian AD, Haas MJ, Wong NC. The effect of select nutrients on serum high-density lipoprotein cholesterol and apolipoprotein A-I levels. Endocr Rev. 2006;27(1):2–16. Epub 2005/10/26.
35. Dattilo AM, Kris-Etherton PM. Effects of weight reduction on blood lipids and lipoproteins: a meta-analysis. Am J Clin Nutr. 1992;56(2):320–8. Epub 1992/08/01.
36. Shaw K, Gennat H, O'Rourke P, Del Mar C. Exercise for overweight or obesity. Cochrane Database Syst Rev. 2006;4, CD003817. Epub 2006/10/21.
37. Kraus WE, Houmard JA, Duscha BD, Knetzger KJ, Wharton MB, McCartney JS, et al. Effects of the amount and intensity of exercise on plasma lipoproteins. N Engl J Med. 2002;347(19):1483–92. Epub 2002/11/08.
38. Axelsson TG, Irving GF, Axelsson J. To eat or not to eat: dietary fat in uremia is the question. Semin Dial. 2010;23(4):383–8. Epub 2010/08/13.
39. Kent PS. Integrating clinical nutrition practice guidelines in chronic kidney disease. Nutr Clin Pract. 2005;20(2):213–7. Epub 2005/10/07.
40. Work Group KDOQI. KDOQI clinical practice guideline for nutrition in children with CKD: 2008 update. Executive summary. Am J Kidney Dis. 2009;53(3 Suppl 2):S11–104.
41. Kris-Etherton PM, Innis S. Ammerican Dietetic A. Dietitians of C Position of the American Dietetic Association and Dietitians of Canada: dietary fatty acids J Am Diet Assoc. 2007;107(9):1599–611. Epub 2007/10/17.

42. Friedman AN. Omega-3 fatty acid supplementation in advanced kidney disease. Semin Dial. 2010;23(4):396–400. Epub 2010/08/13.
43. Kutner NG, Clow PW, Zhang R, Aviles X. Association of fish intake and survival in a cohort of incident dialysis patients. Am J Kidney Dis. 2002;39(5):1018–24. Epub 2002/04/30.
44. Cohen BE, Garg SK, Ali S, Harris WS, Whooley MA. Red blood cell docosahexaenoic acid and eicosapentaenoic acid concentrations are positively associated with socioeconomic status in patients with established coronary artery disease: data from the Heart and Soul Study. J Nutr. 2008;138(6):1135–40. Epub 2008/05/22.
45. Saifullah A, Watkins BA, Saha C, Li Y, Moe SM, Friedman AN. Oral fish oil supplementation raises blood omega-3 levels and lowers C-reactive protein in haemodialysis patients—a pilot study. Nephrol Dial Transplant. 2007;22(12):3561–7. Epub 2007/07/12.
46. Svensson M, Christensen JH, Solling J, Schmidt EB. The effect of n-3 fatty acids on plasma lipids and lipoproteins and blood pressure in patients with CRF. Am J Kidney Dis. 2004;44(1):77–83. Epub 2004/06/24.
47. Svensson M, Schmidt EB, Jorgensen KA, Christensen JH. N-3 fatty acids as secondary prevention against cardiovascular events in patients who undergo chronic hemodialysis: a randomized, placebo-controlled intervention trial. Clin J Am Soc Nephrol. 2006;1(4):780–6. Epub 2007/08/21.
48. KDOQI Work Group. K/DOQI clinical practice guidelines for cardiovascular disease in dialysis patients. Am J Kidney Dis. 2005;45(4 Suppl 3):S1–153. Epub 2005/04/05.
49. Kris-Etherton PM, Harris WS, Appel LJ. Fish consumption, fish oil, omega-3 fatty acids, and cardiovascular disease. Circulation. 2002;106(21):2747–57. Epub 2002/11/20.
50. Howden EJ, Fassett RG, Isbel NM, Coombes JS. Exercise training in chronic kidney disease patients. Sports Med. 2012;42(6):473–88. Epub 2012/05/17.
51. Leehey DJ, Moinuddin I, Bast JP, Qureshi S, Jelinek CS, Cooper C, et al. Aerobic exercise in obese diabetic patients with chronic kidney disease: a randomized and controlled pilot study. Cardiovasc Diabetol. 2009;8:62. Epub 2009/12/17.
52. Balakrishnan VS, Rao M, Menon V, Gordon PL, Pilichowska M, Castaneda F, et al. Resistance training increases muscle mitochondrial biogenesis in patients with chronic kidney disease. Clin J Am Soc Nephrol. 2010;5(6):996–1002. Epub 2010/05/26.
53. Toyama K, Sugiyama S, Oka H, Sumida H, Ogawa H. Exercise therapy correlates with improving renal function through modifying lipid metabolism in patients with cardiovascular disease and chronic kidney disease. J Cardiol. 2010;56(2):142–6. Epub 2010/08/11.
54. Kovesdy CP, Czira ME, Rudas A, Ujszaszi A, Rosivall L, Novak M, et al. Body mass index, waist circumference and mortality in kidney transplant recipients. Am J Transplant. 2010;10(12):2644–51. Epub 2010/11/20.
55. Kovesdy CP, Kalantar-Zadeh K. Introduction: the reverse epidemiology controversy. Semin Dial. 2007;20(6):485. Epub 2007/11/10.
56. Zoccali C, Torino C, Tripepi G, Mallamaci F. Assessment of obesity in chronic kidney disease: what is the best measure? Curr Opin Nephrol Hypertens. 2012;21(6):641–6. Epub 2012/09/27.
57. MacLaughlin HL, Cook SA, Kariyawasam D, Roseke M, van Niekerk M, Macdougall IC. Nonrandomized trial of weight loss with orlistat, nutrition education, diet, and exercise in obese patients with CKD: 2-year follow-up. Am J Kidney Dis. 2010;55(1):69–76. Epub 2009/11/21.
58. Navaneethan SD, Yehnert H, Moustarah F, Schreiber MJ, Schauer PR, Beddhu S. Weight loss interventions in chronic kidney disease: a systematic review and meta-analysis. Clin J Am Soc Nephrol. 2009;4(10):1565–74. Epub 2009/10/08.
59. Morales E, Praga M. The effect of weight loss in obesity and chronic kidney disease. Curr Hypertens Rep. 2012;14(2):170–6. Epub 2012/01/20.
60. Reiner Z, Catapano AL, De Backer G, Graham I, Taskinen MR, Wiklund O, et al. ESC/EAS Guidelines for the management of dyslipidaemias: the Task Force for the management of dyslipidaemias of the European Society of Cardiology (ESC) and the European Atherosclerosis Society (EAS). Eur Heart J. 2011;32(14):1769–818. Epub 2011/06/30.

61. Baigent C, Keech A, Kearney PM, Blackwell L, Buck G, Pollicino C, et al. Efficacy and safety of cholesterol-lowering treatment: prospective meta-analysis of data from 90,056 participants in 14 randomised trials of statins. Lancet. 2005;366(9493):1267–78. Epub 2005/10/11.
62. Baigent C, Blackwell L, Emberson J, Holland LE, Reith C, Bhala N, et al. Efficacy and safety of more intensive lowering of LDL cholesterol: a meta-analysis of data from 170,000 participants in 26 randomised trials. Lancet. 2010;376(9753):1670–81. Epub 2010/11/12.
63. Cannon CP, Steinberg BA, Murphy SA, Mega JL, Braunwald E. Meta-analysis of cardiovascular outcomes trials comparing intensive versus moderate statin therapy. J Am Coll Cardiol. 2006;48(3):438–45. Epub 2006/08/01.
64. Cannon CP, Braunwald E, McCabe CH, Rader DJ, Rouleau JL, Belder R, et al. Intensive versus moderate lipid lowering with statins after acute coronary syndromes. N Engl J Med. 2004;350(15):1495–504. Epub 2004/03/10.
65. LaRosa JC, Grundy SM, Waters DD, Shear C, Barter P, Fruchart JC, et al. Intensive lipid lowering with atorvastatin in patients with stable coronary disease. N Engl J Med. 2005;352(14):1425–35. Epub 2005/03/10.
66. Armitage J, Bowman L, Wallendszus K, Bulbulia R, Rahimi K, Haynes R, et al. Intensive lowering of LDL cholesterol with 80 mg versus 20 mg simvastatin daily in 12,064 survivors of myocardial infarction: a double-blind randomised trial. Lancet. 2010;376(9753):1658–69. Epub 2010/11/12.
67. Rossebo AB, Pedersen TR, Boman K, Brudi P, Chambers JB, Egstrup K, et al. Intensive lipid lowering with simvastatin and ezetimibe in aortic stenosis. N Engl J Med. 2008;359(13):1343–56. Epub 2008/09/04.
68. Toth PP, Morrone D, Weintraub WS, Hanson ME, Lowe RS, Lin J, et al. Safety profile of statins alone or combined with ezetimibe: a pooled analysis of 27 studies including over 22,000 patients treated for 6–24 weeks. Int J Clin Pract. 2012;66(8):800–12. Epub 2012/07/19.
69. Baigent C, Landray MJ, Reith C, Emberson J, Wheeler DC, Tomson C, et al. The effects of lowering LDL cholesterol with simvastatin plus ezetimibe in patients with chronic kidney disease (Study of Heart and Renal Protection): a randomised placebo-controlled trial. Lancet. 2011;377(9784):2181–92. Epub 2011/06/15.
70. Levy P. Review of studies on the effect of bile acid sequestrants in patients with type 2 diabetes mellitus. Metab Syndr Relat Dis. 2010;8 Suppl 1:S9–13. Epub 2010/10/16.
71. Jacobson TA, Armani A, McKenney JM, Guyton JR. Safety considerations with gastrointestinally active lipid-lowering drugs. Am J Cardiol. 2007;99(6A):47C–55. Epub 2007/03/21.
72. Montague T, Murphy B. Lipid management in chronic kidney disease, hemodialysis, and transplantation. Endocrinol Metab Clin North Am. 2009;38(1):223–34. Epub 2009/02/17.
73. Yamada K, Fujimoto S, Tokura T, Fukudome K, Ochiai H, Komatsu H, et al. Effect of sevelamer on dyslipidemia and chronic inflammation in maintenance hemodialysis patients. Renal failure. 2005;27(4):361–5. Epub 2005/08/03.
74. Chertow GM, Burke SK, Raggi P. Sevelamer attenuates the progression of coronary and aortic calcification in hemodialysis patients. Kidney Int. 2002;62(1):245–52. Epub 2002/06/26.
75. Chertow GM, Burke SK, Dillon MA, Slatopolsky E. Long-term effects of sevelamer hydrochloride on the calcium x phosphate product and lipid profile of haemodialysis patients. Nephrol Dial Transplant. 1999;14(12):2907–14. Epub 1999/11/26.
76. Block GA, Spiegel DM, Ehrlich J, Mehta R, Lindbergh J, Dreisbach A, et al. Effects of sevelamer and calcium on coronary artery calcification in patients new to hemodialysis. Kidney Int. 2005;68(4):1815–24. Epub 2005/09/17.
77. Chapman MJ, Redfern JS, McGovern ME, Giral P. Niacin and fibrates in atherogenic dyslipidemia: pharmacotherapy to reduce cardiovascular risk. Pharmacol Ther. 2010;126(3):314–45. Epub 2010/02/16.
78. Zhao XQ, Krasuski RA, Baer J, Whitney EJ, Neradilek B, Chait A, et al. Effects of combination lipid therapy on coronary stenosis progression and clinical cardiovascular events in coronary disease patients with metabolic syndrome: a combined analysis of the Familial Atherosclerosis Treatment Study (FATS), the HDL-Atherosclerosis Treatment Study (HATS), and the Armed Forces Regression Study (AFREGS). Am J Cardiol. 2009;104(11):1457–64. Epub 2009/11/26.

79. Huijgen R, Abbink EJ, Bruckert E, Stalenhoef AF, Imholz BP, Durrington PN, et al. Colesevelam added to combination therapy with a statin and ezetimibe in patients with familial hypercholesterolemia: a 12-week, multicenter, randomized, double-blind, controlled trial. Clin Ther. 2010;32(4):615–25. Epub 2010/05/04.
80. Ballantyne CM, Weiss R, Moccetti T, Vogt A, Eber B, Sosef F, et al. Efficacy and safety of rosuvastatin 40 mg alone or in combination with ezetimibe in patients at high risk of cardiovascular disease (results from the EXPLORER study). Am J Cardiol. 2007;99(5):673–80. Epub 2007/02/24.
81. Sarwar N, Sandhu MS, Ricketts SL, Butterworth AS, Di Angelantonio E, Boekholdt SM, et al. Triglyceride-mediated pathways and coronary disease: collaborative analysis of 101 studies. Lancet. 2010;375(9726):1634–9. Epub 2010/05/11.
82. Frick MH, Elo O, Haapa K, Heinonen OP, Heinsalmi P, Helo P, et al. Helsinki Heart Study: primary-prevention trial with gemfibrozil in middle-aged men with dyslipidemia. Safety of treatment, changes in risk factors, and incidence of coronary heart disease. N Engl J Med. 1987;317(20):1237–45.
83. Rubins HB, Robins SJ, Collins D, Fye CL, Anderson JW, Elam MB, et al. Gemfibrozil for the secondary prevention of coronary heart disease in men with low levels of high-density lipoprotein cholesterol. Veterans Affairs High-Density Lipoprotein Cholesterol Intervention Trial Study Group. N Engl J Med. 1999;341(6):410–8. Epub 1999/08/07.
84. Bezafibrate Infarction Prevention (BIP) study. Secondary prevention by raising HDL cholesterol and reducing triglycerides in patients with coronary artery disease: the Bezafibrate Infarction Prevention (BIP) study. Circulation. 2000;102(1):21–7. Epub 2000/07/06.
85. Keech A, Simes RJ, Barter P, Best J, Scott R, Taskinen MR, et al. Effects of long-term fenofibrate therapy on cardiovascular events in 9795 people with type 2 diabetes mellitus (the FIELD study): randomised controlled trial. Lancet. 2005;366(9500):1849–61. Epub 2005/11/29.
86. Jun M, Foote C, Lv J, Neal B, Patel A, Nicholls SJ, et al. Effects of fibrates on cardiovascular outcomes: a systematic review and meta-analysis. Lancet. 2010;375(9729):1875–84. Epub 2010/05/14.
87. Davidson MH, Armani A, McKenney JM, Jacobson TA. Safety considerations with fibrate therapy. Am J Cardiol. 2007;99(6A):3C–18. Epub 2007/03/21.
88. Taskinen MR, Sullivan DR, Ehnholm C, Whiting M, Zannino D, Simes RJ, et al. Relationships of HDL cholesterol, ApoA-I, and ApoA-II with homocysteine and creatinine in patients with type 2 diabetes treated with fenofibrate. Arterioscler Thromb Vasc Biol. 2009;29(6):950–5. Epub 2009/03/28.
89. McCullough PA, Ahmed AB, Zughaib MT, Glanz ED, Di Loreto MJ. Treatment of hypertriglyceridemia with fibric acid derivatives: impact on lipid subfractions and translation into a reduction in cardiovascular events. Rev Cardiovasc Med. 2011;12(4):173–85. Epub 2012/01/18.
90. Ginsberg HN, Elam MB, Lovato LC, Crouse III JR, Leiter LA, Linz P, et al. Effects of combination lipid therapy in type 2 diabetes mellitus. N Engl J Med. 2010;362(17):1563–74. Epub 2010/03/17.
91. Boden WE, Probstfield JL, Anderson T, Chaitman BR, Desvignes-Nickens P, Koprowicz K, et al. Niacin in patients with low HDL cholesterol levels receiving intensive statin therapy. N Engl J Med. 2011;365(24):2255–67. Epub 2011/11/17.
92. Keane WF, Tomassini JE, Neff DR. Lipid abnormalities in patients with chronic kidney disease: implications for the pathophysiology of atherosclerosis. J Atheroscler Thromb. 2013;20(2):123–33. Epub 2012/10/26.
93. Tonelli M, Collins D, Robins S, Bloomfield H, Curhan GC. Gemfibrozil for secondary prevention of cardiovascular events in mild to moderate chronic renal insufficiency. Kidney Int. 2004;66(3):1123–30. Epub 2004/08/26.
94. Ting RD, Keech AC, Drury PL, Donoghoe MW, Hedley J, Jenkins AJ, et al. Benefits and safety of long-term fenofibrate therapy in people with type 2 diabetes and renal impairment: the FIELD Study. Diabetes Care. 2012;35(2):218–25. Epub 2012/01/03.
95. Slinin Y, Ishani A, Rector T, Fitzgerald P, MacDonald R, Tacklind J, et al. Management of hyperglycemia, dyslipidemia, and albuminuria in patients with diabetes and CKD: a systematic review for a KDOQI clinical practice guideline. Am J Kidney Dis. 2012;60(5):747–69. Epub 2012/09/25.

96. Lee MS, Kim SM, Kim SB, Lee SK, Park JS, Yang WS. Effects of gemfibrozil on lipid and hemostatic factors in CAPD patients. Perit Dial Int. 1999;19(3):280–3. Epub 1999/08/05.
97. Lucatello A, Sturani A, Di Nardo AM, Cocchi R, Fusaroli M. Safe use of gemfibrozil in uremic patients on continuous ambulatory peritoneal dialysis. Nephron. 1998;78(3):338. Epub 1998/04/18.
98. Clouatre Y, Leblanc M, Ouimet D, Pichette V. Fenofibrate-induced rhabdomyolysis in two dialysis patients with hypothyroidism. Nephrol Dial Transplant. 1999;14(4):1047–8. Epub 1999/05/18.
99. Hottelart C, El Esper N, Rose F, Achard JM, Fournier A. Fenofibrate increases creatininemia by increasing metabolic production of creatinine. Nephron. 2002;92(3):536–41. Epub 2002/10/10.
100. Brown WV. Expert commentary: the safety of fibrates in lipid-lowering therapy. Am J Cardiol. 2007;99(6A):19C–21. Epub 2007/03/21.
101. Ansquer JC, Dalton RN, Causse E, Crimet D, Le Malicot K, Foucher C. Effect of fenofibrate on kidney function: a 6-week randomized crossover trial in healthy people. Am J Kidney Dis. 2008;51(6):904–13. Epub 2008/05/27.
102. Hottelart C, el Esper N, Achard JM, Pruna A, Fournier A. [Fenofibrate increases blood creatinine, but does not change the glomerular filtration rate in patients with mild renal insufficiency]. Nephrologie. 1999;20(1):41–4. Epub 1999/03/19. Le fenofibrate augmente la creatininemie mais n'altere pas le debit de filtration glomerulaire chez les patients presentant une insuffisance renale moderee.
103. Devuyst O, Goffin E, Pirson Y, van Ypersele de Strihou C. Creatinine rise after fibrate therapy in renal graft recipients. Lancet. 1993;341(8848):840.
104. Zhao YY, Weir MA, Manno M, Cordy P, Gomes T, Hackam DG, et al. New fibrate use and acute renal outcomes in elderly adults: a population-based study. Ann Intern Med. 2012;156(8):560–9. Epub 2012/04/18.
105. Davis TM, Ting R, Best JD, Donoghoe MW, Drury PL, Sullivan DR, et al. Effects of fenofibrate on renal function in patients with type 2 diabetes mellitus: the Fenofibrate Intervention and Event Lowering in Diabetes (FIELD) Study. Diabetologia. 2011;54(2):280–90. Epub 2010/11/06.
106. Tonelli M, Collins D, Robins S, Bloomfield H, Curhan GC. Effect of gemfibrozil on change in renal function in men with moderate chronic renal insufficiency and coronary disease. Am J Kidney Dis. 2004;44(5):832–9. Epub 2004/10/20.
107. Mychaleckyj JC, Craven T, Nayak U, Buse J, Crouse JR, Elam M, et al. Reversibility of fenofibrate therapy-induced renal function impairment in ACCORD type 2 diabetic participants. Diabetes Care. 2012;35(5):1008–14. Epub 2012/03/21.
108. Lipscombe J, Lewis GF, Cattran D, Bargman JM. Deterioration in renal function associated with fibrate therapy. Clin Nephrol. 2001;55(1):39–44. Epub 2001/02/24.
109. Kamanna VS, Kashyap ML. Mechanism of action of niacin. Am J Cardiol. 2008;101(8A):20B–6. Epub 2008/06/14.
110. Canner PL, Berge KG, Wenger NK, Stamler J, Friedman L, Prineas RJ, et al. Fifteen year mortality in Coronary Drug Project patients: long-term benefit with niacin. J Am Coll Cardiol. 1986;8(6):1245–55. Epub 1986/12/01.
111. Bruckert E, Labreuche J, Amarenco P. Meta-analysis of the effect of nicotinic acid alone or in combination on cardiovascular events and atherosclerosis. Atherosclerosis. 2010;210(2):353–61. Epub 2010/01/19.
112. Lee JM, Robson MD, Yu LM, Shirodaria CC, Cunnington C, Kylintireas I, et al. Effects of high-dose modified-release nicotinic acid on atherosclerosis and vascular function: a randomized, placebo-controlled, magnetic resonance imaging study. J Am Coll Cardiol. 2009;54(19):1787–94. Epub 2009/10/31.
113. Villines TC, Stanek EJ, Devine PJ, Turco M, Miller M, Weissman NJ, et al. The ARBITER 6-HALTS Trial (Arterial Biology for the Investigation of the Treatment Effects of Reducing Cholesterol 6-HDL and LDL Treatment Strategies in Atherosclerosis): final results and the impact of medication adherence, dose, and treatment duration. J Am Coll Cardiol. 2010;55(24):2721–6. Epub 2010/04/20.

114. Lavigne PM, Karas RH. The current state of niacin in cardiovascular disease prevention: a systematic review and meta-regression. J Am Coll Cardiol. 2013;61(4):440–6. Epub 2012/12/26.
115. Niacin causes serious unexpected side-effects, but no worthwhile benefits, for patients who are at increased risk of heart attacks and strokes; 2013 [April 17, 2013]. http://www.thrivestudy.org/press_release.htm.
116. HPS2-THRIVE Collaborative Group. HPS2-THRIVE randomized placebo-controlled trial in 25 673 high-risk patients of ER niacin/laropiprant: trial design, pre-specified muscle and liver outcomes, and reasons for stopping study treatment. Eur Heart J. 2013;34(17):1279–91.
117. Lai E, De Lepeleire I, Crumley TM, Liu F, Wenning LA, Michiels N, et al. Suppression of niacin-induced vasodilation with an antagonist to prostaglandin D2 receptor subtype 1. Clin Pharmacol Ther. 2007;81(6):849–57. Epub 2007/03/30.
118. Alsheikh-Ali AA, Karas RH. The safety of niacin in the US Food and Drug Administration adverse event reporting database. Am J Cardiol. 2008;101(8A):9B–13. Epub 2008/06/14.
119. Ballantyne CM, Davidson MH, McKenney J, Keller LH, Bajorunas DR, Karas RH. Comparison of the safety and efficacy of a combination tablet of niacin extended release and simvastatin vs simvastatin monotherapy in patients with increased non-HDL cholesterol (from the SEACOAST I study). Am J Cardiol. 2008;101(10):1428–36. Epub 2008/05/13.
120. Grundy SM, Vega GL, Yuan Z, Battisti WP, Brady WE, Palmisano J. Effectiveness and tolerability of simvastatin plus fenofibrate for combined hyperlipidemia (the SAFARI trial). Am J Cardiol. 2005;95(4):462–8. Epub 2005/02/08.
121. McKenney JM, Jones PH, Bays HE, Knopp RH, Kashyap ML, Ruoff GE, et al. Comparative effects on lipid levels of combination therapy with a statin and extended-release niacin or ezetimibe versus a statin alone (the COMPELL study). Atherosclerosis. 2007;192(2):432–7. Epub 2007/01/24.
122. Guyton JR, Brown BG, Fazio S, Polis A, Tomassini JE, Tershakovec AM. Lipid-altering efficacy and safety of ezetimibe/simvastatin coadministered with extended-release niacin in patients with type IIa or type IIb hyperlipidemia. J Am Coll Cardiol. 2008;51(16):1564–72. Epub 2008/04/19.
123. Davidson MH, Stein EA, Bays HE, Maki KC, Doyle RT, Shalwitz RA, et al. Efficacy and tolerability of adding prescription omega-3 fatty acids 4 g/d to simvastatin 40 mg/d in hypertriglyceridemic patients: an 8-week, randomized, double-blind, placebo-controlled study. Clin Ther. 2007;29(7):1354–67. Epub 2007/09/11.
124. Castelli WP, Garrison RJ, Wilson PW, Abbott RD, Kalousdian S, Kannel WB. Incidence of coronary heart disease and lipoprotein cholesterol levels. The Framingham Study. JAMA. 1986;256(20):2835–8. Epub 1986/11/28.
125. Gordon DJ, Probstfield JL, Garrison RJ, Neaton JD, Castelli WP, Knoke JD, et al. High-density lipoprotein cholesterol and cardiovascular disease. Four prospective American studies. Circulation. 1989;79(1):8–15. Epub 1989/01/01.
126. Cooney MT, Dudina A, De Bacquer D, Wilhelmsen L, Sans S, Menotti A, et al. HDL cholesterol protects against cardiovascular disease in both genders, at all ages and at all levels of risk. Atherosclerosis. 2009;206(2):611–6. Epub 2009/04/21.
127. Jafri H, Alsheikh-Ali AA, Karas RH. Meta-analysis: statin therapy does not alter the association between low levels of high-density lipoprotein cholesterol and increased cardiovascular risk. Ann Intern Med. 2010;153(12):800–8. Epub 2010/12/22.
128. Chapman MJ, Ginsberg HN, Amarenco P, Andreotti F, Boren J, Catapano AL, et al. Triglyceride-rich lipoproteins and high-density lipoprotein cholesterol in patients at high risk of cardiovascular disease: evidence and guidance for management. Eur Heart J. 2011;32(11):1345–61. Epub 2011/05/03.
129. Rahilly-Tierney C, Sesso HD, Djousse L, Gaziano JM. Lifestyle changes and 14-year change in high-density lipoprotein cholesterol in a cohort of male physicians. Am Heart J. 2011;161(4):712–8. Epub 2011/04/09.
130. Wing RR. Long-term effects of a lifestyle intervention on weight and cardiovascular risk factors in individuals with type 2 diabetes mellitus: four-year results of the Look AHEAD trial. Arch Intern Med. 2010;170(17):1566–75. Epub 2010/09/30.

131. Toth PP. High-density lipoprotein as a therapeutic target: clinical evidence and treatment strategies. Am J Cardiol. 2005;96(9A):50K–8; discussion 34K–5K. Epub 2005/11/18.
132. Kuvin JT, Dave DM, Sliney KA, Mooney P, Patel AR, Kimmelstiel CD, et al. Effects of extended-release niacin on lipoprotein particle size, distribution, and inflammatory markers in patients with coronary artery disease. Am J Cardiol. 2006;98(6):743–5. Epub 2006/09/05.
133. Schaefer EJ, Asztalos BF. Increasing high-density lipoprotein cholesterol, inhibition of cholesteryl ester transfer protein, and heart disease risk reduction. Am J Cardiol. 2007; 100(11 A):n25–31. Epub 2007/12/06.
134. Barter PJ, Kastelein JJ. Targeting cholesteryl ester transfer protein for the prevention and management of cardiovascular disease. J Am Coll Cardiol. 2006;47(3):492–9. Epub 2006/02/07.
135. Forrester JS, Makkar R, Shah PK. Increasing high-density lipoprotein cholesterol in dyslipidemia by cholesteryl ester transfer protein inhibition: an update for clinicians. Circulation. 2005;111(14):1847–54. Epub 2005/04/13.
136. Natarajan P, Ray KK, Cannon CP. High-density lipoprotein and coronary heart disease: current and future therapies. J Am Coll Cardiol. 2010;55(13):1283–99. Epub 2010/03/27.
137. Barter PJ, Caulfield M, Eriksson M, Grundy SM, Kastelein JJ, Komajda M, et al. Effects of torcetrapib in patients at high risk for coronary events. N Engl J Med. 2007;357(21):2109–22. Epub 2007/11/07.
138. Schwartz GG, Olsson AG, Abt M, Ballantyne CM, Barter PJ, Brumm J, et al. Effects of dalcetrapib in patients with a recent acute coronary syndrome. N Engl J Med. 2012;367(22):2089–99. Epub 2012/11/07.
139. Voight BF, Peloso GM, Orho-Melander M, Frikke-Schmidt R, Barbalic M, Jensen MK, et al. Plasma HDL cholesterol and risk of myocardial infarction: a mendelian randomisation study. Lancet. 2012;380(9841):572–80. Epub 2012/05/23.

Chapter 10
Dyslipidemia in Dialysis

Yalcin Solak and Halil Zeki Tonbul

Dyslipidemia is a well-established cardiovascular (CV) risk factor in the general population. However, this is not the case in patients with kidney disease, particularly among end-stage renal disease (ESRD) patients (hemodialysis [HD] and peritoneal dialysis [PD]). HD and PD patients have increased prevalence of dyslipidemia; however, the so-called "ESRD dyslipidemia" shows a number of qualitative and quantitative differences from the dyslipidemia commonly encountered in the general population. Traditional CV risk factors aggregate in dialysis patients [1]. When novel CV risk factors, which are unique to kidney disease and dialysis modalities, are also taken into account, it is not surprising that CV mortality risk is beyond that which can be explained using traditional CV risk factors alone. Actually, dialysis patients are 10–30 times more likely to die from CV disease than the general population [2]. Randomized controlled trials (RCT) in the last 10 years produced disappointing results, in which statin treatment did not translate into conspicuous CV survival advantage. Actually when one looks at the special characteristics of the lipid profile of dialysis patients as well as the cumulative CV risk context in these patients, lack of beneficial effects of statin trials becomes more plausible. In addition, even dialysis modalities differ in the frequency and composition of dyslipidemia. We review dyslipidemia prevalence, characteristics, pathophysiology, and relation to CV morbidity and mortality in dialysis population as well as available treatment choices with a particular emphasis on individual dialysis modalities.

Y. Solak, M.D. (✉)
Department of Nephrology, Karaman State Hospital,
Karaman Devlet Hastanesi, Nefroloji Kliniği 70100 Karaman, Turkey
e-mail: yalcinsolakmd@gmail.com

H.Z. Tonbul, M.D.
Department of Nephrology, Meram School of Medicine Necmettin Erbakan Üniversitesi,
Meram Tıp Fakültesi, Nefroloji Bölümü, Meram, Konya, Turkey
e-mail: htonbul@yahoo.com

A. Covic et al. (eds.), *Dyslipidemias in Kidney Disease*, DOI 10.1007/978-1-4939-0515-7_10,

Prevalence of Dyslipidemia in HD Population

Depending on the definition, dyslipidemia may be present in up to 70 % of patients undergoing chronic hemodialysis [3]. In 20 % of HD patients plasma total cholesterol levels are above 240 mg/dL. Percentage of chronic hemodialysis patients who have elevated levels of LDL and triglycerides, and reduced levels HDL cholesterol are 30, 50 and 45, respectively [4].

Nature of Dyslipidemia in HD Patients

Hemodialysis patients do in part share some of the general characteristics of dyslipidemia observed in predialysis patients [3]. However, HD treatment leads to an attenuation in predialysis dyslipidemia, which is evidenced by slightly lower concentrations of the triglyceride-rich lipoproteins [5]. Alterations in levels of apolipoproteins and lipoprotein cholesterols in patients undergoing long-term HD are summarized in Table 10.1.

The precise mechanisms that are responsible for disturbed lipid profile in HD patients are yet to be elucidated. However, many abnormalities to date have been described in the lipoprotein metabolism in hemodialysis patients:

- Decreased lipoprotein lipase (LPL) activity
- Decreased hepatic triglyceride lipase (HTGL) activity
- Decreased lecithin cholesterol acyltransferase (LCAT)
- Decreased LDL-receptor-related protein
- Reduced cholesterol esterification in HDL
- Inability to form mature HDL particles
- Increased oxidized LDL levels due to oxidative stress and inflammation

HD patients may have an atherogenic lipid profile even in the absence of apparent quantitative hyperlipidemia [6]. A number of qualitative changes in individual parameters of lipid profile have been determined in recent years. These patients have elevated levels of small dense and oxidized LDL and Lp(a), whereas LDL cholesterol levels are within normal limits [7, 8].

Recently, Yamamoto et al. [9] investigated cellular cholesterol efflux and inflammatory response in macrophages that are exposed to HDL of patients undergoing HD and controls. HDL from HD patients was dramatically less effective in accepting cholesterol from macrophages than normal HDL from controls.

Table 10.1 Changes in levels of (apo)lipoproteins and lipoprotein cholesterols in patients undergoing long-term hemodialysis

(Apo) lipoprotein	Apo A-I	Apo A-II	Apo B	Apo E	Apo C-III	Lp(a)	VLDL	IDL
Change in HD patients	↓	↓	↑	↑	↑↑	↑	↑	↑

The authors also showed that in vitro activation of cellular cholesterol transporters increased cholesterol efflux to both normal and uremic HDL. Notably, HDL of patients undergoing HD had reduced anti-chemotactic ability and increased macrophage cytokine response compared with HDL of controls. More importantly, HDL of HD patients on statin therapy had reduced inflammatory response while maintaining impaired cholesterol acceptor function. The authors concluded that dysfunctional HDL may have had more important roles in the pathogenesis of atheroscleroses in uremic subjects than previously thought, as such uremic HDL may be related to impaired reverse cholesterol transport from machrophages and more pronounced inflammation. Holzer et al. [10] also reported altered composition of HDL in uremic patients via mass spectrometry and biochemical analyses. They found that uremic HDL contained reduced phospholipid and increased triglyceride and lysophospholipid content. Mange et al. [11] studied HDL proteomics and reported differences between the HDL-related proteins in HD patients and normal subjects. The investigators found that 40 identified proteins were differentially expressed between the normal subjects and HD patients. These proteins normally play roles in many HDL functions, including lipid metabolism, acute inflammatory response, complement activation, and regulation of lipoprotein oxidation. Among these proteins, apolipoprotein C-II and C-III were significantly increased in the HDL fraction of HD patients, whereas serotransferrin was decreased.

In brief, these studies collectively showed numerous important qualitative alterations in HDL composition and function in HD patients. Thus, it has been speculated that dysfunctional HDL may be responsible for increased CV death and may account for lack of clear-cut benefits of statins in this population.

Hemodialysis-Related Factors and Dyslipidemia

The blood of HD patients is routinely exposed to extracorporeal membranes and contacts with dialysate contents. Thus, compositions of dialysis membranes and dialysate in terms of purity have been investigated as to effects on inflammation, oxidative stress, and dyslipidemia. Normally, a single hemodialysis session has some impact on lipid parameters in uremic patients. In one study, hemodialysis partially improved LDL inflammatory and HDL anti-inflammatory activities and enhanced HDL's ability to suppress LDL inflammatory activity [12]. Another study found that oxidized phospholipids (OxPL) on apolipoprotein B-100 (apoB) (an predictor of CV mortality) particles were significantly reduced during acute hemodialysis [13]. Lippi et al. [14] showed that acute hemodialysis significantly decreased median Lp(a) concentration post-HD, whereas no significant changes were observed for apo A, apo B, and hs-CRP.

Ultrapure dialysate, high-flux membrane, and low-molecular-weight heparin (LMWH) use are among the most commonly studied parameters in terms of impact on uremic dyslipidemia in HD patients.

Ultrapure Dialysate

A small randomized prospective study including patients who were dialyzed with low-flux membrane but with ultrapure dialysate plasma showed that Lp(a) levels did not increase at 12 months in contrast to patients dialyzed with conventional dialysate [15]. Several previous studies and a recent meta-analysis demonstrated beneficial effects of using ultrapure dialysate on inflammation and oxidative stress in hemodialysis patients compared with conventional dialysate [16–19]. Thus, it is plausible to think that reduced inflammation and oxidative stress either by themselves or through reduced oxidation and carbamilation of LDL and HDL may have had salutary effects on atherosclerosis and subsequent cardiovascular events. Actually one study showed that ultrapure dialysate reduced plasma pentosidine levels (a marker of carbonyl stress) and improved plasma triglyceride levels [20]. Another study showed that use of ultrapure dialysate led to reduction in levels of non-HDL cholesterol and apoB at 6 months as well as improvements in inflammation and oxidative stress [21].

High-Flux Dialysis

Several studies showed beneficial effects of high-flux HD on lipid parameters in HD patients. Ingram et al. [22] conducted a blinded cross-over trial of two cellulose acetate dialysers of similar flux but with different clearances of larger molecules. The study showed that low-flux dialysis using a cellulose acetate membrane with a good clearance of higher-molecular-weight molecules may be associated with beneficial changes in plasma lipids and lipoproteins. Seres and colleagues [23] compared high-flux cellulosic and polysulfone dialysis membranes in terms of effects on lipid parameters. The authors found that patients dialyzed with cellulose membrane showed no alteration in serum TG, HDL, LDL, or total cholesterol when predialysis and postdialysis values were compared. On the other hand, patients dialyzed with polysulfone membrane had a significant decrease in TG concentrations as well as a significant rise in HDL cholesterol level. Notably, LPL activity in polysulfone sera was significantly greater than LPL in cellulosic sera. While some studies showed reduction in total cholesterol [24], others showed reductions in LDL cholesterol [24] or triglycerides [25, 26] with use of high-flux membranes. High-flux HD was also shown to improve serum Lp(a) levels as well [27]. In contrast to the aforementioned studies, some other studies did not find any difference between low- and high-flux HD in terms of effects on dyslipidemia [28]. Differences in quantitative and qualitative improvements in uremic dyslipidemia with high-flux membranes may be attributed to differences in membrane characteristics, baseline lipid profile of studied patients, and duration of the studies.

Effects of Heparin

A number of studies have evaluated effects of low-molecular-weight heparin (LMWH) and unfractionated heparin (UFH) on lipid profiles of patients on chronic HD. Most, but not all, studies reported improvements in lipid profile with use of LMWH compared with UFH. Studies found significant decreases in triglycerides [29–31], total cholesterol [31–33], and VLDL [34]. While some studies [35] showed no change in serum LDL and HDL cholesterol levels associated with LMWH use, one study reported increased HDL cholesterol levels in patients undergoing hemodialysis with UFH rather than LMWH [36].

These mixed findings might be due to small sample sizes, using different LMWH preparations in different studies, variability in treatment durations, baseline differences in lipid profiles of studied HD patients, among others. Moreover, no prospective randomized study evaluated effects of different heparin preparations on dyslipidemia in HD patients to date.

Despite presence of evidence showing the contrary [37], it has been suggested that LMWHs release endothelial-bound LPL less efficiently than UFH and thereby cause less impaired lipid metabolism [38].

Reverse Epidemiology of Total Cholesterol and Lipid Parameters to Predict CV Outcomes

In the last decade, as a component of reverse epidemiology concept, several studies showed that low serum total cholesterol level was associated with increased mortality in dialysis patients. Lowrie et al. [39] found that serum total cholesterol level was inversely correlated with the risk of death even after controlled for other biochemical factors and case-mix in a cohort of 12,000 maintenance HD patients. Degoulet and colleagues [40] in the Diaphane Collaborative Study Group showed that a low plasma total cholesterol level was associated with a significantly higher risk of CV death in a cohort of 1,400 HD patients. These observations were in sharp contrast with the case in general population in which high serum total cholesterol level was associated with adverse CV outcomes.

Possible explanations for this reverse association have been suggested. Among these are survival bias, the time discrepancy between competitive risk factors, and the presence of malnutrition inflammation complex syndrome (malnutrition, inflammation, atherosclerosis, MIA) [41]. The latter factor gained popularity to reveal the inverse correlation between total cholesterol level and CV mortality. As a modulator of the relation between cholesterol level and death, MIA is characterized by undernutrition, hypoalbuminemia, increased inflammation, and consequent atherosclerosis. Inflammation per se may lead to hypocholesterolemia in ESRD patients [42, 43]. In a prospective study of maintenance HD patients, Liu et al. [44] showed that average serum cholesterol was lower in the presence of MIA than in its absence.

An increment in baseline total serum cholesterol was associated with decreased overall all-cause mortality. On the other hand, the authors reported that serum cholesterol level was associated with an increased all-cause mortality risk in the absence of inflammation/malnutrition. The authors concluded that the reverse epidemiology of total cholesterol was due to cholesterol-lowering effects of inflammation and malnutrition. Thus, hypercholesterolemia may be a surrogate marker of a better nutritional status, and reduced inflammation and oxidative stress and in turn is associated with better overall CV outcomes.

Since total serum cholesterol level is a marker of general nutritional status rather than a CV risk factor, individual parameters of lipid profile were tested in terms of prediction of CV mortality among HD patients. Kilpatrick and colleagues [45] analyzed data of approximately 15,000 HD patients. The authors reported that both total and LDL hypercholesterolemia showed a paradoxic association with better survival. While hypertriglyceridemia (TG>200 mg/dL) showed a similar trend, HDL cholesterol did not show any association with survival. In subgroup analyses, these trends were more pronounced among patients with hypoalbuminemia and lower dietary protein intake. On the other hand, some other studies did not confirm these results [46].

In an attempt to discover novel lipid targets that can predict mortality in dialysis patients, Noori et al. [47] investigated whether lipoprotein subfraction and size measurement could predict mortality. They found that whereas conventional lipid profile cannot predict mortality in maintenance HD patients, larger novel LDL particle diameter or higher large LDL particle concentrations were predictive of greater survival. Furthermore, higher very small LDL particle concentration was associated with higher death risk after 6 years of follow-up.

In recent years, non-HDL cholesterol attracted interest as a predictor of CV outcomes in dialysis patients. A few prospective studies found that non-HDL cholesterol was a significant and independent predictor of CV death in HD patients [48]. In an observational cohort study in 45,390 HD patients, myocardial and cerebral infarction rates were positively correlated with non-HDL cholesterol levels [49]. On the other hand, death risk was associated with malnutrition/inflammation but not with non-HDL cholesterol levels. Recently, de Oliveira et al. [50] found that there was a positive and significant correlation between non-HDL cholesterol, but not LDL cholesterol, and the anthropometric cardiovascular risk indices. Non-HDL cholesterol also has the advantage of independence from fasting status. One study showed that fasting and nonfasting values were equivalent in HD patients [51].

Given that most apoB-containing lipoproteins including intermediate density lipoprotein (IDL), LDL and VLDL, are atherogenic, total apoB level is considered to be a better predictor than LDL-C level [52]. In one study containing HD and PD patients, non-HDL cholesterol was found to adequately reflect the nontraditional lipid pattern of patients [53]. The authors reported that non-HDL cholesterol >130 mg/dL independent of TG values and HDL cholesterol <40 mg/dL may predict nontraditional lipoprotein risk factors (LDL particle size, LDL particle concentration, small dense LDL, IDL, large HDL, large VLDL and Lp(a)) among dialysis patients.

Treatment of Dyslipidemia in HD Patients

Cholesterol-lowering treatment is widely underutilized among HD patients even before the discouraging results of the recent RCT were published. For example, United States Renal Data System (USRDS) data showed that 8 % of HD patients were receiving cholesterol-lowering treatment [54]. In a HD patient cohort 29.4 % of patients with established atherosclerotic disease were on lipid-lowering treatments, whereas only 9 % of patients without overt prior atherosclerotic disease were receiving cholesterol-lowering treatment [55]. Likely reasons for this underutilization were polypharmacy, cost, compliance, lack of published evidence for efficacy, adverse events, and relatively normal or even low serum LDL cholesterol levels in HD patients [55].

A number of cholesterol-lowering medications and adjunctive measures are available for the treatment of dyslipidemia in HD patients (Table 10.2). However, treatment of dyslipidemia should be considered in a broader context that includes measures to reduce overall CV risk in HD patients. These measures should target traditional as well as novel risk factors for CV disease in HD patients.

Exercise

Only a few studies investigated effects of various exercise modalities on the lipid profile of HD patients. Gordon et al. [56] showed that 16 weeks of yoga exercise improved the lipid profile in HD patients; total and LDL cholesterol as well as triglycerides showed a significant decrease with exercise compared with basal values. Masuda and colleagues [57] showed beneficial effects of physical activity on HDL and apoA1 levels in HD patients. In contrast, Afshar et al. [58] found no change in lipid profile, but a significant decrease in serum CRP levels with aerobic and resistance exercise in HD patients. However, the duration of the study was 8 weeks, and this time might have been too short to reveal the beneficial effects of exercise on dyslipidemia. A recent paper reviewing this issue concluded that the most consistent observation with exercise on blood lipids was a noted decrease in triglycerides and an increase in HDL cholesterol levels as well as improved insulin sensitivity [59].

Table 10.2 Therapeutic options and adjunctive measures for dyslipidemia management in HD patients

Diet and exercise	May have limited efficacy due to malnutrition and chronic disease burden in HD patients
Modification of dialysis-related factors	Synthetic polysulfone membranes High-flux hemodialysis Ultrapure hemodialysate Low-molecular-weight heparin (LMWH)
Pharmacologic treatment	HMG-CoA reductase inhibitors (statins) Fibrates Sevelamer

Statin Treatment

Statin treatment constitutes one of the major therapeutic armamentarium for the treatment of dyslipidemia in HD patients, although there is a lack of evidenced-based beneficial hard outcomes in terms of mortality. Three large-scale RCTs exclusively conducted on HD patients (only SHARP included predialytic patients) have been published to answer the question of whether statin use is associated with improvements in hard CV endpoints in the HD population. The cumulative results of these RCTs were surprising. In contrast to the general population, statin treatment was not found to be associated with a CV risk reduction in HD patients. Table 10.3 summarizes basic characteristics of these RCTs [60–62].

4D trial was the first large-scale trial investigating beneficial effects of statin treatment on CV outcomes in a HD population [60]. The results of this trial showed no difference between atorvastatin and placebo in terms of primary endpoints. Moreover, incidence of fatal stroke was significantly higher in the atorvastatin group. Marz et al. [63] performed a post hoc analysis of 4D trial and showed that baseline LDL cholesterol level was important in predicting CV effects of atorvastatin. Patients with a baseline LDL cholesterol level in the highest quartile only had reduced CV event rate compared with placebo in contrast to patients in other quartiles.

Several points have been emphasized with an attempt to account for the negative results of the 4D trial. First, 15 % of patients receiving atorvastatin required a dose reduction (to 10 mg). Second, 16.6 % of patients on the atorvastatin arm who were free of primary events discontinued atorvastatin treatment. Third, 15 % of patients on the placebo arm received a nonstudy statin. Thus, the decreasing LDC difference between the placebo and study group may have reduced the power of study. In addition, the lack of statin effect in this trial had been attributed to the advanced atherosclerotic state of the patients recruited. Fifty percent of the patients had a past history of diabetes mellitus and had been on HD for at least 2 years [6].

AURORA compared effects of 10 mg rosuvastatin with placebo on CV endpoints [61]. The randomized double-blind study recruited 2,776 patients, 50–80 years of age, who were undergoing maintenance hemodialysis. After 3 months of treatment, mean LDL cholesterol levels showed a 43 % reduction from a mean baseline level of 100 mg/dL in patients receiving rosuvastatin. During a 3.8 years median follow-up period, 396 patients in the rosuvastatin group and 408 patients in the placebo group reached the primary endpoint. The trial showed no benefit of rosuvastatin treatment on primary and secondary endpoints of the study protocol. Rosuvastatin showed no benefit in any subgroup examined, including patients with diabetes. Similar to the results of the Jupiter trial [64], rosuvastatin treatment reduced serum CRP levels but not CV endpoints in contrast to Jupiter. Despite achieving targeted reductions in LDL levels at study planning, lack of beneficial effects had been attributed to high dropout rate, lack of sufficient statistical power [65], and almost statistically significant predominance of diabetes as the cause of ESRD in the statin arm [66]. There was no increase in the incidence of rhabdomyolysis or liver transaminase elevation in the rosuvastatin group as compared with the

Table 10.3 Basic characteristics of RCTs using statin therapy in HD patients

Trial	Lipid-lowering medication and dose	LDL reduction (%)	Median duration of follow-up	Number of HD patients	Primary endpoints	Secondary endpoints	Outcomes
4D (Deutsche Diabetes Dialyse Studie) Wanner et al.	Atorvastatin 20 mg	42	4 years	1,255	Composite outcome (death from cardiac causes, fatal and nonfatal stroke, nonfatal MI)	All-cause mortality, cardiac events, cerebrovascular events	No significant difference in primary endpoints Fatal stroke incidence significantly higher with atorvastatin
AURORA Fellstrom et al.	Rosuvastatin 10 mg	43	3.8 years	2,773	Time to major CV events (fatal and nonfatal MI and stroke)	All-cause mortality, CV event-free survival, Arterial revascularization	No significant differences in primary and secondary endpoints
SHARP Baigent et al.	Simvastatin 20 mg + Ezetimibe 10 mg	77	4.9 years	3,023	Occurrence of major CV events (death due to coronary disease, nonfatal MI, nonhemorrhagic stroke, need for revascularization)		17 % decrease in rate of major atherosclerotic events

placebo group. Holdaas et al. [67] performed a post hoc analysis of AURORA data in which they evaluated effect of rosuvastatin treatment on AURORA composite endpoints and fatal and nonfatal cardiac events. Among the 731 patients with diabetes, assignment to rosuvastatin was associated with a nonsignificant 16.2 % risk reduction for the AURORA trial's composite primary endpoint of cardiac death, nonfatal MI, or fatal or nonfatal stroke. There was no difference in total stroke rate; however, the rosuvastatin group had more frequent hemorrhagic strokes compared with placebo group. Rosuvastatin treatment significantly reduced the rates of cardiac events (when stroke is excluded) by 32 % among diabetic hemodialysis patients (hazard ratio 0.68; 95 % confidence interval 0.51–0.90).

The latest RCT, SHARP trial, had some differences from 4D and AURORA. SHARP included HD patients as well as predialytic CKD and PD patients [62]. It had a larger cohort compared with previous statin trials in HD patients and included patients who had no prior history of CV disease. The study included approximately 9,500 patients (6,245 patients with chronic kidney disease and 3,023 patients on chronic dialysis) that were followed for a median of 4.9 years. The primary endpoint did not comprise CV or all-cause mortality; instead, rate of occurrence of major CV events was established as the primary endpoint of the study. When the whole cohort was evaluated, 20 mg simvastatin plus 10 mg ezetimibe led to significant reductions in major atherosclerotic events, nonhemorrhagic stroke, and arterial revascularization. On the other hand, subgroup analysis did not demonstrate any statistically significant reduction in mortality or CV event rate in HD patients. In dialysis patients there was an insignificant reduction of relative risk in all cardiovascular events with the simvastatin and ezetimibe group compared with placebo arm (15 % versus 16.5 %). The primary limitation of the study is that one-third of the patients were nonadherent to study drugs and there was not a group receiving only simvastatin, enabling comparison with placebo. SHARP trial did not have sufficient power to assess the effects on major atherosclerotic events separately in dialysis and nondialysis patients, but the proportional effects in dialysis patients did not significantly differ from those seen in patients not on dialysis. Furthermore, since about a third of the patients who were not on dialysis at baseline began dialysis during the trial (about one-third of those started dialysis within the first year), the effects of simvastatin plus ezetimibe in the dialysis subgroup are reinforced by the favorable results in the nondialysis subgroup (the effects of lowering LDL cholesterol with simvastatin plus ezetimibe in patients with chronic kidney disease) [62]. Dialysis patients had lower baseline LDL cholesterol concentrations and average use of LDL cholesterol-lowering therapy was lower compared with nondialysis patients. Thus, these factors led to absolute reductions in LDL cholesterol that were about a third smaller in dialysis patients (0.60 mmol/L) compared with patients not on dialysis (0.96 mmol/L). The investigators found that the proportional reductions in major atherosclerotic events per 1 mmol/L LDL cholesterol reduction were similar in dialysis patients with nondialysis patients.

In sum, the results of these RCTs showed that HD patients do not apparently benefit from statin treatment in terms of CV morbidity and mortality.

A very recent meta-analysis [68] investigating effect of statin treatment on CV and renal outcomes in patients with CKD included 31 trials providing data for almost 48,000 patients with CKD, including 6,690 major CV events and 6,653 deaths. Statin treatment led to a 23 % relative risk reduction for major CV events and 9 % reduction in CV or all-cause death. Subgroup analysis revealed that relative effects of statin treatment in CKD were significantly reduced in patients with ESRD; nonetheless, absolute risk reductions were comparable. The authors concluded that statin treatment reduces the risk of major CV events in dialysis patients.

Guideline Recommendations for Statin Use

K/DOQI guidelines [69] had been published long before the publication of results of major RCTs studying various statins in HD patients. Thus, recommendations had been done without the knowledge of RCTs showing long-term hard outcomes of lowering LDL cholesterol with use of statins in HD patients. K/DOQI recommended treatment of patients whose serum fasting triglycerides level >500 mg/dL by removing the underlying cause, treatment with therapeutic lifestyle changes, and a triglyceride-lowering agent. K/DOQI also recommended that treatment should be considered to reduce LDL to <100 mg/dL with a statin starting with a low dose and titrate upward to attain target levels. For adults with stage 5 CKD and LDL <100 mg/dL, fasting triglycerides >200 mg/dL, and non-HDL cholesterol (total cholesterol minus HDL) >130 mg/dL, treatment should be considered to reduce non-HDL cholesterol to <130 mg/dL. The 2012 update of KDOQI Clinical Practice Guideline for Diabetes and CKD [70] recommended not to use statins in diabetic dialysis patients based on the data derived from 4D, AURORA, and SHARP trials.

KDIGO Clinical Practice Guideline for Lipid Management in Chronic Kidney Disease was still under preparation during the writing of this chapter. However, KDIGO 2012 Clinical Practice Guideline for the Evaluation and Management of Chronic Kidney Disease [71] reported that the key aspects of the draft recommendations include treating those at high risk for atherosclerotic disease with lipid-lowering therapies, regardless of LDL levels, in those 50 years of age and above.

Carnitine and Sevelamer

Although individual studies [72, 73] showed beneficial effects of L-carnitine supplementation on lipid profile, a systematic review found that there was no effect of L-carnitine on triglycerides, total cholesterol, or any of its fractions [74].

A meta-analysis [75] investigating the effect of sevelamer on mineral metabolism parameters and serum lipids showed that sevelamer treatment was associated with a significant reduction in total cholesterol (30 mg/dL), LDL cholesterol (31 mg/dL), triglycerides (20 mg/dL), and a significant increase in HDL cholesterol (4 mg/dL).

Why Do Statins Seem Ineffective in HD Patients?

Several hypotheses have been proposed to explain the disappointing results of RCT that tested statins in HD patients. Some authors emphasized the different nature of atherosclerotic plaques as well as lipid profile [76] in patients undergoing dialysis treatment. Arterial calcification with prominent thickening of the intima and media layers of the vessel wall is the characteristic of the arterial lesions in ESRD patients and differs from general structure of atherosclerotic plaques [77]. Others explained lack of efficiency of statins due to presence of excess CV mortality, particularly sudden cardiac death, in HD population. In fact most CV deaths taking place in HD population is due to sudden cardiac death rather than coronary artery occlusion. Several factors influence the heightened risk of sudden cardiac death including left ventricular hypertrophy, vascular calcification, electrolyte abnormalities and rapid fluctuations in electrolytes with hemodialysis treatment, and cardiomyocyte fibrosis, among others [78]. Hence, even if statins were beneficial in terms of curbing deaths related to coronary artery occlusion due to atherosclerotic plaques, this benefit might have been masked by the high prevalence of sudden cardiac death against which statins may not be that effective. It has also been argued that HD patients have advanced atherosclerotic disease, and in addition to traditional risk factors, several novel risk factors unique to ESRD population are also at work to affect CV mortality [79]. Thus, merely manipulating a single CV risk factor, namely dyslipidemia, would not suffice to impact CV survival in this high CV risk patient group. To our opinion, comprehensive risk reduction strategies that also take novel risk factors into account is needed to significantly reduce CV risk in this special patient group.

Dyslipidemia in Peritoneal Dialysis

Compared with hemodialysis, peritoneal dialysis (PD) has been studied less in terms of dyslipidemia and associated cardiovascular disease burden. Patients starting PD as part of the renal replacement therapy carry their "renal dyslipidemia," which starts to emerge from the early stages of chronic kidney disease, with them. However, some alterations occur in the lipid profile of CKD due to factors unique to PD modality.

Cardiovascular Disease in Peritoneal Dialysis

Cardiovascular disease is the leading cause of death in PD patients as in predialysis CKD and HD patients. The risk of cardiovascular mortality in patients on dialysis is almost ninefold higher than in the general population [80]. The overall adjusted probability of survival in incident PD patients at 1 year is 86.8 %, but only 11.3 % at 10 years [81]. Just as in the HD patients, a constellation of traditional and nontraditional risk factors plays a role in these mortality rates [82].

Dyslipidemia and CV Morbidity/Mortality in PD

Dyslipidemia is regarded as one of the nontraditional CV risk factors in PD patients. Most of the studies examining the association of dyslipidemia and CV events or death have been conducted on HD patients. The reverse epidemiologic pattern seen in the HD population has also been demonstrated in PD patients, as low serum cholesterol and malnutrition are associated with increased mortality [83, 84]. Habib et al. [85] evaluated the relationship between lipid levels and mortality on data of 1,053 PD patients from the USRDS prospective Dialysis Morbidity and Mortality Study Wave 2. Patients with total cholesterol levels ≤125 mg/dL had a statistically significant increased risk of all-cause mortality, including those on or not on lipid-modifying medications, compared with the reference value of 176–225 mg/dL. On the other hand, some other studies showed positive correlation between dyslipidemia and CV mortality in PD patients [86, 87]. There exists observational data showing the association between elevated serum lipoprotein a (Lp(a)) with increased CV disease or mortality in PD patients [88].

Prevalence of Dyslipidemia in PD

Dyslipidemia is common among PD patients. One study examining 168 Continuous Ambulatory Peritoneal Dialysis (CAPD) patients found that elevated total cholesterol, triglycerides and Lp(a) concentrations were present in 67 %, 47 % and 37 % of the patients, respectively. About two-thirds of the patients LDL cholesterol was above 100 mg/dL and HDL cholesterol below 40 mg/dL [8]. In other studies, 20–40 % of PD patients had elevated total cholesterol and LDL cholesterol, whereas 25–50 % of them had elevated levels of triglycerides and low HDL cholesterol [55].

Lipid and Lipoprotein Profile in PD

The most commonly encountered lipid profile in PD patients includes elevated total cholesterol, LDL cholesterol, triglycerides, and low HDL cholesterol levels. In addition, these patients usually have elevated Lp(a) and apolipoprotein B (apoB) as well as low apolipoprotein B1 levels [89].

Classic lipid profiles including total, LDL, and HDL cholesterols and triglycerides have limited value in terms of risk stratification in PD patients. These individual components of the classic lipid profile are affected by fasting state. It is practically cumbersome to attain a true fasting state in PD patients, particularly in patients whose night dwell is dextrose-based solutions rather than icodextrin. Besides this practical difficulty, recent studies have shown that novel parameters of the lipoprotein family are of better predictive ability in the general population [90]. Not all of these novel lipoproteins have been shown to be associated with adverse CV events in PD patients. However, when inert actions of statins regarding CV events are taken into account in dialysis patients, as shown in recent randomized controlled studies, it would not be wrong to think that evaluation and targeting of these lipoproteins would be beneficial in this particularly high-risk group.

In addition to quantitative changes, some qualitative alterations take place in the lipid profile of PD patients. There is an increased concentration of small dense LDL particles together with the increased apoB level [91]. One study showed that small dense LDL percentage and concentration was increased in patients undergoing PD [7]. In another study, 48 % of PD patients had small LDL particle size [92]. In addition, oxidized LDL level has been reported to be increased in PD patients [93]. A recent study including 24 CAPD patients found that oxidized LDL was increased in these patients compared with control subjects [94].

Effects of Peritoneal Dialysis Modality on Lipid Profile

While lipid profiles of ESRD patients starting hemodialysis generally do not differ qualitatively from renal dyslipidemia observed in CKD, patients starting on PD acquire a qualitatively distinct type of dyslipidemia. Thus, some factors related to PD modality per se have been implicated for these changes in dyslipidemia of CKD. The main mechanisms that are held responsible for the atherogenic lipid profile observed in PD patients follow:

1. Insulin resistance coupled with glucose load from dextrose-based dialysis fluids
2. Peritoneal protein clearance
3. Defects in lipid metabolism and micronutrient deficiency

Absorption of glucose from the dialysate solution may stimulate hepatic lipoprotein synthesis and increase insulin levels and, consequently, triglyceride synthesis [95]. Peritoneal dialysis patients have insulin resistance as a typical feature of CKD patients. Consequently, in these patients increased delivery of free fatty acids (FFAs) to liver occurs [96]. Liver oxidizes or esterifies these FFAs either to cytozolic triglycerides or VLDL [4]. The abundant availability of FFAs in PD patients due to insulin resistance and de novo lipogenesis lead to increased production of VLDL. Another defect that contributes to elevated serum VLDL levels in PD patients is decreased catabolism of VLDL and triglycerides [96]. The high level of intermediate-density lipoprotein (IDL) may be due to overproduction of VLDL and dysfunctional LPL enzyme activity [89]. Despite the failure of demonstration of the relation between absorbed glucose level and the severity of dyslipidemia [95], indirect confirmation of this mechanism comes from the studies in which glucose-based dialysate solutions were switched to icodextrine. After the switch, patients showed significant decreases in total and LDL cholesterol and triglyceride levels [97, 98].

Most PD patients lose 1–2 g of protein per liter of drained dialysate [96]. Some authors proposed an analogy between protein loss through urine in nephrotic syndrome and protein loss through peritoneal effluents in PD patients. Thus, mechanisms operative in nephrotic syndrome-related dyslipidemia may also in part be responsible for dyslipidemia of PD patients. Loss of apolipoproteins and

Table 10.4 Comparison of lipid profiles of PD and HD

Dialysis modality	Total cholesterol	LDL cholesterol	HDL cholesterol	VLDL cholesterol	Triglyceride
PD	↑	↑	↓	↑	↑
HD	↑ ↔ ↓	↔ ↓	↓	↑	↑

lipoproteins through peritoneal exchange has been well documented [99, 100]. In spite of clearance of a number of (apo)lipoproteins through peritoneal membrane, the impact on serum levels of these (apo)lipoproteins and clinical consequences is yet to be elucidated. Despite high peritoneal clearance of apoAIV, levels are comparable in PD and HD patients [99]. Smaller-sized proteins, including several lipoproteins, are preferentially lost by means of peritoneal sieving [6]. As an example of the latter, HDL is lost through peritoneal exchanges at a rate equivalent to 34 % of its synthetic rate, whereas apoB-containing lipoprotein loss is negligible [100, 101].

Some other defects in lipid metabolism have been identified in PD patients. Cholesterol ester transfer protein (CETF) has been found to be increased in children undergoing PD [102]. Elevated levels of this enzyme have been linked with increased atherosclerosis risk in the general population [103]. Loss of carnitene through peritoneal membrane may also contribute dyslipidemia [104]. Confirmation of this has been come from the studies that showed beneficial effects of L-carnitene supplementation on lipid profiles of PD patients [105].

Differences in Dyslipidemias of Peritoneal Dialysis and Hemodialysis

Dyslipidemia is more prevalent in PD patients when compared with hemodialysis counterparts [5, 8, 91]. In addition to difference in frequency, there exist qualitative differences in dyslipidemia seen in HD and PD patients (Table 10.4). Furthermore, PD patients have a higher incidence of multiple dyslipidemic factors simultaneously [8, 91]. One comparative study found that the CAPD group had a markedly higher number of patients with three or four concurrent dyslipidemic factors than HD patients [8]. Generally, PD patients have a more atherogenic lipid profile compared with HD patients [106, 107].

Treatment of Dyslipidemia in PD Patients

Few studies evaluated treatment of dyslipidemia in PD patients. In contrast to the general population, diet therapy may not be reasonable or achievable because these patients are already under dietary restrictions. Further restriction in calories and protein intake parallel to dietary lipids may worsen protein energy malnutrition and inflammation. Studies investigating the effects of an exercise program on individual lipid parameters in PD patients are lacking. One study showed that serum HDL

Table 10.5 Therapeutic options and adjunctive measures for dyslipidemia management in PD patients

Treatment modality	Comments
Diet and exercise	Insufficiently studied Exercise is difficult to accomplish due to physical disability and heavy burden of chronic diseases Strict diet may worsen protein energy malnutrition
Statin treatment	No randomized controlled studies in PD patients Generally safe and effective in PD patients Additional pleiotropic effects beyond lipid lowering
Sevelamer hydrochloride	May be beneficial in retarding atherosclerosis by means of salutary effects on serum lipids and phosphorus Carbonate salt should be preferable to prevent acidosis
L-Carnitine supplementation	Limited data available
Modification of dialysate types	Use of amino acid-based and icodextrine solutions instead of overuse of glucose-based dialysate solutions

cholesterol level was positively correlated with physical activity, which was estimated as the average number of steps taken per day [57]. Again in contrast to the general population, strenuous exercise programs may not be feasible in the PD population due to increased burden of other chronic diseases.

Sevelamer hydrochloride (SH) is a nonabsorbed calcium and aluminum-free phosphate binder [108]. Several studies showed improvements in lipid profile with use of SH as a phosphate binder in PD patients [109–111]. Evenepoel et al. [110], in a multi-center, open-label prospective study, randomized 143 CAPD patients to SH or calcium acetate treatment for 12 weeks. SH treatment was associated with decreases in total and LDL cholesterol levels. In all these aforementioned studies, SH treatment decreased serum phosphorus levels along with a neutral effect on calcium levels. When it is considered that hyperphosphatemia is also associated with coronary artery calcification in uremic patients [112], SH may have a dual favorable effect on atherosclerosis progression in these patients, namely, improvements in both dyslipidemia and hyperphosphatemia while averting hypercalcemia. However, no study has yet evaluated effects of SH treatment on hard CV outcomes in the PD population.

Carnitine, 3-hydroxy-4-trimethylaminobutyrate, is a small, water-soluble molecule that is essential for mitochondrial fatty acid oxidation. Levels are usually found to be reduced in dialysis patients [113]. A small study in PD patients [114] did not show a significant change in lipid levels with L-carnitine supplementation, whereas another study [105] found a significant decrease in apolipoprotein B levels in pediatric CAPD patients with oral supplementation. Considering the importance of apoB in atherogenesis, larger studies are warranted to investigate the effects of L-carnitine supplementation in PD patients. Table 10.5 summarizes available treatment modalities for treatment of dyslipidemia in PD patients.

A few studies conducted on PD patients showed improved survival with statin use. Lee et al. [115] found that statins were prescribed for 37.8 % of incident PD patients. Cumulative survival probabilities for statin user versus nonuser were 87 % versus 80 % and 76 % versus 69 % at 3 and 5 years, respectively ($P=0.01$).

Goldfarb-Rumyantzev et al. [116] evaluated data from 1,053 incident PD patients from the US Renal Data System prospective Dialysis Morbidity and Mortality Wave 2 study. The authors showed that use of lipid-modifying medications was associated with decreased all-cause and cardiovascular mortality compared with no use of lipid-modifying medications.

Unfortunately, no large RCT has been conducted specifically on PD patients to investigate the effects of statin treatment on clinical CV outcomes and death. A few small RCT included PD patients to evaluate the safety and efficacy of statin treatment. While in three of these trials [117–119] simvastatin was used (10–20 mg/day), one study evaluated the efficacy of atorvastatin at doses of 10–20 mg/day [120]. Cumulatively, these trials recruited only 160 CAPD patients. Overall, these trials showed significant reductions in total and LDL cholesterol and triglyceride concentrations. Only two trials showed modest but significant increase in HDL cholesterol levels compared with placebo. In all these trials adverse events, mainly alterations in liver function tests and creatine kinase levels, were comparable between statin and placebo groups.

In a recent study, Clementi et al. [121] showed that statin treatment reduced LDL as well as small dense LDL, more atherogenic subtype of LDL, in chronic PD patients.

Two small noncontrolled trials [122, 123] evaluated the efficacy and safety of ezetimibe in combination with low-dose simvastatin. In one of these trials, simvastatin 10 mg/day plus ezetimibe 10 mg/day significantly reduced levels of total cholesterol (by a mean of 27 %), triglycerides (by 9 %), and LDL-C (by 33 %) and increased levels of high-density lipoprotein cholesterol (by 15 %).

Pleiotropic effects of statins beyond lipid lowering have also been evaluated in PD patients. Carrion et al. [124] evaluated toxic effects of high glucose (50 and 83 mmol/L) and its reversal by atorvastatin on cultures of rat peritoneal mesothelial cells. Atorvastatin blocked the increase in intracellular reactive oxygen species and prevented glucose-induced increase in caspase-3 activity. In another experimental study, Duman and colleagues [125] showed that atorvastatin improves peritoneal sclerosis induced by hypertonic PD solution in rats. Another study also confirmed beneficial effects of atorvastatin on structural changes in rat peritoneal membrane [126]. Statin therapy in PD patients decreased serum CRP [127, 128] and TNF-alpha [129].

In brief, despite comparable CV mortality rates in PD and HD patients, significantly less data regarding benefits of statin use are present in the PD population compared with HD counterparts. More robust clinical trial data are needed before recommending use of statins in PD patients.

References

1. Longenecker JC, Coresh J, Powe NR, Levey AS, Fink NE, Martin A, et al. Traditional cardiovascular disease risk factors in dialysis patients compared with the general population: the CHOICE Study. J Am Soc Nephrol. 2002;13(7):1918–27.
2. Tonelli M, Wiebe N, Culleton B, House A, Rabbat C, Fok M, et al. Chronic kidney disease and mortality risk: a systematic review. J Am Soc Nephrol. 2006;17(7):2034–47.

3. Attman PO, Samuelsson O, Johansson AC, Moberly JB, Alaupovic P. Dialysis modalities and dyslipidemia. Kidney Int Suppl. 2003;84:S110–2.
4. Liu J, Rosner MH. Lipid abnormalities associated with end-stage renal disease. Semin Dial. 2006;19(1):32–40.
5. Attman PO, Samuelsson OG, Moberly J, Johansson AC, Ljungman S, Weiss LG, et al. Apolipoprotein B-containing lipoproteins in renal failure: the relation to mode of dialysis. Kidney Int. 1999;55(4):1536–42.
6. Shurraw S, Tonelli M. Statins for treatment of dyslipidemia in chronic kidney disease. Perit Dial Int. 2006;26(5):523–39.
7. Deighan CJ, Caslake MJ, McConnell M, Boulton-Jones JM, Packard CJ. Atherogenic lipoprotein phenotype in end-stage renal failure: origin and extent of small dense low-density lipoprotein formation. Am J Kidney Dis. 2000;35(5):852–62.
8. Kronenberg F, Lingenhel A, Neyer U, Lhotta K, Konig P, Auinger M, et al. Prevalence of dyslipidemic risk factors in hemodialysis and CAPD patients. Kidney Int Suppl. 2003;84:S113–6.
9. Yamamoto S, Yancey PG, Ikizler TA, Jerome WG, Kaseda R, Cox B, et al. Dysfunctional high-density lipoprotein in patients on chronic hemodialysis. J Am Coll Cardiol. 2012;60(23): 2372–9.
10. Holzer M, Birner-Gruenberger R, Stojakovic T, El-Gamal D, Binder V, Wadsack C, et al. Uremia alters HDL composition and function. J Am Soc Nephrol. 2011;22(9):1631–41.
11. Mange A, Goux A, Badiou S, Patrier L, Canaud B, Maudelonde T, et al. HDL proteome in hemodialysis patients: a quantitative nanoflow liquid chromatography-tandem mass spectrometry approach. PLoS One. 2012;7(3):e34107.
12. Vaziri ND, Navab K, Gollapudi P, Moradi H, Pahl MV, Barton CH, et al. Salutary effects of hemodialysis on low-density lipoprotein proinflammatory and high-density lipoprotein anti-inflammatory properties in patient with end-stage renal disease. J Natl Med Assoc. 2011;103(6):524–33.
13. Bossola M, Tazza L, Merki E, Giungi S, Luciani G, Miller ER, et al. Oxidized low-density lipoprotein biomarkers in patients with end-stage renal failure: acute effects of hemodialysis. Blood Purif. 2007;25(5–6):457–65.
14. Lippi G, Tessitore N, Salvagno GL, Bedogna V, Bassi A, Montagnana M, et al. Influence of haemodialysis on high-sensitivity C-reactive protein, lipoprotein(a), apolipoproteins A and B. Clin Biochem. 2007;40(16–17):1336–8.
15. Tao J, Sun Y, Li X, Li H, Liu S, Wen Y, et al. Conventional versus ultrapure dialysate for lowering serum lipoprotein(a) levels in patients on long-term hemodialysis: a randomized trial. Int J Artif Organs. 2010;33(5):290–6.
16. Schiffl H, Lang SM, Stratakis D, Fischer R. Effects of ultrapure dialysis fluid on nutritional status and inflammatory parameters. Nephrol Dial Transplant. 2001;16(9):1863–9.
17. Lederer SR, Schiffl H. Ultrapure dialysis fluid lowers the cardiovascular morbidity in patients on maintenance hemodialysis by reducing continuous microinflammation. Nephron. 2002;91(3): 452–5.
18. Susantitaphong P, Riella C, Jaber BL. Effect of ultrapure dialysate on markers of inflammation, oxidative stress, nutrition and anemia parameters: a meta-analysis. Nephrol Dial Transplant. 2013;28(2):438–46.
19. Hsu PY, Lin CL, Yu CC, Chien CC, Hsiau TG, Sun TH, et al. Ultrapure dialysate improves iron utilization and erythropoietin response in chronic hemodialysis patients—a prospective cross-over study. J Nephrol. 2004;17(5):693–700.
20. Izuhara Y, Miyata T, Saito K, Ishikawa N, Kakuta T, Nangaku M, et al. Ultrapure dialysate decreases plasma pentosidine, a marker of "carbonyl stress". Am J Kidney Dis. 2004;43(6): 1024–9.
21. Honda H, Suzuki H, Hosaka N, Hirai Y, Sanada D, Nakamura M, et al. Ultrapure dialysate influences serum myeloperoxidase levels and lipid metabolism. Blood Purif. 2009;28(1):29–39.
22. Ingram AJ, Parbtani A, Churchill DN. Effects of two low-flux cellulose acetate dialysers on plasma lipids and lipoproteins—a cross-over trial. Nephrol Dial Transplant. 1998;13(6):1452–7.

23. Seres DS, Strain GW, Hashim SA, Goldberg IJ, Levin NW. Improvement of plasma lipoprotein profiles during high-flux dialysis. J Am Soc Nephrol. 1993;3(7):1409–15.
24. Kitamura Y, Kamimura K, Yoshioka N, Hosotani Y, Tsuchida K, Koremoto M, et al. The effect of vitamin E-bonded polysulfone membrane dialyzer on a new oxidative lipid marker. J Artif Organs. 2013;16(2):206–10.
25. Goldberg IJ, Kaufman AM, Lavarias VA, Vanni-Reyes T, Levin NW. High flux dialysis membranes improve plasma lipoprotein profiles in patients with end-stage renal disease. Nephrol Dial Transplant. 1996;11 Suppl 2:104–7.
26. Josephson MA, Fellner SK, Dasgupta A. Improved lipid profiles in patients undergoing high-flux hemodialysis. Am J Kidney Dis. 1992;20(4):361–6.
27. Diop ME, Viron B, Bailleul S, Lefevre G, Fessi H, Maury J, et al. Lp(a) is increased in hemodialysis patients according to the type of dialysis membrane: a 2-year follow-up study. Clin Nephrol. 2000;54(3):210–7.
28. House AA, Wells GA, Donnelly JG, Nadler SP, Hebert PC. Randomized trial of high-flux vs low-flux haemodialysis: effects on homocysteine and lipids. Nephrol Dial Transplant. 2000;15(7):1029–34.
29. Elisaf MS, Bairaktari H, Germanos N, Pappas M, Koulouridis E, Papagalanis N, et al. Long-term effects of low molecular weight heparin on lipid parameters in hemodialysis patients. Int Angiol. 1996;15(3):252–6.
30. Vlassopoulos D, Noussias C, Hadjipetrou A, Arvanitis D, Logothetis E, Magana P, et al. Long-term effect of low molecular weight heparin on serum lipids in hypertriglyceridemic chronic hemodialysis patients. J Nephrol. 1997;10(2):111–4.
31. Elisaf MS, Germanos NP, Bairaktari HT, Pappas MB, Koulouridis EI, Siamopoulos KC. Effects of conventional vs. low-molecular-weight heparin on lipid profile in hemodialysis patients. Am J Nephrol. 1997;17(2):153–7.
32. Deuber HJ, Schulz W. Reduced lipid concentrations during four years of dialysis with low molecular weight heparin. Kidney Int. 1991;40(3):496–500.
33. Lai KN, Ho K, Cheung RC, Lit LC, Lee SK, Fung KS, et al. Effect of low molecular weight heparin on bone metabolism and hyperlipidemia in patients on maintenance hemodialysis. Int J Artif Organs. 2001;24(7):447–55.
34. Yang C, Wu T, Huang C. Low molecular weight heparin reduces triglyceride, VLDL and cholesterol/HDL levels in hyperlipidemic diabetic patients on hemodialysis. Am J Nephrol. 1998;18(5):384–90.
35. Wiemer J, Winkler K, Baumstark M, Marz W, Scherberich JE. Influence of low molecular weight heparin compared to conventional heparin for anticoagulation during haemodialysis on low density lipoprotein subclasses. Nephrol Dial Transplant. 2002;17(12):2231–8.
36. Kronenberg F, Konig P, Neyer U, Auinger M, Pribasnig A, Meisl T, et al. Influence of various heparin preparations on lipoproteins in hemodialysis patients: a multicentre study. Thromb Haemost. 1995;74(4):1025–8.
37. Nasstrom B, Stegmayr B, Gupta J, Olivecrona G, Olivecrona T. A single bolus of a low molecular weight heparin to patients on haemodialysis depletes lipoprotein lipase stores and retards triglyceride clearing. Nephrol Dial Transplant. 2005;20(6):1172–9.
38. Persson E. Lipoprotein lipase, hepatic lipase and plasma lipolytic activity. Effects of heparin and a low molecular weight heparin fragment (Fragmin). Acta Med Scand Suppl. 1988;724:1–56.
39. Lowrie EG, Lew NL. Death risk in hemodialysis patients: the predictive value of commonly measured variables and an evaluation of death rate differences between facilities. Am J Kidney Dis. 1990;15(5):458–82.
40. Degoulet P, Legrain M, Reach I, Aime F, Devries C, Rojas P, et al. Mortality risk factors in patients treated by chronic hemodialysis. Report of the Diaphane collaborative study. Nephron. 1982;31(2):103–10.
41. Kalantar-Zadeh K, Block G, Humphreys MH, Kopple JD. Reverse epidemiology of cardiovascular risk factors in maintenance dialysis patients. Kidney Int. 2003;63(3):793–808.
42. Iseki K, Yamazato M, Tozawa M, Takishita S. Hypocholesterolemia is a significant predictor of death in a cohort of chronic hemodialysis patients. Kidney Int. 2002;61(5):1887–93.

43. Bologa RM, Levine DM, Parker TS, Cheigh JS, Serur D, Stenzel KH, et al. Interleukin-6 predicts hypoalbuminemia, hypocholesterolemia, and mortality in hemodialysis patients. Am J Kidney Dis. 1998;32(1):107–14.
44. Liu Y, Coresh J, Eustace JA, Longenecker JC, Jaar B, Fink NE, et al. Association between cholesterol level and mortality in dialysis patients: role of inflammation and malnutrition. JAMA. 2004;291(4):451–9.
45. Kilpatrick RD, McAllister CJ, Kovesdy CP, Derose SF, Kopple JD, Kalantar-Zadeh K. Association between serum lipids and survival in hemodialysis patients and impact of race. J Am Soc Nephrol. 2007;18(1):293–303.
46. Bowden RG, La Bounty P, Shelmadine B, Beaujean AA, Wilson RL, Hebert S. Reverse epidemiology of lipid-death associations in a cohort of end-stage renal disease patients. Nephron Clin Pract. 2011;119(3):c214–9.
47. Noori N, Caulfield MP, Salameh WA, Reitz RE, Nicholas SB, Molnar MZ, et al. Novel lipoprotein subfraction and size measurements in prediction of mortality in maintenance hemodialysis patients. Clin J Am Soc Nephrol. 2011;6(12):2861–70.
48. Echida Y, Ogawa T, Otsuka K, Ando Y, Nitta K. Serum non-high-density lipoprotein cholesterol (non-HDL-C) levels and cardiovascular mortality in chronic hemodialysis patients. Clin Exp Nephrol. 2012;16(5):767–72.
49. Shoji T, Masakane I, Watanabe Y, Iseki K, Tsubakihara Y. Elevated non-high-density lipoprotein cholesterol (non-HDL-C) predicts atherosclerotic cardiovascular events in hemodialysis patients. Clin J Am Soc Nephrol. 2011;6(5):1112–20.
50. de Oliveira CM, Melo SR, Mota AM, Kubrusly M. Non-high-density lipoprotein cholesterol and its correlation with anthropometric markers of cardiovascular risk in hemodialysis. J Ren Nutr. 2012;22(2):251–7.
51. Desmeules S, Arcand-Bosse JF, Bergeron J, Douville P, Agharazii M. Nonfasting non-high-density lipoprotein cholesterol is adequate for lipid management in hemodialysis patients. Am J Kidney Dis. 2005;45(6):1067–72.
52. Executive Summary of The Third Report of The National Cholesterol Education Program (NCEP). Expert panel on detection, evaluation, and treatment of high blood cholesterol in adults (adult treatment panel III). JAMA. 2001;285(19):2486–97.
53. Belani SS, Goldberg AC, Coyne DW. Ability of non-high-density lipoprotein cholesterol and calculated intermediate-density lipoprotein to identify nontraditional lipoprotein subclass risk factors in dialysis patients. Am J Kidney Dis. 2004;43(2):320–9.
54. The USRDS Dialysis Morbidity and Mortality Study: Wave 2. United States Renal Data System. Am J Kidney Dis. 1997;30(2 Suppl 1):S67–85.
55. Prichard SS. Impact of dyslipidemia in end-stage renal disease. J Am Soc Nephrol. 2003;14(9 Suppl 4):S315–20.
56. Gordon L, McGrowder DA, Pena YT, Cabrera E, Lawrence-Wright M. Effect of exercise therapy on lipid parameters in patients with end-stage renal disease on hemodialysis. J Lab Physicians. 2012;4(1):17–23.
57. Masuda R, Imamura H, Mizuuchi K, Miyahara K, Kumagai H, Hirakata H. Physical activity, high-density lipoprotein cholesterol subfractions and lecithin:cholesterol acyltransferase in dialysis patients. Nephron Clin Pract. 2009;111(4):c253–9.
58. Afshar R, Shegarfy L, Shavandi N, Sanavi S. Effects of aerobic exercise and resistance training on lipid profiles and inflammation status in patients on maintenance hemodialysis. Indian J Nephrol. 2010;20(4):185–9.
59. Imamura H, Mizuuchi K, Oshikata R. Physical activity and blood lipids and lipoproteins in dialysis patients. Int J Nephrol. 2012;2012:106914.
60. Wanner C, Krane V, Marz W, Olschewski M, Mann JF, Ruf G, et al. Atorvastatin in patients with type 2 diabetes mellitus undergoing hemodialysis. N Engl J Med. 2005;353(3):238–48.
61. Fellstrom BC, Jardine AG, Schmieder RE, Holdaas H, Bannister K, Beutler J, et al. Rosuvastatin and cardiovascular events in patients undergoing hemodialysis. N Engl J Med. 2009;360(14):1395–407.

62. Baigent C, Landray MJ, Reith C, Emberson J, Wheeler DC, Tomson C, et al. The effects of lowering LDL cholesterol with simvastatin plus ezetimibe in patients with chronic kidney disease (Study of Heart and Renal Protection): a randomised placebo-controlled trial. Lancet. 2011;377(9784):2181–92.
63. Marz W, Genser B, Drechsler C, Krane V, Grammer TB, Ritz E, et al. Atorvastatin and low-density lipoprotein cholesterol in type 2 diabetes mellitus patients on hemodialysis. Clin J Am Soc Nephrol. 2011;6(6):1316–25.
64. Ridker PM, Danielson E, Fonseca FA, Genest J, Gotto Jr AM, Kastelein JJ, et al. Rosuvastatin to prevent vascular events in men and women with elevated C-reactive protein. N Engl J Med. 2008;359(21):2195–207.
65. Epstein M, Vaziri ND. Statins in the management of dyslipidemia associated with chronic kidney disease. Nat Rev Nephrol. 2012;8(4):214–23.
66. Strippoli GF, Craig JC. Sunset for statins after AURORA? N Engl J Med. 2009;360(14):1455–7.
67. Holdaas H, Holme I, Schmieder RE, Jardine AG, Zannad F, Norby GE, et al. Rosuvastatin in diabetic hemodialysis patients. J Am Soc Nephrol. 2011;22(7):1335–41.
68. Hou W, Lv J, Perkovic V, Yang L, Zhao N, Jardine MJ, et al. Effect of statin therapy on cardiovascular and renal outcomes in patients with chronic kidney disease: a systematic review and meta-analysis. Eur Heart J. 2013;34(24):1807–17.
69. K/DOQI. K/DOQI clinical practice guidelines for management of dyslipidemias in patients with kidney disease. Kidney Disease Outcomes Quality Initiative (K/DOQI) Group. Am J Kidney Dis. 2003;41(4 Suppl 3):I–IV, S1–91.
70. KDOQI clinical practice guideline for diabetes and CKD: 2012 update. National Kidney Foundation. Am J Kidney Dis. 2012;60(5):850–86. Erratum in: Am J Kidney Dis. 2013;61(6): 1049.
71. Stevens PE, Levin A. Evaluation and management of chronic kidney disease: synopsis of the kidney disease: improving global outcomes 2012 clinical practice guideline. Ann Intern Med. 2013;158(11):825–30.
72. Argani H, Rahbaninoubar M, Ghorbanihagjo A, Golmohammadi Z, Rashtchizadeh N. Effect of L-carnitine on the serum lipoproteins and HDL-C subclasses in hemodialysis patients. Nephron Clin Pract. 2005;101(4):c174–9.
73. Vesela E, Racek J, Trefil L, Jankovy'ch V, Pojer M. Effect of L-carnitine supplementation in hemodialysis patients. Nephron. 2001;88(3):218–23.
74. Hurot JM, Cucherat M, Haugh M, Fouque D. Effects of L-carnitine supplementation in maintenance hemodialysis patients: a systematic review. J Am Soc Nephrol. 2002;13(3):708–14.
75. Burke SK, Dillon MA, Hemken DE, Rezabek MS, Balwit JM. Meta-analysis of the effect of sevelamer on phosphorus, calcium, PTH, and serum lipids in dialysis patients. Adv Ren Replace Ther. 2003;10(2):133–45.
76. Sniderman AD, Solhpour A, Alam A, Williams K, Sloand JA. Cardiovascular death in dialysis patients: lessons we can learn from AURORA. Clin J Am Soc Nephrol. 2010;5(2):335–40.
77. Schwarz U, Buzello M, Ritz E, Stein G, Raabe G, Wiest G, et al. Morphology of coronary atherosclerotic lesions in patients with end-stage renal failure. Nephrol Dial Transplant. 2000;15(2):218–23.
78. Parfrey PS, Foley RN. The clinical epidemiology of cardiac disease in chronic renal failure. J Am Soc Nephrol. 1999;10(7):1606–15.
79. Ortiz A, Massy ZA, Fliser D, Lindholm B, Wiecek A, Martinez-Castelao A, et al. Clinical usefulness of novel prognostic biomarkers in patients on hemodialysis. Nat Rev Nephrol. 2012;8(3):141–50.
80. Krediet RT, Balafa O. Cardiovascular risk in the peritoneal dialysis patient. Nat Rev Nephrol. 2010;6(8):451–60.
81. U.S. Renal Data System, USRDS 2008 Annual Data Report: Atlas of Chronic Kidney Disease and End-Stage Renal Disease in the United States, National Institutes of Health, National Institute of Diabetes and Digestive and Kidney Diseases, Bethesda, MD; 2008.

82. Kendrick J, Teitelbaum I. Strategies for improving long-term survival in peritoneal dialysis patients. Clin J Am Soc Nephrol. 2010;5(6):1123–31.
83. Piccoli GB, Quarello F, Salomone M, Iadarola GM, Funaro L, Marciello A, et al. Are serum albumin and cholesterol reliable outcome markers in elderly dialysis patients? Nephrol Dial Transplant. 1995;10 Suppl 6:72–7.
84. Sreedhara R, Avram MM, Blanco M, Batish R, Mittman N. Prealbumin is the best nutritional predictor of survival in hemodialysis and peritoneal dialysis. Am J Kidney Dis. 1996;28(6):937–42.
85. Habib AN, Baird BC, Leypoldt JK, Cheung AK, Goldfarb-Rumyantzev AS. The association of lipid levels with mortality in patients on chronic peritoneal dialysis. Nephrol Dial Transplant. 2006;21(10):2881–92.
86. Gault MH, Longerich L, Prabhakaran V, Purchase L. Ischemic heart disease, serum cholesterol, and apolipoproteins in CAPD. ASAIO Trans. 1991;37(3):M513–4.
87. Gamba G, Mejia JL, Saldivar S, Pena JC, Correa-Rotter R. Death risk in CAPD patients. The predictive value of the initial clinical and laboratory variables. Nephron. 1993;65(1):23–7.
88. Iliescu EA, Marcovina SM, Morton AR, Lam M, Koschinsky ML. Apolipoprotein(a) phenotype and lipoprotein(a) level predict peritoneal dialysis patient mortality. Perit Dial Int. 2002;22(4):492–9.
89. Prichard SS. Management of hyperlipidemia in patients on peritoneal dialysis: current approaches. Kidney Int Suppl. 2006;103:S115–7.
90. Walldius G, Jungner I. The apoB/apoA-I ratio: a strong, new risk factor for cardiovascular disease and a target for lipid-lowering therapy—a review of the evidence. J Intern Med. 2006;259(5):493–519.
91. Moberly JB, Attman PO, Samuelsson O, Johansson AC, Knight-Gibson C, Alaupovic P. Alterations in lipoprotein composition in peritoneal dialysis patients. Perit Dial Int. 2002;22(2):220–8.
92. O'Neal D, Lee P, Murphy B, Best J. Low-density lipoprotein particle size distribution in end-stage renal disease treated with hemodialysis or peritoneal dialysis. Am J Kidney Dis. 1996;27(1):84–91.
93. Maggi E, Bellazzi R, Gazo A, Seccia M, Bellomo G. Autoantibodies against oxidatively-modified LDL in uremic patients undergoing dialysis. Kidney Int. 1994;46(3):869–76.
94. Samouilidou EC, Karpouza AP, Kostopoulos V, Bakirtzi T, Pantelias K, Petras D, et al. Lipid abnormalities and oxidized LDL in chronic kidney disease patients on hemodialysis and peritoneal dialysis. Ren Fail. 2012;34(2):160–4.
95. Johansson AC, Samuelsson O, Attman PO, Haraldsson B, Moberly J, Knight-Gibson C, et al. Dyslipidemia in peritoneal dialysis—relation to dialytic variables. Perit Dial Int. 2000;20(3):306–14.
96. Shoji T, Nishizawa Y, Nishitani H, Yamakawa M, Morii H. Roles of hypoalbuminemia and lipoprotein lipase on hyperlipoproteinemia in continuous ambulatory peritoneal dialysis. Metabolism. 1991;40(10):1002–8.
97. Babazono T, Nakamoto H, Kasai K, Kuriyama S, Sugimoto T, Nakayama M, et al. Effects of icodextrin on glycemic and lipid profiles in diabetic patients undergoing peritoneal dialysis. Am J Nephrol. 2007;27(4):409–15.
98. Hiramatsu T, Furuta S, Kakuta H. Favorable changes in lipid metabolism and cardiovascular parameters after icodextrin use in peritoneal dialysis patients. Adv Perit Dial. 2007;23:58–61.
99. Kandoussi A, Cachera C, Reade R, Pagniez D, Fruchart JC, Tacquet A. Apo AIV in plasma and dialysate fluid of CAPD patients: comparison with other apolipoproteins. Nephrol Dial Transplant. 1992;7(10):1026–9.
100. Kagan A, Bar-Khayim Y, Schafer Z, Fainaru M. Kinetics of peritoneal protein loss during CAPD: II. Lipoprotein leakage and its impact on plasma lipid levels. Kidney Int. 1990;37(3):980–90.

101. Steele J, Billington T, Janus E, Moran J. Lipids, lipoproteins and apolipoproteins A-I and B and apolipoprotein losses in continuous ambulatory peritoneal dialysis. Atherosclerosis. 1989;79(1):47–50.
102. Asayama K, Hayashibe H, Mishiku Y, Honda M, Ito H, Nakazawa S. Increased activity of plasma cholesteryl ester transfer protein in children with end-stage renal disease receiving continuous ambulatory peritoneal dialysis. Nephron. 1996;72(2):231–6.
103. Barter PJ, Rye KA. Cholesteryl ester transfer protein inhibition as a strategy to reduce cardiovascular risk. J Lipid Res. 2012;53(9):1755–66.
104. Chatzidimitriou C, Pliakogiannis T, Evangeliou A, Tsalkidou T, Bohles HJ, Kalaitzidis K. Evaluation of carnitine levels according to the peritoneal equilibration test in patients on continuous ambulatory peritoneal dialysis. Perit Dial Int. 1993;13 Suppl 2:S444–7.
105. Kosan C, Sever L, Arisoy N, Caliskan S, Kasapcopur O. Carnitine supplementation improves apolipoprotein B levels in pediatric peritoneal dialysis patients. Pediatr Nephrol. 2003;18(11):1184–8.
106. Kronenberg F, Konig P, Neyer U, Auinger M, Pribasnig A, Lang U, et al. Multicenter study of lipoprotein(a) and apolipoprotein(a) phenotypes in patients with end-stage renal disease treated by hemodialysis or continuous ambulatory peritoneal dialysis. J Am Soc Nephrol. 1995;6(1):110–20.
107. Siamopoulos KC, Elisaf MS, Bairaktari HT, Pappas MB, Sferopoulos GD, Nikolakakis NG. Lipid parameters including lipoprotein (a) in patients undergoing CAPD and hemodialysis. Perit Dial Int. 1995;15(8):342–7.
108. Raggi P, Vukicevic S, Moyses RM, Wesseling K, Spiegel DM. Ten-year experience with sevelamer and calcium salts as phosphate binders. Clin J Am Soc Nephrol. 2010;5 Suppl 1:S31–40.
109. Katopodis KP, Andrikos EK, Gouva CD, Bairaktari ET, Nikolopoulos PM, Takouli LK, et al. Sevelamer hydrochloride versus aluminum hydroxide: effect on serum phosphorus and lipids in CAPD patients. Perit Dial Int. 2006;26(3):320–7.
110. Evenepoel P, Selgas R, Caputo F, Foggensteiner L, Heaf JG, Ortiz A, et al. Efficacy and safety of sevelamer hydrochloride and calcium acetate in patients on peritoneal dialysis. Nephrol Dial Transplant. 2009;24(1):278–85.
111. Ramos R, Moreso F, Borras M, Ponz E, Buades JM, Teixido J, et al. Sevelamer hydrochloride in peritoneal dialysis patients: results of a multicenter cross-sectional study. Perit Dial Int. 2007;27(6):697–701.
112. Qunibi WY. Dyslipidemia and progression of cardiovascular calcification (CVC) in patients with end-stage renal disease (ESRD). Kidney Int Suppl. 2005;95:S43–50.
113. Calo LA, Vertolli U, Davis PA, Savica V. L carnitine in hemodialysis patients. Hemodial Int. 2012;16(3):428–34.
114. Verrina E, Caruso U, Calevo MG, Emma F, Sorino P, De Palo T, et al. Effect of carnitine supplementation on lipid profile and anemia in children on chronic dialysis. Pediatr Nephrol. 2007;22(5):727–33.
115. Lee JE, Oh KH, Choi KH, Kim SB, Kim YS, Do JY, et al. Statin therapy is associated with improved survival in incident peritoneal dialysis patients: propensity-matched comparison. Nephrol Dial Transplant. 2011;26(12):4090–4.
116. Goldfarb-Rumyantzev AS, Habib AN, Baird BC, Barenbaum LL, Cheung AK. The association of lipid-modifying medications with mortality in patients on long-term peritoneal dialysis. Am J Kidney Dis. 2007;50(5):791–802.
117. Saltissi D, Morgan C, Rigby RJ, Westhuyzen J. Safety and efficacy of simvastatin in hypercholesterolemic patients undergoing chronic renal dialysis. Am J Kidney Dis. 2002;39(2):283–90.
118. Baigent C, Landray M, Leaper C, Altmann P, Armitage J, Baxter A, et al. First United Kingdom Heart and Renal Protection (UK-HARP-I) study: biochemical efficacy and safety of simvastatin and safety of low-dose aspirin in chronic kidney disease. Am J Kidney Dis. 2005;45(3):473–84.

119. Robson R, Collins J, Johnson R, Kitching R, Searle M, Walker R, et al. Effects of simvastatin and enalapril on serum lipoprotein concentrations and left ventricular mass in patients on dialysis. The Perfect Study Collaborative Group. J Nephrol. 1997;10(1):33–40.
120. Harris KP, Wheeler DC, Chong CC. A placebo-controlled trial examining atorvastatin in dyslipidemic patients undergoing CAPD. Kidney Int. 2002;61(4):1469–74.
121. Clementi A, Kim JC, Floris M, Cruz DN, Garzotto F, Zanella M, et al. Statin therapy is associated with decreased small, dense low-density lipoprotein levels in patients undergoing peritoneal dialysis. Contrib Nephrol. 2012;178:111–5.
122. Suzuki H, Inoue T, Watanabe Y, Kikuta T, Sato T, Tsuda M. Efficacy and safety of ezetimibe and low-dose simvastatin as primary treatment for dyslipidemia in peritoneal dialysis patients. Adv Perit Dial. 2010;26:53–7.
123. Landray M, Baigent C, Leaper C, Adu D, Altmann P, Armitage J, et al. The second United Kingdom Heart and Renal Protection (UK-HARP-II) Study: a randomized controlled study of the biochemical safety and efficacy of adding ezetimibe to simvastatin as initial therapy among patients with CKD. Am J Kidney Dis. 2006;47(3):385–95.
124. Carrion B, Perez-Martinez FC, Monteagudo S, Perez-Carrion MD, Gomez-Roldan C, Cena V, et al. Atorvastatin reduces high glucose toxicity in rat peritoneal mesothelial cells. Perit Dial Int. 2011;31(3):325–31.
125. Duman S, Sen S, Sozmen EY, Oreopoulos DG. Atorvastatin improves peritoneal sclerosis induced by hypertonic PD solution in rats. Int J Artif Organs. 2005;28(2):170–6.
126. Yenicerioglu Y, Uzelce O, Akar H, Kolatan E, Yilmaz O, Yenisey C, et al. Effects of atorvastatin on development of peritoneal fibrosis in rats on peritoneal dialysis. Ren Fail. 2010;32(9):1095–102.
127. Doh FM, Chang TI, Koo HM, Lee MJ, Shin DH, Kim CH, et al. The effect of HMG-CoA reductase inhibitor on insulin resistance in patients undergoing peritoneal dialysis. Cardiovasc Drugs Ther. 2012;26(6):501–9.
128. Kumar S, Raftery M, Yaqoob M, Fan SL. Anti-inflammatory effects of 3-hydroxy-3-methylglutaryl coenzyme a reductase inhibitors (statins) in peritoneal dialysis patients. Perit Dial Int. 2007;27(3):283–7.
129. Sezer MT, Katirci S, Demir M, Erturk J, Adana S, Kaya S. Short-term effect of simvastatin treatment on inflammatory parameters in peritoneal dialysis patients. Scand J Urol Nephrol. 2007;41(5):436–41.

Chapter 11
Dyslipidemia in the Kidney Transplant Patient

Rajan Kantilal Patel and Alan G. Jardine

Introduction

Renal transplantation (RT) is the optimal treatment for patients with end-stage renal disease (ESRD). Transplant recipients have significantly improved all-cause and cardiovascular (CV) morbidity and mortality compared to patients who receive maintenance hemo- or peritoneal dialysis [1, 2], establishing transplantation as the most desirable method of renal replacement therapy. Over the last 40 years, short- and long-term survival of renal transplant recipients (RTRs) and grafts has improved significantly due to improved surgical techniques and aggressive management of infections [3]. Furthermore, rejection of the transplant is more likely to be recognized and treated with augmentation and optimization of immunosuppressant therapy. Most recent data from the United States Renal Database System (USRDS) for 2012 demonstrated this improved outcome of RTRs with 1-year graft and patient survival rates of 90.9 % and 96.6 %, respectively [4].

Nonetheless, premature CV death remains the commonest cause of mortality in RTRs. According to USRDS data from 2006 to 2010, CV disease was the commonest cause of death (30 % of cases) in patients with a functioning renal transplant (Fig. 11.1) [4]. This greater prevalence of CV disease compared to the general population has been attributed to greater burden of preexisting morbidities (e.g., diabetes mellitus, peripheral vascular and coronary artery disease), and higher prevalence of traditional and novel CV risk factors [5].

R.K. Patel, M.B.Ch.B., Ph.D.
Renal Research Group, Institute of Cardiovascular and Medical Sciences, University of Glasgow, Glasgow, UK

A.G. Jardine, Bs.C., M.D., F.E.S.C., F.E.B.S. (✉)
Institute of Cardiovascular and Medical Sciences, University of Glasgow, 129 University Place, Glasgow G128TA, UK
e-mail: alan.jardine@glasgow.ac.uk

A. Covic et al. (eds.), *Dyslipidemias in Kidney Disease*, DOI 10.1007/978-1-4939-0515-7_11,

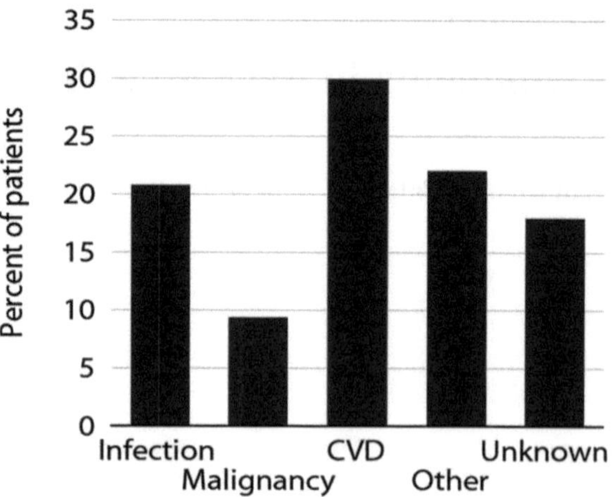

Fig. 11.1 Main causes of death of renal transplant recipients between 2006 and 2010. Data from USRDS [4]

Dyslipidemia is common in RTRs, even when transplant function is normal or reduced, and a result of multiple factors. Moreover, there is good evidence demonstrating an association between dyslipidemia and CV disease in RTRs. Although lipid-lowering agents have been shown to significantly improve all-cause and CV survival in primary and secondary interventional studies of the general population, there is a paucity of studies investigating the effect of treating dyslipidemias in RTRs.

Dyslipidemia in Renal Transplant Recipients

Abnormalities of lipoprotein profiles are common in RTRs. The causes are multifactorial (Fig. 11.2) and the commonest patterns detected are elevated total cholesterol (TC), low-density lipoprotein cholesterol (LDL-C), and triglyceride (TG) levels. Most observational studies have estimated TC levels above 200 mg/dL (5.2 mmol/L) at 12 months after transplantation in 60–90 % of patients. TC levels reach their peak at 3–6 months after transplantation and remain elevated after 12 months. Similarly, LDL-C levels are commonly high (above 100 mg/dL) in greater than 90 % of RTRs after 12 months from their operation. These levels have reduced considerably with the use of newer immunosuppressive regimens and statin therapy. High-density lipoprotein cholesterol (HDL-C) levels vary, and observational studies have demonstrated increased, unchanged, and reduced levels after transplantation. Other changes observed include elevated lipoprotein (a) and apolipoprotein B levels, and altered oxidation of LDL [6].

The causes of dyslipidemia in RTRs can be categorized according to patient and pharmacological features (see Fig. 11.2). Recipient characteristics associated with

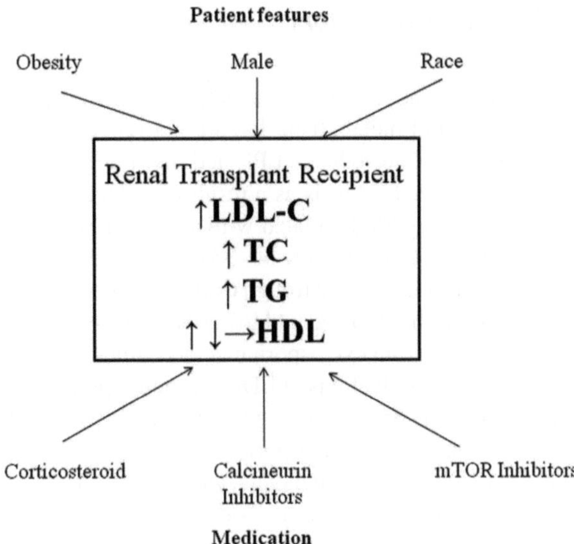

Fig. 11.2 Causes of dyslipidemia and lipid fraction abnormalities found in renal transplant recipients

elevated TC and LDL-C include obesity, African ethnicity, and male sex. Common comorbidities in RTRs, including diabetes mellitus, hypothyroidism, nephrotic syndrome, and chronic liver disease, are also associated with dyslipidemia. Immunosuppressive agents linked with lipid abnormalities include corticosteroids (CS), calcineurin inhibitors (CNIs), and rapamycin.

Corticosteroids

CS induce secondary hyperinsulinemia as a result of impaired insulin sensitivity, which in turn causes reduced lipoprotein lipase (LPL) activity, elevated very low-density lipoprotein (VLDL) synthesis and secretion, and excess TG production. In a number of observational studies, there are significant associations between elevated CS dose and greater levels of TC and LDL-C. Furthermore, immunosuppressive regimens that rapidly withdraw CS therapy have demonstrated improvement in TC and TG levels. In a large ($n=500$), double-blinded study of steroid reduction followed by withdrawal after 12 weeks compared to normal CS dose in RTRs, patients in the withdrawal arm developed lower post-transplant TC (after 12 months withdrawal group 5.60 ± 1.8 vs. control 6.27 ± 1.7, $p<0.01$) and TG compared to the normal CS treatment arm (12 months withdrawal group 1.88 ± 1.1 vs. control 2.16 ± 1.2, $p<0.01$). Unfortunately, biopsy-proven acute rejection (BPAR) was more significantly common in the withdrawal group (at 12 months withdrawal group 25 % vs. control 14 %, $p<0.01$) [7].

Calcineurin Inhibitors

Cyclosporine and, to a lesser extent, tacrolimus therapy are associated with abnormalities of lipid metabolism that are not related to concomitant use of corticosteroid. Cyclosporine reduces LPL activity, bile salt production, and secretion, and increases serum TC levels as a result of reduced LDL-C receptor production. In a study comparing RTRs treated with azathioprine and prednisolone with or without cyclosporine, TC levels were 30–35 mL/dL higher in patients treated with cyclosporine. In addition, elevated trough cyclosporine levels in RTRs are significantly associated with higher LDL-C and lower HDL-C levels [8].

Conversion from cyclosporine to tacrolimus may improve dyslipidemia in RTRs with significant reductions of LDL-C, apolipoprotein B, and TG levels demonstrated [9]. The ELITE-Symphony study compared over 1,600 RTRs randomized to four arms: standard-dose cyclosporine, mycophenolate, and corticosteroids, or daclizumab induction, mycophenolate, and corticosteroids in combination with low-dose tacrolimus, low-dose sirolimus, or low-dose cyclosporine. In this study, patients in the low-dose tacrolimus arm demonstrated significantly reduced development of dyslipidemia compared to low- and standard-dose cyclosporine arms [10].

Mammalian Targets of Rapamycin Inhibitors

Dyslipidemia, especially hypertriglyceridemia, is one of the significant side effects of mammalian targets of rapamycin (mTOR) inhibitor therapy. Sirolimus causes alteration in LPL activity resulting in higher serum levels of TG and VLDL. In RTRs with sirolimus-induced hypertriglyceridemia, there is often reduced catabolism of apoB100-containing lipoprotein. The effect of sirolimus on lipid levels is dose-dependent and is usually highest early after transplantation, when trough levels require to be higher [11]. A number of studies comparing CNI therapy with sirolimus in RTRs have demonstrated significant dyslipidemias that peak around 2 months from conversion/transplantation, with the effect lessening as trough levels fall thereafter. For example, in the CONVERT trial, which compared continuing CNI therapy with conversion from CNI to sirolimus in 830 RTRs with stable graft function, hyperlipidemia was found in 53.5 % of patients in the sirolimus arm compared to 26.4 % of patients who remained on CNIs [12]. Similarly, elevated TC levels were demonstrated in 41.9 % of patients in the sirolimus arm compared to 12.1 % in the CNI one.

Cardiovascular Events and Dyslipidemia in Renal Transplant Recipients

Although recipients of renal transplants have significantly lower rates of CV morbidity and mortality compared to patients who remain on the transplant waiting list [1], RTRs continue to have reduced life expectancy compared to the general population, despite excellent transplant function [2]. Premature CV death remains the leading cause of mortality in RTR, and this has been demonstrated in a number of observational studies from European, US, and CARI renal registries [4, 13]. It is estimated that 50–60 % of deaths with a functioning transplant are due to CV disease, and the commonest cause of graft loss is death with a functioning transplant. Population-based studies from the Australia and New Zealand Dialysis and Transplant registry have demonstrated rates of CV death of 5 per 1,000 patients, which increase with advancing patient age [14].

Studies have attempted to determine associations between dyslipidemia and adverse outcome in RTRs. In a study of 403 RTRs followed for 10 years, independent predictors of developing coronary artery disease included hypercholesterolemia, high LDL-C, male sex, obesity, and smoking [15]. In a similar study of 2,071 RTRs with stable function after a year, higher TG levels were independently associated with adverse cardiac events (fatal and nonfatal; HR 1.122 per 100 mg/dL; 95 % CI 1.033–1.219; $p=0.007$) [16].

The Assessment of Lescol in Renal Transplant (ALERT) trial was a prospective randomized study comparing RTRs, with mean baseline cholesterol of between 154 and 347 mg/dL, treated with fluvastatin or placebo (see below). Post hoc analysis of 1,052 patients recruited to the placebo arm demonstrated a rate of CV death or nonfatal myocardial infarction (MI) of 21.5 per 1,000 patient-years. In addition, independent predictors of myocardial infarction, cardiac death, and non-cardiac death in these patients included serum TC level (HR 1.55 per 50 mg/dL; $p=0.0045$). Taken together, these studies indicate a significant association between dyslipidemia and adverse CV outcome [17, 18].

Treatment of Dyslipidemia in Renal Transplant Recipients

Evidence from the general population has demonstrated improvement of dyslipidemia using lifestyle modifications (e.g., dietary changes, increased physical activity). However, this approach does not improve lipid abnormalities of RTRs, necessitating use of pharmacological agents [19].

Statins

Current evidence suggests that lowering LDL-C can be achieved using HMG Co-A reductase inhibitors. In an early study investigating the effect of fluvastatin on lipid profiles of RTRs, treatment with these statins was associated with an 18 % reduction of TC and 34 % reduction of LDL-C [20]. Similarly, in the fluvastatin treatment arm of the ALERT study, mean LDL-C levels fell by 32 % (38 mg/dL) after a mean follow-up of 5.1 years [17]. In a recent Cochrane review of 16 studies that recruited 3,229 RTRs, statin therapy was significantly associated with a 42.2 mg/dL reduction in TC, 46.2 mg/dL reduction in LDL-C, and 25.5 mg/dL reduction in TGs when compared to placebo. Statin therapy was not associated with significant alteration in HDL-C levels [21].

Cholesterol Uptake Inhibitors

Given the results of the SHARP study, ezetimibe has also been investigated for use in RTRs. In a study of 40 RTRs with stable transplant function, treatment with ezetimibe alone has been associated with reduction in LDL-C and TC by 33 % and 23 %, respectively, with a greater effect if used in combination with statins (reduction of LDL-C of 41 %). In a study of RTRs with poorly controlled TC levels despite maximum-dose statin therapy, addition of ezetimibe therapy significantly reduced TC, LDL-C, and TG levels during 6 months of therapy. However, 14 of the 77 (18.1 %) patients recruited withdrew from the study due to transaminitis or muscle pains [22, 23].

Nicotinic Acid Derivatives

In a small, open-labeled cross-over study of 12 RTRs already receiving lovastatin, 16 weeks of nicotinic acid therapy was associated with a significant reduction in TC, LDL-C, and TG levels, and elevation of HDL-C compared to control values. Unfortunately, these agents are not popular given the high frequency of adverse side effects, including flushing and impaired glucose tolerance [24].

In general, there is a reluctance to prescribe lipid-lowering agents given the high prevalence of drug interactions and subsequent side effects in RTRs. For example, bile acid sequestrants significantly alter the pharmacokinetic properties of CNIs (particularly cyclosporine) while fibrates are associated with an unacceptably high prevalence of rhabdomyolysis and myositis. Hopefully, practice will change with the publication of national and international guidelines directing care of kidney transplant recipients including reducing risk of CV events.

Outcomes of Lowering Lipids in Renal Transplant Recipients

The benefits of lipid-lowering therapy have been clearly demonstrated for primary and secondary CV morbidity and mortality in the general population and cardiac transplant recipients. However, the effect of treating dyslipidemia in RTRs is not clear [25, 26].

Some retrospective studies have demonstrated benefit in treating dyslipidemia in RTRs. In a single-center study of 1,574 RTRs, statin use was significantly associated with patients survival (HR 0.76; CI 0.6–0.96; $p=0.02$) after correction for patient age, transplant age, and serum cholesterol. Similarly, in an observational study of 2,041 first-time RTRs, treatment with statins was independently associated with improved survival (HR 0.64; 95 % CI 0.48–0.86; $p=0.003$) with a significantly improved 12-year patient survival rate (73 % statin users vs. 64 % nonusers = 0.055) [27, 28].

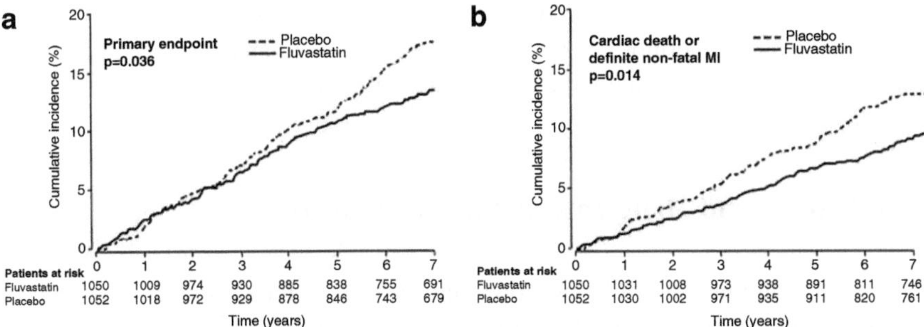

Fig. 11.3 The ALERT study [18] showing the impact of fluvastatin therapy on major cardiac events (primary endpoint) and cardiac death and myocardial infarction (secondary endpoint) in a cohort of renal transplant recipients with stable graft function

The ALERT study remains the largest ($n=2,012$) study to date that prospectively evaluates the benefit of statin therapy in RTRs. This was a randomized, double-blind trial investigating the effect of fluvastatin compared to placebo on the primary endpoint of number of major adverse cardiac events (MACE, defined as cardiac death, nonfatal myocardial infarction, or coronary intervention procedure). After a mean follow-up of 5.1 years, there was a 17 % relative risk reduction in MACE in the treatment arm compared to placebo (Fig. 11.3a; RR 0.83; 95 % CI 0.64–1.06), although this did not reach statistical significance. However, fluvastatin led to a statistically significant relative reduction in the risk of cardiac death or definite nonfatal myocardial infarction (see Fig. 11.3b; HR 0.65; 95 % CI 0.48–0.88). An unblinded extension study demonstrated that fluvastatin therapy was associated with significant reduction of the primary outcome (HR 0.79; 95 % CI 0.63–0.99; $p=0.036$) and cardiac death or nonfatal MI after 6.7 years [17, 18].

Cochrane database review of statin therapy in RTRs included 16 studies comparing treatment with placebo (15 studies) or another statin. Statin therapy did not decrease all-cause mortality (14 studies: RR 1.30; 95 % CI 0.54–3.12). However, CV mortality (13 studies: RR 0.68; 95 % CI 0.46–1.03) and nonfatal cardiovascular events (1 study: RR 0.70; 95 % CI 0.48–1.01) were improved after treatment compared to placebo, although this did not reach statistical significance [21].

Other markers of CV morbidity have been shown to improve after statin therapy, such as carotid artery intimal thickness, brachial artery flow-mediated vasodilatation, and prevalence of transplant vasculopathy on biopsy [29, 30]. The time of statin commencement is associated with different CV outcome. Post hoc analyses of the ALERT cohort demonstrated enhanced benefit of reducing risk of cardiac death and nonfatal MI if statins were started up to 2 years from transplantation compared to commencement greater than 6 years post-op (RR 0.41; 95 % CI 0.2–0.9; $p=0.03$) [31].

There is a weak association between dyslipidemia and adverse transplant function possibly due to development of atherosclerotic vascular disease or reduced acute rejection rates. There is little evidence to suggest preservation of transplant function with statin therapy. Data from the ALERT study did not demonstrate any benefit in statin therapy compared to placebo for graft loss or doubling of serum creatinine [32]. Furthermore, results from Cochrane meta-analysis (see above) did not demonstrate a significant reduction in rates of BPAR (five studies).

Side Effects and Drug Interactions of Statins

In general, administration of lipid-lowering therapy to RTRs remains low due to potential interactions with other medications (especially immunosuppressive agents) and possible poor tolerability.

Most statins (namely atorvastatin, simvastatin, and lovastatin) are metabolized solely by cytochrome P450 (CYP) 3A4 in the liver, which also metabolizes cyclosporine, tacrolimus, and rapamycin. Pravastatin is also a substrate for CYP3A4 but is partially excreted by the kidneys, whereas rosuvastatin is metabolized by CYP2C9 in addition to CYP3A4 [33]. When cyclosporine and statins are used concomitantly, statin levels tend to increase rather than CNI levels. In one study, concomitant use of atorvastatin and cyclosporine was associated with a near sixfold increase in atorvastatin plasma levels [34]. Levels of lovastatin and pravastatin have been shown to increase up to 20-fold when administered with cyclosporine, whereas simvastatin and fluvastatin levels increase to a lesser degree [35]. Although data are limited, tacrolimus has not been shown to significantly affect the levels of statin when they are used together.

In the general population, statin-related side effects include liver toxicity, rhabdomyolysis, and myositis. Initial studies of statin use in RTRs suggested increased rates of adverse side effects, particularly muscular, neoplastic, and infective ones. However, data from the ALERT study demonstrated no significant difference in rates of adverse side effects between statin treatment and placebo arms and demonstrated good tolerability in RTRs [17, 18].

Conclusion

RTRs have significantly poorer CV prognosis compared to the general population and attempts to reduce event rates have targeted traditional and novel CV risk factors. Lipid fractions associated with atherosclerotic cardiovascular disease are also associated with adverse outcome on RTRs. Statin therapy effectively lowers atherogenic lipid levels of RTRs with few drug interactions and good tolerability compared to placebo. Data from the ALERT trial demonstrate benefit to CV survival after treatment of RTR with fluvastatin during the long-term follow-up compared to controls, and are consistent with the effects of statins in the general populations. In general, these agents are well tolerated by RTRs and should be administered to all RTRs with dyslipidemia.

References

1. Wolfe RA, Ashby VB, Milford EL, Ojo AO, Ettenger RE, Agodoa LY, et al. Comparison of mortality in all patients on dialysis, patients on dialysis awaiting transplantation, and recipients of a first cadaveric transplant. N Engl J Med. 1999;341(23):1725–30.
2. Meier-Kriesche HU, Schold JD, Srinivas TR, Reed A, Kaplan B. Kidney transplantation halts cardiovascular disease progression in patients with end-stage renal disease. Am J Transplant. 2004;4(10):1662–8.
3. Nankivell BJ, Alexander SI. Rejection of the kidney allograft. N Engl J Med. 2010;363(15): 1451–62.
4. USRDS 2012 Annual Data Report. 2013. www.usrds.org
5. Jardine AG, Gaston RS, Fellstrom BC, Holdaas H. Prevention of cardiovascular disease in adult recipients of kidney transplants. Lancet. 2011;378(9800):1419–27.
6. Moore R, Thomas D, Morgan E, Wheeler D, Griffin P, Salaman J, et al. Abnormal lipid and lipoprotein profiles following renal transplantation. Transplant Proc. 1993;25(1 Pt 2):1060–1.
7. Vanrenterghem Y, Lebranchu Y, Hene R, Oppenheimer F, Ekberg H. Double-blind comparison of two corticosteroid regimens plus mycophenolate mofetil and cyclosporine for prevention of acute renal allograft rejection. Transplantation. 2000;70(9):1352–9.
8. Kuster GM, Drexel H, Bleisch JA, Rentsch K, Pei P, Binswanger U, et al. Relation of cyclosporine blood levels to adverse effects on lipoproteins. Transplantation. 1994;57(10):1479–83.
9. Artz MA, Boots JM, Ligtenberg G, Roodnat JI, Christiaans MH, Vos PF, et al. Improved cardiovascular risk profile and renal function in renal transplant patients after randomized conversion from cyclosporine to tacrolimus. J Am Soc Nephrol. 2003;14(7):1880–8.
10. Ekberg H, Tedesco-Silva H, Demirbas A, Vitko S, Nashan B, Gurkan A, et al. Reduced exposure to calcineurin inhibitors in renal transplantation. N Engl J Med. 2007;357(25):2562–75.
11. Hoogeveen RC, Ballantyne CM, Pownall HJ, Opekun AR, Hachey DL, Jaffe JS, et al. Effect of sirolimus on the metabolism of apo. Transplantation. 2001;72(7):1244–50.
12. Schena FP, Pascoe MD, Alberu J, del Carmen RM, Oberbauer R, Brennan DC, et al. Conversion from calcineurin inhibitors to sirolimus maintenance therapy in renal allograft recipients: 24-month efficacy and safety results from the CONVERT trial. Transplantation. 2009;87(2): 233–42.
13. Renal Association. 2009. http://www.renal.org/
14. Pilmore H, Dent H, Chang S, McDonald SP, Chadban SJ. Reduction in cardiovascular death after kidney transplantation. Transplantation. 2010;89(7):851–7.
15. Kasiske BL. Risk factors for accelerated atherosclerosis in renal transplant recipients. Am J Med. 1988;84(6):985–92.
16. Vanrenterghem YF, Claes K, Montagnino G, Fieuws S, Maes B, Villa M, et al. Risk factors for cardiovascular events after successful renal transplantation. Transplantation. 2008;85(2):209–16.
17. Holdaas H, Fellstrom B, Jardine AG, Holme I, Nyberg G, Fauchald P, et al. Effect of fluvastatin on cardiac outcomes in renal transplant recipients: a multicentre, randomised, placebo-controlled trial. Lancet. 2003;361(9374):2024–31.
18. Holdaas H, Fellstrom B, Cole E, Nyberg G, Olsson AG, Pedersen TR, et al. Long-term cardiac outcomes in renal transplant recipients receiving fluvastatin: the ALERT extension study. Am J Transplant. 2005;5(12):2929–36.
19. Ong CS, Pollock CA, Caterson RJ, Mahony JF, Waugh DA, Ibels LS. Hyperlipidemia in renal transplant recipients: natural history and response to treatment. Medicine (Baltimore). 1994;73(4):215–23.
20. Ghods AJ, Milanian I, Arghani H, Ghadiri G. The efficacy and safety of fluvastatin in hypercholesterolemia in renal transplant recipients. Transplant Proc. 1995;27(5):2579–80.
21. Navaneethan SD, Perkovic V, Johnson DW, Nigwekar SU, Craig JC, Strippoli GF. HMG CoA reductase inhibitors (statins) for kidney transplant recipients. Cochrane Database Syst Rev. 2009;2, CD005019.

22. Puthenparumpil JJ, Keough-Ryan T, Kiberd M, Lawen J, Kiberd BA. Treatment of hypercholesterolemia with ezetimibe in the kidney transplant population. Transplant Proc. 2005;37(2): 1033–5.
23. Langone AJ, Chuang P. Ezetimibe in renal transplant patients with hyperlipidemia resistant to HMG-CoA reductase inhibitors. Transplantation. 2006;81(5):804–7.
24. Lal SM, Hewett JE, Petroski GF, Van Stone JC, Ross Jr G. Effects of nicotinic acid and lovastatin in renal transplant patients: a prospective, randomized, open-labeled crossover trial. Am J Kidney Dis. 1995;25(4):616–22.
25. Shepherd J, Cobbe SM, Ford I, Isles CG, Lorimer AR, Macfarlane PW, et al. Prevention of coronary heart disease with pravastatin in men with hypercholesterolemia. West of Scotland Coronary Prevention Study Group. N Engl J Med. 1995;333(20):1301–7.
26. Randomised trial of cholesterol lowering in 4444 patients with coronary heart disease: the Scandinavian Simvastatin Survival Study (4S). Lancet. 1994;344(8934):1383–9.
27. Cosio FG, Pesavento TE, Pelletier RP, Henry M, Ferguson RM, Kim S, et al. Patient survival after renal transplantation III: the effects of statins. Am J Kidney Dis. 2002;40(3):638–43.
28. Wiesbauer F, Heinze G, Mitterbauer C, Harnoncourt F, Horl WH, Oberbauer R. Statin use is associated with prolonged survival of renal transplant recipients. J Am Soc Nephrol. 2008;19(11):2211–8.
29. Hausberg M, Kosch M, Stam F, Heidenreich S, Kisters K, Rahn KH, et al. Effect of fluvastatin on endothelium-dependent brachial artery vasodilation in patients after renal transplantation. Kidney Int. 2001;59(4):1473–9.
30. Seron D, Oppenheimer F, Pallardo LM, Lauzurica R, Errasti P, Gomez-Huertas E, et al. Fluvastatin in the prevention of renal transplant vasculopathy: results of a prospective, randomized, double-blind, placebo-controlled trial. Transplantation. 2008;86(1):82–7.
31. Holdaas H, Fellstrom B, Jardine AG, Nyberg G, Gronhagen-Riska C, Madsen S, et al. Beneficial effect of early initiation of lipid-lowering therapy following renal transplantation. Nephrol Dial Transplant. 2005;20(5):974–80.
32. Holdaas H, Fellstrom B, Holme I, Nyberg G, Fauchald P, Jardine A, et al. Effects of fluvastatin on cardiac events in renal transplant patients: ALERT (Assessment of Lescol in Renal Transplantation) study design and baseline data. J Cardiovasc Risk. 2001;8(2):63–71.
33. Kasiske B, Cosio FG, Beto J, Bolton K, Chavers BM, Grimm Jr R, et al. Clinical practice guidelines for managing dyslipidemias in kidney transplant patients: a report from the Managing Dyslipidemias in Chronic Kidney Disease Work Group of the National Kidney Foundation Kidney Disease Outcomes Quality Initiative. Am J Transplant. 2004;4 Suppl 7:13–53.
34. Asberg A, Hartmann A, Fjeldsa E, Bergan S, Holdaas H. Bilateral pharmacokinetic interaction between cyclosporine A and atorvastatin in renal transplant recipients. Am J Transplant. 2001;1(4):382–6.
35. Launay-Vacher V, Izzedine H, Deray G. Statins' dosage in patients with renal failure and cyclosporine drug-drug interactions in transplant recipient patients. Int J Cardiol. 2005;101(1):9–17.

Chapter 12
Dyslipidemia in Nephrotic Syndrome

Minso Kim and Howard Trachtman

Introduction

Kidney disease causes many metabolic disturbances, including abnormal serum lipid levels. These alterations are both the result of the underlying disorder and a contributing factor to the progression of the renal disease (see chapter on this topic in this book). The mechanism and manifestations of dyslipidemia vary depending upon the underlying kidney problem. In this chapter, we review the characteristics, pathophysiology, and treatment of the dyslipidemia observed in patients with nephrotic syndrome (NS), chronic kidney disease (CKD), and diabetic nephropathy.

Nephrotic Syndrome

Characteristics

Hypercholesterolemia is a key characteristic of the nephrotic syndrome. Free and total cholesterol, low-density lipoprotein (LDL), very low-density lipoprotein (VLDL), triglycerides (TG), free fatty acid, and lipoprotein A have been shown

M. Kim, M.D.
Department of Pediatrics, NYU Langone Medical Center, New York, NY, USA
e-mail: Minso.Kim@med.nyu.edu

H. Trachtman, M.D. (✉)
Division of Pediatric Nephrology, Department of Pediatrics, NYU Langone Medical Center, CTSI, Room 110, 227 East 30th Street, New York, NY 10016, USA
e-mail: Howard.Trachtman@nyumc.org

A. Covic et al. (eds.), *Dyslipidemias in Kidney Disease*, DOI 10.1007/978-1-4939-0515-7_12,

Table 12.1 Serum lipid profile in kidney disease

	Nephrotic syndrome	Chronic kidney disease	Diabetic nephropathy
Total cholesterol	↑↑↑	↑	↑
LDL	↑↑↑	↑	±↑
VLDL	↑↑↑	↑	±↑
HDL	↓	↓	↓
TG	↑↑↑	↑↑	↑

to be elevated in animal models of nephrotic syndrome and in patients with NS. Serum high-density lipoprotein (HDL) concentration is decreased, and the proportion of nascent HDL and mature HDL also changes with decreased level of HDL2 and elevated HDL3. The lipid abnormalities associated with nephrotic syndrome can persist even after the patient achieves remission [1, 2] (Table 12.1).

Pathophysiology

Total serum cholesterol concentration in patients with nephrotic syndrome is increased by dysregulation of enzymes and receptors of lipid metabolism pathway at each step of biosynthesis, trafficking, and catabolism of cholesterol.

Biosynthesis of cholesterol is increased by upregulation of acyl-coenzyme A (CoA) cholesterol acyl transferase (ACAT) and subsequent upregulation of 3-hydroxy-3-methylglutaryl-CoA (HMG-CoA) reductase. ACAT catalyzes free cholesterol esterification and subsequent sequestration, which reduces the local free cholesterol pool. This reduction leads to upregulation of HMG-CoA reductase, which enhances cholesterol biosynthesis [3].

The uptake of plasma cholesterol by the liver in nephrotic mice is compromised due to deficiency in the hepatic LDL receptor. Instead of being taken up by the LDL receptors, the cholesterol-containing particles from LDL are increasingly taken up by macrophages. This is enabled by the upregulation of the two key enzymes in the macrophage uptake pathway of fatty acid and oxidized LDL—scavenger receptor class, A-1 (SR-A1) and CD36 [4].

The catabolism of cholesterol is also closely related to the activity of ACAT described above. Cholesterol 7α-hydroxylase, the rate-limiting enzyme in biliary cholesterol secretion, is unchanged in nephrotic syndrome. However, the reduced local free cholesterol pool (from elevated ACAT activity—see above) leads to downregulation of cholesterol 7α-hydroxylase, leading to decreased clearance of cholesterol.

In addition to the overall elevation of the total serum cholesterol concentration, TG and LDL levels are also elevated in nephrotic syndrome. TG metabolism is disrupted in mice with nephrotic syndrome due to impaired clearance of chylomicrons and other TG-rich lipoproteins. Chylomicron and VLDL undergo lipolysis of fatty acids, which is catalyzed by lipoprotein lipase and hepatic lipase. Both lipases are impaired in nephrotic syndrome [5, 6], leading to hypertriglyceridemia. Nephrotic syndrome also upregulates hepatic diacylglyceride acyl transferase (DGAT), which increases endogenous production of TG and compounds the disturbance in TG levels [7].

Similarly, the conversion from intermediate-density lipoproteins (IDL) to LDL involves removal of TG and lipolysis by hepatic lipase. The TG in IDL are exchanged for cholesterol ester on mature HDL by cholesterol ester transfer protein (CETP), and the TG removed from IDL are hydrolyzed by the hepatic lipase. The activity of CETP is elevated in nephrotic syndrome, which leads to increased transformation of IDL to LDL. In addition to the increased production, clearance of LDL is compromised in nephrotic syndrome due to the hepatic LDL receptor deficiency.

The level of HDL may be normal or even slightly elevated in nephrotic syndrome; however, the function and composition of HDL are disrupted. Reverse cholesterol transport is one of the major protective mechanisms of HDL against atherosclerosis and this process is impaired at multiple levels in nephrotic syndrome. Reverse cholesterol transport is a pathway by which cholesterol is taken up from the vessel wall, transported to the liver, and finally excreted by the hepatic cells. It begins with cholesterol efflux where cholesterol is taken up from macrophages in the vessel wall and then collected by nascent HDL. Lecithin-cholesterol acyl transferase (LCAT) is essential in esterification of the cholesterol so that it can be carried by HDL. Nascent HDL (HDL3), once loaded with cholesterol ester, becomes mature HDL (HDL2). Cholesterol ester-rich HDL2 then docks itself to the docking receptor of liver, scavenger receptor B-1 (SRB-1), to unload its lipid cargo [8].

In nephrotic syndrome, LCAT is excreted with other proteins to urine, resulting in diminished concentration and activities of LCAT. This leads to impaired esterification of cholesterol and decreased cholesterol uptake by nascent HDL. This results in reduced mature HDL concentration. This is evidenced by the reduced ratio of mature-to-nascent HDL (HDL2/HDL3) found in multiple studies of patients with nephrotic syndrome. This relative decrease in HDL2 leads to reduced sequestration of intracellular cholesterol.

Moreover, HDL2 is involved in transport of apolipoprotein (apo) C and apoE to nascent VLDL and chylomicrons so that the apolipoproteins can activate lipoprotein lipase and consequent catabolism of VLDL and chylomicrons. The reduction in HDL2 in nephrotic syndrome diminishes this conversion from nascent to mature VLDL, leading to overall increased VLDL level.

In addition, the hepatic HDL receptor SRB-1 is significantly decreased in nephrotic syndrome, which makes it difficult for the remaining mature HDL to unload its cholesterol ester to the liver [8]. The mRNA of SRB-1 is not affected by the nephrotic syndrome; however, expression of PDZK1, a molecule essential for transport and anchoring of SRB-1 to the hepatocyte plasma membrane, is downregulated in nephrotic syndrome, resulting in decreased SRB-1 abundance [9]. The pathways involved in the pathogenesis of dyslipidemia in nephrotic syndrome are illustrated in Fig. 12.1.

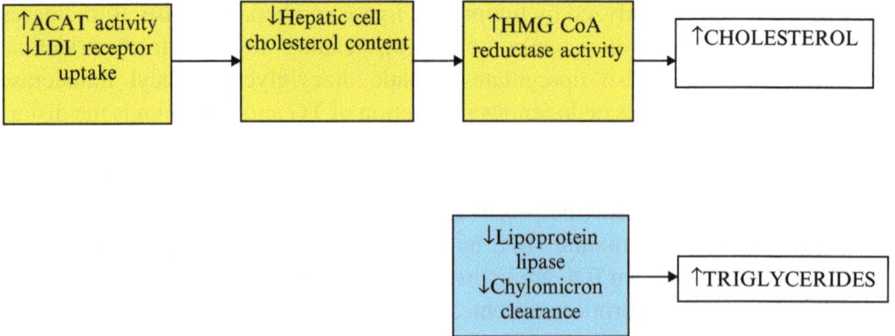

Fig. 12.1 Illustration of mechanisms involved in the pathogenesis of dyslipidemia in patients with nephrotic syndrome. *Yellow fill* indicates alterations in synthesis and *blue fill* indicates defects in clearance. *ACAT* acyl-coenzyme A cholesterol acyl transferase, *HMG CoA* 3-hydroxy-3-methylglutaryl-coenzyme A

Table 12.2 Treatment of dyslipidemias in kidney disease

	Nephrotic syndrome	Chronic kidney disease	Diabetic nephropathy
Diet	+	+	+
Statins	+++	++ Benefit uncertain with ESKD	++
Fibrates	?	+ Caution in advanced stages due to drug accumulation and muscle toxicity	+ May lower risk of CV events and slow progression of nephropathy
Niacin	?	?	?

Symbols: +, mild effect; ++, moderate effect; +++, strong effect; ?, unknown effect

Treatment

Based on the pathophysiology outlined above, the treatment of dyslipidemia in patients with nephrotic syndrome has been largely targeted at the key enzymes of the lipid metabolism (Table 12.2).

Statins are generally used as a first line of treatment. As discussed above, nephrotic syndrome upregulates the hepatic HMG-CoA reductase. In normal physiologic status, HMG-CoA reductase would be expected to be downregulated in response to hypercholesterolemia. HMG-CoA reductase inhibition improves hepatic LDL and HDL receptor deficiencies documented in animals with nephrotic syndrome and ameliorated the associated hyperlipidemia [10].

HMG-CoA reductase inhibitors have been shown to be effective in lowering the lipids in multiple studies, including 2-week treatment of nephrotic mice with rosuvastatin [11] and 6-week treatment of mice with simvastatin [12]. Statin therapy has been repeatedly demonstrated to lower plasma cholesterol, TG, LDL, and VLDL in nephrotic syndrome. Lp(a)-derived cholesterol was an exception to this therapeutic effect, although the mechanism of which is unclear. Thus, Valdivielso et al. showed that in a small group of ten patients with primary or secondary nephrotic syndrome, the addition of 10 mg atorvastatin daily for 6 months resulted in a 41 % reduction in LDL-cholesterol and 31 % in triglycerides (both $P<0.05$), and a 15 % increase in HDL-cholesterol (NS) [13].

Statins have demonstrated short-term safety and efficacy in the pediatric patients with nephrotic syndrome. Implementing treatment with this class of drugs is capable of safely reducing total cholesterol up to 42 %, LDL-C up to 46 %, and triglyceride levels up to 44 % [14]. Pravastatin effectively lowers LDL in adult patients with nephrotic syndrome who have isolated hypercholesterolemia or in combination with high triglyceride levels [15]. Extended treatment with the liver-selective agent, fluvastatin, resulted in a 31 % reduction in total cholesterol and 29 % in LDL-cholesterol [16]. This indicates that the beneficial effect of statins in nephrotic syndrome can be safely sustained for an extended period without incurring significant side effects. In addition, the beneficial changes in serum lipids achieved with statin therapy are paralleled by improved endothelial vasodilation, assessed by post-ischemia brachial artery flow-mediated dilation [17].

The pleiotropic effects of statins in patients with nephrotic syndrome are vast and a full review is beyond the depth of this particular chapter. In brief, statins inhibit proliferation of the mesangial cells, which confers protection of kidney from glomerulosclerosis and any renal injury secondary to inflammation from hypercholesterolemia. Some of the other non-lipid effects include inhibition of renal tubular epithelial, smooth muscle, and mesangial cell proliferation; anti-inflammation by reducing glutathione peroxidase and superoxide dismutase; immunomodulation by inhibiting production of tumor necrosis factor (TNF)-α and eNOS; neovascularization; reduction of endothelial fibrinolytic potential; improvement of endothelial vasodilation; reduction of arterial blood pressure; and inhibition of osteoclastic activities [18].

An ACAT inhibitor may be useful in the treatment of dyslipidemia in nephrotic syndrome. In rats with puromycin aminonucleoside nephropathy, 2 weeks of treatment with ACAT inhibitor CI-976 versus placebo yielded reduced plasma cholesterol, TG, total cholesterol–HDL ratio, hepatic ACAT activity, near-normalized plasma LCAT, hepatic SRB-1, LDL receptor, and amelioration of proteinuria and hypoalbuminemia [8].

Administration of antithrombin for 10 days resulted in a decreased TG, total cholesterol, LDL, and VLDL levels, improvement in tubular cast and tubular expansion, suppression of tubular epithelial apoptosis, and decrease in renal cytokine in this same model. L-Carnitine given orally for 15 days resulted in a partial reduction in serum TG and cholesterol levels without complete normalization.

Dietary changes are a key element in the treatment of dyslipidemia in patients who have normal kidney function and have been prescribed for those with nephrotic syndrome. In animals with nephrotic syndrome, soy protein intake reduced HMG-CoA reductase and LDL receptor while lowering total cholesterol, TG, VLDL-TG, and LDL-cholesterol in comparison to the control nephrotic mice fed with 20 % casein diet [19].

This intervention also reduced the gene expression of SREBP-1 [19]. However, the effect of soy protein intake has not been evaluated in the treatment of patients with nephrotic syndrome and dyslipidemia.

A variety of herbs and natural compounds have been prescribed to lower hyperlipidemia in patients with nephrotic syndrome. Macrothelypteris torresiana was administered for 9 weeks with modest effect [20]. Probucol is another agent used to treat dyslipidemia in nephrotic syndrome in a study of 14 children with nephrotic syndrome; this drug yielded a decline in mean serum triglycerides (−15 %), total cholesterol (−25 %), VLDL-cholesterol (−27 %), LDL-cholesterol (−23 %), and HDL-cholesterol (−24 %), as well as apoA-1 (−19 %), apoB (−21 %), and MDA (−32 %) that were maintained over 24 weeks of treatment [21]. The positive effects of probucol on the lipoprotein profile were not associated with any significant change in either proteinuria or GFR.

Antiproteinuric therapy has been proposed to ameliorate hyperlipidemia in patients with nephrotic syndrome by reducing the extent of the defect in glomerular permselectivity. Treatment of Imai rats that develop spontaneous FSGS and nephrotic syndrome with the angiotensin converting enzyme inhibitor, losartan, and pravastatin results in complete resolution of proteinuria and hypercholesterolemia [22]. Similarly, a robust reduction in proteinuria with renoprotective agents, such as losartan, can result in a reduction in LDL-cholesterol due to a decrease in CETP mass [23]. In a study of 28 patients with nondiabetic kidney disease, upward titration of dose of the angiotensin converting enzyme inhibitor, lisinopril, to maximum tolerated doses safely ameliorated hypercholesterolemia through amelioration of the nephrotic syndrome, particularly in patients with more severe hypoalbuminemia and lowered hypertriglyceridemia in a dose-dependent manner [24].

A number of miscellaneous treatments have been tried to correct the dyslipidemia in nephrotic syndrome. Activation of lipoprotein lipase corrects hyperlipidemia and preserves renal function in experimental adriamycin nephropathy [25]. However, this approach to therapy is unavailable in clinical practice. LDL apheresis, originally used for the management of familial hyperlipidemia, has been used in Japan for the treatment of patients with nephrotic syndrome and dyslipidemia due to steroid-resistant focal segmental glomerulosclerosis (FSGS) [26]. The device has been safely utilized and achieved complete or partial remission of disease with restoration of normal serum cholesterol and triglyceride concentrations in 62 % and 87 % of patients after 2 and 5 years of follow-up, respectively [27].

A wide range of alternative and complementary medications have been used to correct the hyperlipidemia observed in nephrotic syndrome. These include ginger given as a capsule 3 g/day to adults [28].

Chronic Kidney Disease

Characteristics

Dyslipidemia in patients with CKD shows differing patterns based on their stage and accompanying proteinuria [29]. However, there is no consistent pattern of lipid abnormalities among the different clinical strata of CKD. With decreasing kidney function there is generally a consistent rise in serum TG levels due to the accumulation of TG-enriched apoB particles and a decrease in serum HDL. Moreover, the lipid levels change if there is concomitant nephrotic-range proteinuria or if renal replacement therapy is initiated (hemodialysis or peritoneal dialysis). Patients with mild to moderate CKD and proteinuria have elevated total cholesterol and LDL levels. However, total and LDL-cholesterol levels are not as uniformly elevated in patients with CKD as in those with nephrotic-range proteinuria. Patients with end-stage kidney disease (ESKD) on peritoneal dialysis also show the same pattern, likely due to the large-volume protein loss similar to proteinuria. The level of LDL and total cholesterol normalizes in ESKD patients on hemodialysis, while TG, VLDL, small dense LDL, and IDL are elevated. HDL and serum apoA-1 are significantly reduced in all stages of CKD [30]. However, there is a poor correlation between absolute HDL levels and clinical outcomes in patients with CKD. This has raised the possibility that alteration in HDL composition, metabolism, and function may contribute more to cardiovascular (CV) risk associated with CKD compared to otherwise healthy patients [31]. For example, HDL isolated from patients with CKD has reduced capacity to promote reverse cholesterol transport and efflux from cells compared to the fraction obtained from healthy controls [32]. Similarly, HDL samples from CKD patients promote an inflammatory response in macrophages with enhanced release of interleukin-1β, IL-6, and TNF-α [33]. These functional disturbances are not consistently normalized by statin treatment and may account for the limited therapeutic efficacy of these agents in patients with CKD (see below) (see Table 12.1).

With advanced CKD, mortality is often associated with low cholesterol levels that may reflect concomitant malnutrition and ongoing low-grade systemic inflammation. It is unlikely that high cholesterol levels are actually protective in patients with advanced CKD and more work is needed to clarify the interaction between serum cholesterol, inflammation, and nutritional status and mortality.

Pathophysiology

Unlike in nephrotic syndrome, where cholesterol production is increased and clearance is decreased, cholesterol levels in CKD depend solely on the degree of impairment of lipid clearance as cholesterol production remains unchanged [34]. The serum concentrations of TG, VLDL, and LDL in CKD are determined by their clearance rate.

In VLDL and chylomicron metabolism of CKD, lipoprotein lipase, hepatic lipase, VLDL receptor, and LDL receptor-related protein are all downregulated. Under physiologic conditions, lipoprotein lipase binds to capillary endothelium where it catalyzes lipolysis of VLDL. Glycosylphosphatidylinositol-anchored binding protein 1 (GPIHBP1) anchors lipoprotein lipase to the capillary endothelium and facilitates attachment of chylomicron as well. This key protein is downregulated in CKD, which may contribute to lipoprotein lipase deficiency [35].

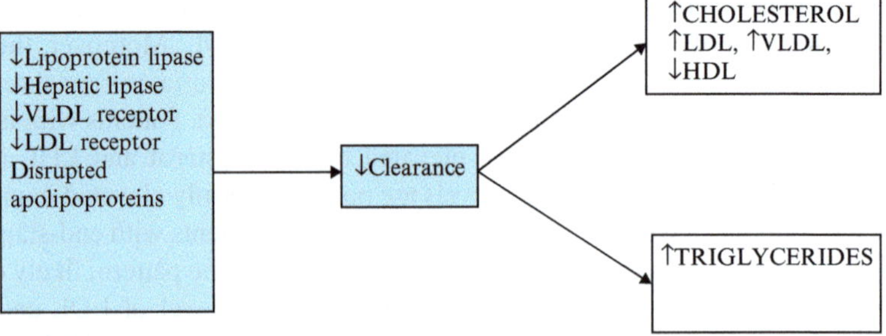

Fig. 12.2 Illustration of mechanisms involved in the pathogenesis of dyslipidemia in patients with chronic kidney disease. *Blue fill* indicates defect in clearance. *LDL* low-density lipoprotein, *VLDL* very low-density lipoprotein, *HDL* high-density lipoprotein

Apolipoproteins are also disrupted in CKD, partaking in the impaired clearance. apoCIII is increased while apoCII is decreased in VLDL, resulting in decreased activation of lipoprotein lipase. apoE is also reduced in VLDL, which makes it difficult to bind to the capillary endothelium and VLDL receptor [29].

LDL metabolism in CKD is affected by the change in hepatic lipase. The expression and activity of hepatic lipase are reduced in CKD, leading to accumulation of IDL and triglyceride.

As mentioned above, the concentration and function of HDL are both severely impaired in CKD. The principal constituent in HDL is apoA-1, which normally participates in disposal of oxidized fatty acids and phospholipids in conjunction with LCAT. The deficiency of apoA-1 found in CKD decreases HDL production [36]. LCAT activity and concentration are also decreased in CKD similar to those of nephrotic kidneys, where HDL maturation is impaired due to diminished esterification of cholesterol by LCAT [29]. In addition to the impaired reverse cholesterol transport, HDL's function as antioxidant is also compromised in CKD [36]. Key antioxidant components of HDL—paraoxonase and glutathione peroxidase—activities are both decreased in CKD patients. The pathophysiological pathways involved in the pathogenesis of dyslipidemia in CKD are illustrated in Fig. 12.2.

In addition to derangements caused by the underlying disease process, iatrogenic problems such as repeated heparinization during hemodialysis treatments can degrade and deplete lipoprotein lipase, worsening hypertriglyceridemia.

Treatment

Statins are generally the first line of therapy for treatment of dyslipidemia in patients with CKD because of their confirmed ability to lower LDL and their safety and tolerability in the general population [37] (see Table 12.2). A recent meta-analysis involving 21,295 participants in studies done between 1966 and 2013 has confirmed that use of statins in patients with CKD who are not on dialysis resulted in a significant reduction in all-cause mortality (relative risk 0.66), cardiac deaths (relative risk 0.69), cardiovascular events (relative risk 0.55), and stroke (relative risk 0.66) [38].

Atorvastatin is the most widely prescribed agent in this class. Both atorvastatin and rosuvostatin have a longer half-life compared to other statins, which provides pharmacokinetic justification for preferred use of these drugs [39]. Newer agents have also been utilized in clinical practice and pitavastatin has been administered safely to lower serum lipid levels. Interestingly, it also resulted in a 5 mL/min/1.73 m^2 increase in GFR when prescribed for a 2-year period to a subgroup of 958 adults with initial GFR <60 mL/min/1.73 m^2 [40]. Although they are generally effective for this indication, the reduction in serum cholesterol and TG levels is generally lower in patients with renal disease compared to primary prevention in otherwise healthy patients [41]. The major controversy surrounding use of statins is whether they reduce cardiovascular (CV) and all-cause mortality in the CKD subgroup as effectively as in the general population and in patients with cardiovascular disease (CVD). In these latter two groups, clinical trials of statins have achieved a 30 % reduction in the relative risk of major coronary events. CV risk gradually increases with increasing stages of CKD and is highest in patients receiving renal replacement therapy. The uncertainty about statins in CKD stems from generally negative studies of statin use to correct hyperlipidemia and reduce the risk of CVD in patients on dialysis. Thus, in the 4D and AURORA studies, lipid lowering with atorvastatin or rosuvostatin, or simvastatin, respectively, lowered LDL levels but had no favorable impact on the primary cardiovascular end point in each study [42, 43].

In the SHARP clinical trial, which evaluated the efficacy of a combination of simvastatin and ezetimibe in a broad spectrum of patients with CKD (3,023 on dialysis and 6,247 who were not on dialysis), there was a significant decline in LDL levels and a 17 % reduction in major cardiovascular events. However, there was no favorable impact on mortality. The protective effect against cardiovascular events was primarily observed in patients not yet on dialysis, but there was minimal effect on the rate of progression of CKD. Finally, it is unclear if the benefit documented in the SHARP trial was due to the statin, ezetimibe, or the drug combination [44, 45]. Therefore, it is imperative to identify whether CKD patients benefit from alteration of lipid fractions and how to best achieve this objective. However, there is recent evidence that pretreatment LDL-cholesterol levels and changes in response to therapy may be less useful as a marker of CVD in patients with CKD than in the general population [46].

In light of experimental evidence suggesting that dyslipidemia is a factor promoting worsening renal function, treatment with statins may be worthwhile in patients with CKD for their renoprotective effects [47]. This would be consistent with the hypothesis that lipid nephrotoxicity contributes to the progressive decline in kidney function in a wide range of conditions including obesity, hypertension, and atherosclerosis [30]. The Lipid lowering and Onset of Renal Disease (LORD) study, which enrolled 132 patients, documented a trend towards a slower rate of progressive decline in renal function in patients with CKD who received atorvastatin for 2.5 years [48]. Additional studies will be needed to clarify this important aspect of the optimal clinical management of CKD.

Fibrates have been used as an alternative to statins in patients with CKD. Although gemfibrozil can lower serum TG levels as effectively as atorvastatin, neither drug had a favorable effect on endothelial dysfunction and only the stain reduced small artery stiffness [49]. However, fibrates are eliminated by the kidney and some authorities suggest not using fibrates in patients with reduced GFR, specifically those with CKD stage 4 to avoid drug accumulation and muscle toxicity [50]. Despite this caution, fibrates are a useful adjunctive treatment when used with proper precautions such as avoidance of statin–fibrate combination therapy and appropriate dose modification as GFR declines [51]. A recent meta-analysis concluded that administration of fibrates has a place in the management of patients with CKD (GFR <60 mL/min/1.73 m^2). The treatment leads to an improvement in lipid profiles and prevents cardiovascular events. A beneficial effect on clinically relevant renal endpoints remains to be proven [52].

Niacin is another alternative to treat the lipid abnormalities and to treat hyperphosphatemia in CKD. There is preclinical evidence to support this therapy as a lipid-lowering, anti-inflammatory, and renoprotective agent [53]. However, there is a paucity of data and well-designed studies are needed to assess the efficacy of niacin for this indication in patients with CKD [54]. The pharmacokinetics of niacin are altered in patients with CKD and dose modification is required to minimize the risk of side effects like flushing [55].

Diabetic Nephropathy

Characteristics

Hyperglycemia results in hypercholesterolemia and accentuates its subsequent damage to kidney [56]. Unlike nephrotic and nephritic disease, the overall level of LDL may be normal or slightly high; however, the proportion of small dense LDL is increased which hold higher risk for atherosclerosis. TG levels are also elevated while HDL is decreased (see Table 12.1).

Pathophysiology

Hyperglycemia causes glycation, namely posttranslational attachment of glucose to protein or lipid molecules. The resulting products of this attachment are called advanced glycation end-products (AGEs). When apolipoproteins and LDL undergo glycation, the resulting modified lipids become more susceptible to oxidation [56]. AGE-modified protein in itself exacerbates inflammation and vascular remodeling, which will be further discussed in detail later in this chapter. When this is applied to lipids, its kinetics of clearance is significantly changed as described below.

Glycation of LDL occurs near its receptor binding site, leading to lower affinity to LDL receptor. AGE peptides also bind to LDL, further impairing LDL receptor-mediated clearance and resulting in elevated serum LDL concentration. Aside from glycation, LDL particle sizes also become smaller. These small, dense LDL particles are known to be more atherogenic [57]. A similar pattern occurs in VLDL. Glycated VLDL does not bind to lipoprotein lipase as well and, as a result, lipolysis

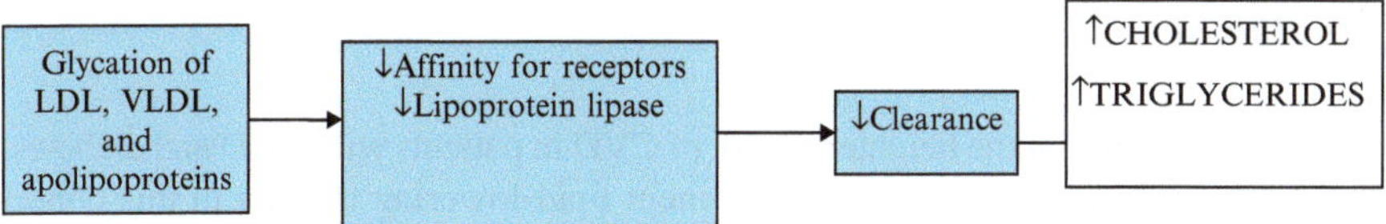

Fig. 12.3 Illustration of mechanisms involved in the pathogenesis of dyslipidemia in patients with diabetic nephropathy. *Blue fill* indicates defect in clearance. *LDL* low-density lipoprotein, *VLDL* very low-density lipoprotein

of triglyceride is compromised and serum VLDL and triglyceride levels increase [56]. This is confirmed by human studies which showed decreased lipoprotein lipase activities and hypertriglyceridemia in diabetics [58]. As the TG-rich lipoprotein is increased, more cholesterol is required to be transferred from HDL, resulting in decreased HDL level.

For diabetic nephropathy, it is vital to understand the vicious cyclical nature of renal disease and dyslipidemia. We have discussed how renal disease leads to dyslipidemia thus far; in addition, dyslipidemia causes further renal injury via inflammation and subsequent vascular remodeling. This secondary injury is particularly accentuated in diabetic kidneys.

In nephrotic syndrome or CKD, renal damage mediated by dyslipidemia occurs at the level of tubulointerstitial cells and mesangium [47, 59]. Reabsorption of the lipids—fatty acids, phospholipids, and cholesterol—with lipoprotein by tubulointerstitial cells leads to tubulointerstitial inflammation. Accumulation of lipoprotein in glomerular mesangium leads to glomerulosclerosis via matrix formation. Similar changes occur in diabetic kidneys at an accelerated pace.

Oxidized lipoproteins are abundant in diabetic nephropathy due to the impaired LDL clearance as discussed above. Exposure to such lipoproteins promotes cytokine and chemokine secretion by mesangial cells and subsequent recruitment of macrophages [60]. The recruited macrophages take up oxidized LDLs and become foam cells, which release more cytokines such as TGF-β1 and platelet-derived growth factor-AB. These proliferative and prosclerotic cytokines lead to extracellular matrix protein production, resulting in mesangial expansion and thickening of the glomerular basement membrane. The TGF-β1 and macrophage infiltration also damage the tubular interstitium via inflammation in local area. Angiotensin II contributes to this process [60]. Angiotensin II increases pressure at the glomerular capillary level, which increases the glomerular permeability of macromolecules including mesangial lipids. Chemokines and cytokines, also released via angiotensin II-triggered pathway, help infiltration of macrophages and accumulation of the permeated lipids to macrophages.

AGE-receptors for AGE (RAGE) play a unique role in diabetic nephropathy by amplifying the renal injury. AGEs that are formed on lipids and proteins bind to receptors, activate growth factors and cytokines, and promote extracellular matrix synthesis and inhibit its degradation. The pathways involved in the pathogenesis of dyslipidemia in diabetic nephropathy are illustrated in Fig. 12.3.

Treatment

In general, because of the heightened risk of CVD in patients with CKD and diabetes, the general recommendation is to implement lipid-lowering therapy in this cohort with a target LDL concentration of 70 mg/dL [61]. This guideline is reinforced because hyperlipidemia contributes to the microvascular complications of diabetes including nephropathy [62]. Similar to other patients with CKD, statins are generally the first-line therapy in these patients (see Table 12.2). In a study of 40 patients with type 2 diabetes, rosuvastatin lowered serum LDL-cholesterol levels in conjunction with a reduction in serum retinol-binding protein (RBP)-4, an insulin-resistant adipokine [63]. Fluvastatin is an alternative agent that is effective and well tolerated in patients with CKD and diabetic nephropathy [64]. Simvastatin treatment reduces serum lipoprotein-phospholipase A2 and lyso-phosphatidylcholine content in LDL. This may be important because lipoprotein-phospholipase A2 may have enhanced pro-atherogenic activity in patients with diabetic nephropathy by promoting the production of lyso-phosphatidylcholine in circulating LDL [65]. The limited efficacy of statins in patients with diabetic nephropathy may be because statins are unable to completely correct hypertriglyceridemia and low HDL-cholesterol. This has justified clinical use of peroxisome proliferator-activated receptor (PPAR)-α agonists, which include fibrates [66]. In a study of 314 patients with type 2 diabetes and early nephropathy with microalbuminuria, treatment with fenofibrate for over 3 years reduced the rate percentage of patients who progressed to macroalbuminuria from 18 to 8 % [67]. The Fenofibrate Intervention and Event Lowering in Diabetes (FIELD) study evaluated 9,795 participants aged 50–75 years with type 2 diabetes who were treated with fenofibrate 200 mg daily or matching placebo for a median of 5 years [68]. Treatment with fenofibrate (versus placebo) resulted in significantly fewer total cardiovascular events, the pre-specified secondary outcome for subgroup analyses. Fenofibrate treatment also was associated with a significant reduction in the proportion of participants who had progression of albuminuria, from normal to micro- or macroalbuminuria. However, patients with renal impairment, defined as a plasma creatinine level >130 μmol/L, were excluded from the study. The ACCORD study also examined the impact of fibrates in patients with type 2 diabetes but excluded patients with CKD [69]. The further addition of polyunsaturated n-3 fatty acids to a statin–fibrate combination yielded an incremental 28 % reduction in serum TG levels [70]. Overall, at present based on the available published information, it is not possible to confirm the safety of fibrates in patients with diabetes and CKD.

Colestimide, a new anion exchange resin, has been used successfully to lower lipid levels in a 12-week study of patients with type 2 diabetes [63]. Diacylglycerol oil has been tested to treat dyslipidemias in patients with diabetes but the results have not been confirmed [71]. A soy protein diet has been used in short-term studies (14 weeks) and effectively lowers total and LDL-cholesterol and TG levels [72]. Interestingly, in contrast to other causes of CKD, there are no published reports describing the use of niacin to treat hyperlipidemia in patients with diabetic nephropathy.

Disordered sphingolipid metabolism has been documented in patients with diabetes and future interventions that target this pathway may lead to improvements in dyslipidemia and renal function [73].

Conclusion

Dyslipidemia is a prominent feature in the full spectrum of kidney disease. However, it is important to recognize the differences in pathogenesis of the lipid disturbances in specific renal conditions because this impacts on the exact phenotype of the abnormal serum lipid profile and the anticipated response to treatment. Improved approaches to the management of dyslipidemia in kidney may be beneficial to both slow the rate of progressive decline in kidney function and prevent the serous cardiovascular consequences of chronic renal disease.

Hypercholesterolemia in nephrotic syndrome is associated with and largely due to acquired LDL receptor (LDLR) deficiency. PCSK9 (proprotein convertase subtilisin/kexin type 9) promotes degradation of LDLR, raising the possibility that elevation of LDL cholesterol levels in patients with nephrotic syndrome and PD patients may be due to increased PCSK9 levels. In a study of 15 patients with nephrotic syndrome, the mean serum total and LDL cholesterol levels in patients with nephrotic syndrome (317.9 ± 104.2 [SD] and 205.9 ± 91.1 mg/dL) were significantly ($P<0.05$) higher than in the control group (166.5 ± 26.5 and 95.9 ± 25.2 mg/dL). This was associated with significantly ($P<0.05$) higher plasma PCSK9 levels in patients with nephrotic syndrome (15.13 ± 4.99 ng/mL) than in the control (9.19 ± 0.60 ng/mL) patients. Plasma PCSK9 level was directly related to total and LDL cholesterol concentrations in the study population ($r=0.559$ [$P<0.001$] and $r=0.497$ [$P<0.001$], respectively). Thus, the nephrotic syndrome is associated with a higher plasma PCSK9 concentration, which can contribute to elevation of LDL levels by promoting LDLR deficiency [74].

References

1. Mérouani A, Lévy E, Mongeau JG, Robitaille P, Lambert M, Delvin EE. Hyperlipidemic profiles during remission in childhood idiopathic nephrotic syndrome. Clin Biochem. 2003;36: 571–4.
2. Kronenberg F. Dyslipidemia and nephrotic syndrome: recent advances. J Ren Nutr. 2005;15(2):195–203.
3. Vaziri ND, Liang K. Up-regulation of acyl coenzyme A:cholesterol acyltransferase (ACAT) in nephrotic syndrome. Kidney Int. 2002;61:1769–75.
4. Kim HJ, Vaziri ND. Sterol regulatory element-binding proteins, liver X receptor, ABCA1 transporter, CD36, scavenger receptors A1 and B1 in nephrotic kidney. Am J Nephrol. 2009;29:607–14.
5. Liang K, Vaziri ND. Gene expression of lipoprotein lipase in experimental nephrosis. J Lab Clin Med. 1997;130(4):387–94.

6. Liang K, Vaziri ND. Down-regulation of hepatic lipase expression in experimental nephrotic syndrome. Kidney Int. 1997;51(6):1933–7.
7. Vaziri ND, Kim CH, Phan D, Kim S, Liang K. Up-regulation of hepatic acyl CoA: diacylglycerol acyltransferase-1 (DGAT-1) expression in nephrotic syndrome. Kidney Int. 2004;66:262–7.
8. Vaziri ND, Liang KH. Acyl-coenzyme A: cholesterol acyltransferase inhibition ameliorates proteinuria, hyperlipidemia, lecithin-cholesterol acyltransferase, SRB-1, and low-density lipoprotein receptor deficiencies in nephrotic syndrome. Circulation. 2004;110:419–25.
9. Vaziri ND, Gollapudi P, Han S, Farahmand G, Yuan J, Rahimi A, Moradi H. Nephrotic syndrome causes upregulation of HDL endocytic receptor and PDZK-1-dependent downregulation of HDL docking receptor. Nephrol Dial Transplant. 2011;26:3118–23.
10. Vaziri ND, Liang K. Effects of HMG-CoA reductase inhibition on hepatic expression of key cholesterol-regulatory enzymes and receptors in nephrotic syndrome. Am J Nephrol. 2004;24:606–13.
11. Kim S, Kim CH, Vaziri ND. Upregulation of hepatic LDL receptor-related protein in nephrotic syndrome: response to statin therapy. Am J Physiol Endocrinol Metab. 2004;288:E813–7.
12. Sonmez A, Yilmaz MI, Korkmaz A, Topal T, Caglar K, Kaya A, et al. Hyperbaric oxygen treatment augments the efficacy of cilazapril and simvastatin regimens in an experimental nephrotic syndrome model. Clin Exp Nephrol. 2008;12(2):110–8.
13. Valdivielso P, Moliz M, Valera A, Corrales MA, Sanchez-Chaparro MA, Gonzalez-Santos P. Atorvastatin in dyslipidaemia of the nephrotic syndrome. Nephrology (Carlton). 2003;8:61–4.
14. Prescott Jr WA, Streetman DA, Streetman DS. The potential role of HMG-CoA reductase inhibitors in pediatric nephrotic syndrome. Ann Pharmacother. 2004;38:2105–14.
15. Toto RD, Grundy SM, Vega GL. Pravastatin treatment of very low density, intermediate density and low density lipoproteins in hypercholesterolemia and combined hyperlipidemia secondary to the nephrotic syndrome. Am J Nephrol. 2000;20:12–7.
16. Matzkies FK, Bahner U, Teschner M, Hohage H, Heidland A, Schaefer RM. Efficiency of 1-year treatment with fluvastatin in hyperlipidemic patients with nephrotic syndrome. Am J Nephrol. 1999;19(4):492–4.
17. Dogra GK, Watts GF, Herrmann S, Thomas MA, Irish AB. Statin therapy improves brachial artery endothelial function in nephrotic syndrome. Kidney Int. 2002;62:550–7.
18. Buemi M, Nostro L, Crascì E, Barillà A, Cosentini V, Aloisi C, Sofi T, Campo S, Frisina N. Statins in nephrotic syndrome: a new weapon against tissue injury. Med Res Rev. 2005;25(6):587–609.
19. Tovar AR, Murguía F, Cruz C, Hernández-Pando R, Aguilar-Salinas CA, Pedraza-Chaverri J, et al. A soy protein diet alters hepatic lipid metabolism gene expression and reduces serum lipids and renal fibrogenic cytokines in rats with chronic nephrotic syndrome. J Nutr. 2002;132:2562–9.
20. Chen J, Lei Y, Wu G, Zhang Y, Fu W, Xiong C, Ruan J. Renoprotective potential of Macrothelypteris torresiana via ameliorating oxidative stress and proinflammatory cytokines. J Ethnopharmacol. 2012;139(1):207–13.
21. Querfeld U, Kohl B, Fiehn W, Minor T, Michalk D, Schärer K, et al. Probucol for treatment of hyperlipidemia in persistent childhood nephrotic syndrome. Report of a prospective uncontrolled multicenter study. Pediatr Nephrol. 1999;13:7–12.
22. Rodríguez-Iturbe B, Sato T, Quiroz Y, Vaziri ND. AT-1 receptor blockade prevents proteinuria, renal failure, hyperlipidemia, and glomerulosclerosis in the Imai rat. Kidney Int. 2004;66:668–75.
23. Krikken JA, Waanders F, Dallinga-Thie GM, Dikkeschei LD, Vogt L, Navis GJ, et al. Antiproteinuric therapy decreases LDL-cholesterol as well as HDL-cholesterol in non-diabetic proteinuric patients: relationships with cholesteryl ester transfer protein mass and adiponectin. Expert Opin Ther Targets. 2009;13:497–504.
24. Ruggenenti P, Mise N, Pisoni R, Arnoldi F, Pezzotta A, Perna A, et al. Diverse effects of increasing lisinopril doses on lipid abnormalities in chronic nephropathies. Circulation. 2003;107:586–92.
25. Nakayama K, Hara T, Kusunoki M, Tsutsumi K, Minami A, Okada K, et al. Effect of the lipoprotein lipase activator NO-1886 on adriamycin-induced nephrotic syndrome in rats. Metabolism. 2000;49:588–93.

26. Kobayashi S. Applications of LDL-apheresis in nephrology. Clin Exp Nephrol. 2008;12:9–15.
27. Muso E, Mune M, Yorioka N, Nishizawa Y, Hirano T, Hattori M, et al. Beneficial effect of low-density lipoprotein apheresis (LDL-A) on refractory nephrotic syndrome (NS) due to focal glomerulosclerosis (FSGS). Clin Nephrol. 2007;67:341–4.
28. Alizadeh-Navaei R, Roozbeh F, Saravi M, Pouramir M, Jalali F, Moghadamnia AA. Investigation of the effect of ginger on the lipid levels. A double blind controlled clinical trial. Saudi Med J. 2008;29:1280–4.
29. Vaziri ND, Norris K. Lipid disorders and their relevance to outcomes in chronic kidney disease. Blood Purif. 2011;31:189–96.
30. Heymann EP, Kassimatis TI, Goldsmith DJA. Dyslipidemia, statins, and CKD patients' outcomes—review of the evidence in the post-sharp era. J Nephrol. 2012;25(4):460–72.
31. Kon V, Ikizler TA, Fazio S. Importance of high-density lipoprotein quality: evidence from chronic kidney disease. Curr Opin Nephrol Hypertens. 2013;22:259–65.
32. Yamamoto S, Yancey PG, Ikizler TA, Jerome WG, Kaseda R, Cox B, et al. Dysfunctional high-density lipoprotein in patients on chronic hemodialysis. J Am Coll Cardiol. 2012;60(23): 2372–9.
33. Weichhart T, Kopecky C, Kubicek M, Haidinger M, Döller D, Katholnig K, et al. Serum amyloid A in uremic HDL promotes inflammation. J Am Soc Nephrol. 2012;23(5):934–47.
34. Vaziri ND, Dang B, Zhan CD, Liang K. Downregulation of hepatic acyl-CoA:diglycerol acyltransferase (DGAT) in chronic renal failure. Am J Physiol Renal Physiol. 2004;287:F90–4.
35. Vaziri ND, Yuan J, Ni Z, Nicholas SB, Norris KC. Lipoprotein lipase deficiency in chronic kidney disease is accompanied by down-regulation of endothelial GPIHBP1 expression. Clin Exp Nephrol. 2012;16:238–43.
36. Moradi H, Phal MV, Elahimehr R, Vaziri ND. Impaired antioxidant activity of high-density lipoprotein in chronic kidney disease. Transl Res. 2009;153(2):77–85.
37. Olyaei A, Greer E, Delos Santos R, Rueda J. The efficacy and safety of the 3-hydroxy-3-methylglutaryl-CoA reductase inhibitors in chronic kidney disease, dialysis, and transplant patients. Clin J Am Soc Nephrol. 2011;6(3):664–78.
38. Barylski M, Nikfar S, Mikhailidis DP, Toth PP, Salari P, Ray KK, et al. Lipid and Blood Pressure Meta-Analysis Collaboration Group. Statins decrease all-cause mortality only in CKD patients not requiring dialysis therapy—a meta-analysis of 11 randomized controlled trials involving 21,295 participants. Pharmacol Res. 2013;72:35–44.
39. Neuvonen PJ, Backman JT, Niemi M. Pharmacokinetic comparison of the potential over-the-counter statins simvastatin, lovastatin, fluvastatin and pravastatin. Clin Pharmacokinet. 2008;47(7):463–74.
40. Kimura K, Shimano H, Yokote K, Urashima M, Teramoto T. Effects of pitavastatin (LIVALO tablet) on the estimated glomerular filtration rate (eGFR) in hypercholesterolemic patients with chronic kidney disease. Sub-analysis of the LIVALO Effectiveness and Safety (LIVES) Study. J Atheroscler Thromb. 2010;17(6):601–9.
41. Sheng X, Murphy MJ, MacDonald TM, Wei L. The comparative effectiveness of statin therapy in selected chronic diseases compared with the remaining population. BMC Public Health. 2012;12:712. doi:10.1186/1471-2458-12-712.
42. Wanner C, Krane V, März W, Olschewski M, Mann JF, Ruf G, Ritz E. German Diabetes and Dialysis Study Investigators. Atorvastatin in patients with type 2 diabetes mellitus undergoing hemodialysis. N Engl J Med. 2005;353(3):238–48.
43. Fellström BC, Jardine AG, Schmieder RE, Holdaas H, Bannister K, Beutler J, et al. AURORA Study Group. Rosuvastatin and cardiovascular events in patients undergoing hemodialysis. N Engl J Med. 2009;360(14):1395–407.
44. Sharp Collaborative Group. Study of Heart and Renal Protection (SHARP): randomized trial to assess the effects of lowering low-density lipoprotein cholesterol among 9,438 patients with chronic kidney disease. Am Heart J. 2010;160(5):785–94.
45. Baigent C, Landray MJ, Reith C, Emberson J, Wheeler DC, Tomson C, et al. SHARP Investigators. The effects of lowering LDL cholesterol with simvastatin plus ezetimibe in patients with chronic kidney disease (Study of Heart and Renal Protection): a randomised placebo-controlled trial. Lancet. 2011;377(9784):2181–92.

46. Tonelli M, Muntner P, Lloyd A, Manns B, Klarenbach S, Pannu N, et al.; for the Alberta Kidney Disease Network. Association between LDL-C and risk of myocardial infarction in CKD. J Am Soc Nephrol. 2013;24:979–86.
47. Gyebi L, Soltani Z, Reisin E. Lipid nephrotoxicity: new concept for an old disease. Curr Hypertens Rep. 2012;14:177–81.
48. Fassett RG, Robertson IK, Ball MJ, Geraghty DP, Coombes JS. Effect of atorvastatin on kidney function in chronic kidney disease: a randomised double-blind placebo-controlled trial. Atherosclerosis. 2010;213(1):218–24.
49. Dogra G, Irish A, Chan D, Watts G. A randomized trial of the effect of statin and fibrate therapy on arterial function in CKD. Am J Kidney Dis. 2007;49(6):776–85.
50. Lewis D, Wanner C. Diabetes: should we use fibrates in patients with diabetes and mild CKD? Nat Rev Nephrol. 2012;8(4):201–2.
51. Harper CR, Jacobson TA. Managing dyslipidemia in chronic kidney disease. J Am Coll Cardiol. 2008;51(25):2375–84.
52. Jun M, Zhu B, Tonelli M, Jardine MJ, Patel A, Neal B, et al. Effects of fibrates in kidney disease: a systematic review and meta-analysis. J Am Coll Cardiol. 2012;60(20):2061–71.
53. Cho KH, Kim HJ, Rodriguez-Iturbe B, Vaziri ND. Niacin ameliorates oxidative stress, inflammation, proteinuria, and hypertension in rats with chronic renal failure. Am J Physiol Renal Physiol. 2009;297(1):F106–13.
54. Ahmed MH. Niacin as potential treatment for dyslipidemia and hyperphosphatemia associated with chronic renal failure: the need for clinical trials. Ren Fail. 2010;32(5):642–6.
55. Reiche I, Westphal S, Martens-Lobenhoffer J, Tröger U, Luley C, Bode-Böger SM. Pharmacokinetics and dose recommendations of Niaspan® in chronic kidney disease and dialysis patients. Nephrol Dial Transplant. 2011;26(1):276–82.
56. Veiraiah A. Hyperglycemia, lipoprotein glycation, and vascular disease. Angiology. 2005;56(4):431–8.
57. Hahr AJ, Molitch ME. Diabetes, cardiovascular risk and nephropathy. Cardiol Clin. 2010;28(3):467–75.
58. Pruneta-Deloche V, Sassolas A, Dallinga-Thie GM, Berthezene F, Ponsin G, Moulin P. Alteration in lipoprotein lipase activity bound to triglyceride-rich lipoproteins in the postprandial state in type 2 diabetes. J Lipid Res. 2004;45(5):859–65.
59. Vaziri ND. Dyslipidemia of chronic renal failure: the nature, mechanisms, and potential consequences. Am J Physiol Renal Physiol. 2006;290:F262–72.
60. Rosario RF, Prabhakar S. Lipids and diabetic nephropathy. Curr Diab Rep. 2006;6:455–62.
61. Molitch ME. Management of dyslipidemias in patients with diabetes and CKD. Clin J Am Soc Nephrol. 2006;1(5):1090–9.
62. Misra A, Kumar S, Kishore Vikram N, Kumar A. The role of lipids in the development of diabetic microvascular complications: implications for therapy. Am J Cardiovasc Drugs. 2003;3(5):325–38.
63. Takebayashi K, Suetsugu M, Matsumoto S, Aso Y, Inukai T. Effects of rosuvastatin and colestimide on metabolic parameters and urinary monocyte chemoattractant protein-1 in type 2 diabetic patients with hyperlipidemia. South Med J. 2009;102(4):361–8.
64. Yasuda G, Kuji T, Hasegawa K, Ogawa N, Shimura G, Ando D, et al. Safety and efficacy of fluvastatin in hyperlipidemic patients with chronic renal disease. Ren Fail. 2004;26(4):411–8.
65. Iwase M, Sonoki K, Sasaki N, Ohdo S, Higuchi S, Hattori H, et al. Lysophosphatidylcholine contents in plasma LDL in patients with type 2 diabetes mellitus: relation with lipoprotein-associated phospholipase A2 and effects of simvastatin treatment. Atherosclerosis. 2008;196(2):931–6.
66. Staels B, Maes M, Zambon A. Fibrates and future PPARalpha agonists in the treatment of cardiovascular disease. Nat Clin Pract Cardiovasc Med. 2008;5(9):542–53.
67. Ansquer JC, Foucher C, Rattier S, Taskinen MR, Steiner G. DAIS Investigators. Fenofibrate reduces progression to microalbuminuria over 3 years in a placebo-controlled study in type 2 diabetes: results from the Diabetes Atherosclerosis Intervention Study (DAIS). Am J Kidney Dis. 2005;45(3):485–93.

68. Keech AC, Simes RJ, Barter P, Best J, Scott R, Taskinen MR, et al. FIELD Study Investigators. Effects of long-term fenofibrate therapy on cardiovascular events in 9795 people with type 2 diabetes mellitus (the FIELD study): randomized controlled trial. Lancet. 2005;366:1849–61.
69. The ACCORD Study Group. Effects of combination lipid therapy in type 2 diabetes mellitus. N Engl J Med. 2010;362:1563–74.
70. Zeman M, Zák A, Vecka M, Tvrzická E, Písaríková A, Stanková B. N-3 fatty acid supplementation decreases plasma homocysteine in diabetic dyslipidemia treated with statin-fibrate combination. J Nutr Biochem. 2006;17(6):379–84.
71. Yamamoto K, Tomonobu K, Asakawa H, Tokunaga K, Hase T, Tokimitsu I, et al. Diet therapy with diacylglycerol oil delays the progression of renal failure in type 2 diabetic patients with nephropathy. Diabetes Care. 2006;29(2):417–9.
72. Azadbakht L, Shakerhosseini R, Atabak S, Jamshidian M, Mehrabi Y, Esmaill-Zadeh A. Beneficiary effect of dietary soy protein on lowering plasma levels of lipid and improving kidney function in type II diabetes with nephropathy. Eur J Clin Nutr. 2003;57(10):1292–4.
73. Fox TE, Kester M. Therapeutic strategies for diabetes and complications: a role for sphingolipids. Adv Exp Med Biol. 2010;688:206–16.
74. Jin K, Park BS, Kim YW, Vaziri ND. Plasma PCSK9 in nephrotic syndrome and in peritoneal dialysis: a cross-sectional study. Am J Kidney Dis. 2013. doi:10.1053/j.ajkd.2013.10.042. [Epub ahead of print].

Chapter 13
Dyslipidemias in the Pediatric Chronic Kidney Disease Patient

Zeynep Birsin Özçakar and Fatoş Yalçınkaya

Dyslipidemias in Patients with Nephrotic Syndrome

Introduction

Nephrotic syndrome (NS) is among the most common types of kidney diseases seen in children, and its incidence varies with age, race, and geography. The annual incidence in children in the United States and in Europe has been estimated to be 1–3 per 100,000 with a cumulative prevalence of 16 per 100,000 children [1, 2]. It is characterized by massive proteinuria, hypoalbuminemia, hyperlipidemia, and edema. Although NS most often occurs as a primary disorder in children, it can also be associated with systemic illnesses. Structural and functional abnormalities in the glomerular filtration barrier resulting in severe proteinuria are responsible for the clinical manifestations of NS. Minimal change NS is the most common form of idiopathic NS, accounting for more than 90 % of cases; other types, such as focal segmental glomerulosclerosis (FSGS) and membranoproliferative glomerulonephritis, are seen rarely [3]. It is more appropriate to categorize childhood NS according to response to steroid therapy, because renal biopsy is usually not performed in patients who respond to steroid therapy. Response to steroid therapy carries a greater prognostic weight than the histological findings on initial biopsy. Thus, two types of NS can be defined in the childhood period: steroid-responsive NS, in which the proteinuria rapidly resolves with therapy, and steroid-resistant NS, in which steroids do not induce remission [4]. It is estimated that about 80 % of children with idiopathic NS will respond to corticosteroid treatment with complete resolution of

Z.B. Özçakar (✉) • F. Yalçınkaya
Division of Pediatric Nephrology and Rheumatology, Department of Pediatrics, Ankara University School of Medicine, Ankara Üniversitesi Tıp Fakültesi, Cebeci Kampüsü, Çocuk Sağlığı ve Hastalıkları A.D. Dikimevi, Ankara 06100, Turkey
e-mail: zbozcakar@yahoo.com; fyalcin@medicine.ankara.edu.tr

A. Covic et al. (eds.), *Dyslipidemias in Kidney Disease*, DOI 10.1007/978-1-4939-0515-7_13,

proteinuria and edema. Among this steroid-responsive group, the clinical course is variable, with up to 60 % having frequent relapses or becoming dependent on steroid therapy to maintain them in remission. Both of these groups are at increased risk of developing complications of NS and complications from frequent use of steroid and other immunosuppressive agents. On the other hand, the steroid-resistant group had significantly higher risk for development of complications of the disease, as well as progression of the disease to chronic kidney disease (CKD) and end-stage renal failure [5].

Hyperlipidemia is an almost universal finding in children with NS. In plasma, lipids are bound to lipoproteins, and the disturbances in lipid metabolism in NS result in increased levels of lipoproteins (hyperlipoproteinemia) and remodeling of the composition of lipoproteins (dyslipoproteinemia). The lipid profile is characterized by elevations in total plasma cholesterol, very low-density lipoprotein (VLDL), and low-density lipoprotein (LDL) cholesterol, and often triglyceride levels, as well as variable alterations (more often decreased) in high-density lipoprotein (HDL) cholesterol [6]. In addition, significant increases in plasma levels of lipoprotein(a), which is known to be both atherogenic and thrombogenic, are also often seen in children with proteinuria [7].

The definition of dyslipidemia differs in children and adults. The National Cholesterol Education Program pediatric report recommended that in order to identify children and adolescents with abnormal lipid and lipoprotein concentrations, total cholesterol concentrations of >200 mg/dL and LDL concentrations of >130 mg/dL be considered elevated [8]. The American Heart Association has recommended that triglyceride concentrations of >150 mg/dL and HDL concentrations of <35 mg/dL be considered abnormal for children and adolescents [9]. Owing to the concerns for using the same cut points for all children, percentile values for total cholesterol, triglycerides, LDL, and HDL cholesterol concentrations according to age and gender were developed in the 1981 prevalence study of the Lipid Research Clinics Program from the National Institute of Health [10]. Hyperlipidemia in children is defined as lipid levels greater than the 95th percentile for age and gender. For example, LDL concentrations greater than the 95th percentile (or HDL concentration less than the 5th percentile) would be considered abnormal, particularly if the abnormality was insistent. LDL concentrations between the 90th and 95th percentiles (5th–10th for HDL concentration) would be considered borderline. Clinical effects of natural changes in lipid and lipoprotein concentrations with age will be reduced with the use of these tables and percentiles [11].

Epidemiology

Almost all patients with NS or nephrotic range proteinuria have elevated total cholesterol levels, although some exceptions do occur (e.g., in glomerulonephritis). The plasma cholesterol concentration shows an inverse hyperbolic correlation with plasma albumin, accompanied by a steep rise in triglycerides in patients with severe hypoalbuminemia [12]. In patients with steroid-sensitive NS, hyperlipidemia resolves gradually upon developing a remission, whereas children with steroid-resistant NS who are refractory to therapy are often exposed to prolonged hyperlipidemia and its associated risks [13]. Moreover, it was shown that children with frequently relapsing NS have prolonged periods of hypercholesterolemia, even during clinical remission [14]. Merouani et al. [15] compared plasma lipid profiles of 25 children with NS at remission, with or without active prednisone treatment, with those of an age-matched population. Plasma total and LDL cholesterol were above normal in 12 of the 25 patients (48 %), with 7 of them having apolipoprotein B and triglyceride concentrations above normal. Hyperlipidemic profiles correlated significantly with number of relapse episodes.

Causes and Pathogenesis

Pathophysiology of nephrotic dyslipoproteinemia is multifactorial, including both an increased hepatic synthesis and a diminished plasma catabolism of lipoproteins [6]. Since its details have been mentioned in the "Dyslipidemia in Nephrotic Syndrome" chapter, herein, we do not further discuss the pertinent pathophysiology.

Clinical Implications

As early as 1969, Berlyne and Mallick reported an 85 times greater incidence of ischemic heart disease in adult patients with NS [16]. The question whether nephrotic hyperlipidemia is a cardiovascular (CV) risk factor for the patients is studied further exclusively in adults. In nephrotic children, there is only anecdotal evidence of myocardial infarction or documented atherosclerosis [17–19]. Antikainen et al. [20] investigated the arterial pathologies in renal arteries collected at nephrectomy in congenital NS of Finnish-type patients. They concluded that the vascular pathology, together with altered lipoprotein metabolism, indicates that children with congenital NS might have early atherosclerotic arterial disease risk. In an autopsy study of 40 children with NS due to mixed renal disease, a significantly increased incidence of mild to severe atherosclerotic changes were found when compared with 29 matched controls who died of non-renal causes [21]. These patients frequently have additional risk factors for ischemic events besides hyperlipidemia, such as hypertension, steroid-induced obesity, and insulin resistance, which may act together to produce atherosclerotic vascular lesions. Lechner et al. [22] evaluated if relapsing childhood NS would predispose patients to develop cardiovascular (CV) disease as young adults, in 62 patients between 25 and 53 years of age who had steroid responsive-dependent NS during childhood. They found that the occurrence of cardiovascular mortality is similar to that of the general population; and suggest that steroid-responsive NS during childhood is not a risk factor for cardiovascular events in early adulthood in the absence of traditional risk factors.

Therapy-resistant NS almost invariably leads to progressive renal insufficiency, which is histologically characterized by progressive glomerulosclerosis and tubulointersititial fibrosis. This development is driven by pathological mechanisms analogous to atherosclerosis, regarded by many investigators as an active process [23–25]. There is also evidence that hyperlipidemia contributes to the progression of renal insufficiency in nephrotic patients. This was first shown in animal experiments with cholesterol-rich diets that induced focal sclerosis in strains of guinea pigs, rats, and rabbits [26]. Lipid-lowering drugs reduced proteinuria and the development of focal sclerosis, and retarded the progression of established glomerular disease in rats [27]. Muntner et al. [28] studied the relationship between plasma lipids and decreasing renal function in 12,728 patients in their Atherosclerosis Risk in Communities Study and found that HDL, HDL-2 cholesterol, and triglycerides appeared to be predictors of creatinine increase. Thus, experimental and clinical evidence demonstrates that hyperlipidemia could cause renal injury.

Treatment

Healthy-eating dietary advice is advocated in steroid-responsive NS, where the hyperlipidemia usually resolves as proteinuria abates. Dietary fat restriction is usually recommended in hyperlipidemic states of steroid-resistant NS. Dietary supplementation with fish oil has some lipid-lowering effects, mainly decreasing triglycerides [29].

There are some major classes of lipid-lowering drugs: bile acid sequestrants (cholestyramine, colestipol), fibric acid derivatives (gemfibrozil, bezafibrate), nicotinic acid derivatives (niacin), probucol, hydroxymethylglutaryl CoA (HMG-CoA) reductase inhibitors (lovastatin, fluvastatin, pravastatin, simvastatin), and cholesterol absorption inhibitors such as ezetimibe [6, 30]. In general, these drugs are widely used in adult patients, but experience in patients with childhood NS is limited.

Bile acid-binding resins act by binding the cholesterol in bile acids in the intestinal lumen, which prevents their reuptake as part of the enterohepatic circulation. Average lowering of cholesterol is 10–20 % below baseline. Although these drugs do not have systemic effects, the side effect of gastrointestinal discomfort and difficulties in the administration of the medicines limit their use for young patients [11].

Fibrates are used for elevated triglyceride concentration; however, these drugs have not been extensively studied in children. Fibric acid derivatives lead to a decrease in VLDL production by inhibiting the synthesis and increasing the clearance of the VLDL apoprotein B. These medications also impede peripheral lipolysis and decrease hepatic extraction of free fatty acids, which reduces hepatic triglyceride production. The risk of myopathy and rhabdomyolysis is markedly increased when fibrates are used together with statins or in patients with renal insufficiency [11]. Büyükçelik et al. [31] evaluated the effects of gemfibrozil on hyperlipidemia in 12 children with persistent NS and found that at the end of the fourth month, gemfibrozil reduced total cholesterol by 34 %, LDL by 30 %, apolipoprotein

B by 21 %, and triglycerides by 53 % without any side effects. HDL cholesterol and apolipoprotein A levels were not significantly altered.

Niacin or nicotinic acid lowers LDL and triglyceride concentrations while increasing HDL concentration. The mechanism of action is by decreasing hepatic production of VLDL. Niacin may also lower lipoprotein(a) levels. Niacin is a potentially attractive medication for management of dyslipidemia. However, adverse effects, including flushing, hepatic failure, myopathy, glucose intolerance, and hyperuricemia, were impediments to recommending niacin for routine use in the treatment of pediatric dyslipidemia [11].

Probucol is a diphenolic compound with anti-oxidant and anti-inflammatory properties that reduces atherosclerosis and lipid-lowering effects [32]. Querfeld et al. [33], in a prospective uncontrolled multicenter study, found that probucol treatment decreased serum concentrations of triglycerides (15 %), total cholesterol (25 %), VLDL cholesterol (27 %), LDL cholesterol (23 %), and HDL cholesterol (24 %), as well as apolipoprotein A-I, apolipoprotein B, and malondialdehyde levels after 12 weeks of treatment in persistent childhood NS. The positive effects of probucol on the lipoprotein profile persisted over 24 weeks; however, there was no significant effect on either proteinuria or glomerular filtration rate (GFR). The drug was well tolerated but had to be discontinued because of prolonged QT interval in some patients.

Statins inhibit the rate-limiting enzyme 3-hydroxy-3-methyl-glutaryl coenzyme A (HMG-CoA) reductase for endogenous synthesis of cholesterol, which lowers the intracellular cholesterol level and upregulates the LDL receptors, resulting in increased clearance of LDL from the circulation. The adverse effects of statins are increased hepatic transaminase and also creatine kinase levels, which may be associated with rare but clinically important episodes of rhabdomyolysis. Patients should be instructed to report symptoms of muscle aches or cramping, and they should be monitored with periodic measurement of liver transaminase and creatine kinase levels [11]. The US Food and Drug Administration has approved the use of pravastatin for children with familial hypercholesterolemia who are 8 years and older, and lovastatin, simvastatin, fluvastatin, atorvastatin, and rosuvastatin for children ≥10 years, regardless of pubertal status. Coleman et al. [34] have assessed the efficacy and tolerability of diet prior to and in combination with HMG-CoA reductase inhibitor, simvastatin, in seven children with steroid-resistant NS with a mean age of 8 years. They found that dietary advice alone had little impact on lipid levels of children with persistent NS, whereas simvastatin produced a significant and sustained reduction in lipid levels. On a median simvastatin dose of 10 mg/day, there was a 41 % reduction in cholesterol level and 44 % reduction in triglyceride level at 6 months that was sustained at 12 months in five patients. The drug was well tolerated with no clinical side effects noted. Similarly, Sanjad et al. [35] evaluated the efficacy and safety of statins (lovastatin and simvastatin) in 12 children with steroid-resistant NS followed prospectively for 1–5 years. A marked reduction in their total cholesterol (40 %), LDL cholesterol (44 %), and triglyceride levels (33 %) was observed, but there was no appreciable change in HDL cholesterol. Statin therapy was well tolerated without clinical and laboratory adverse effects. No changes were observed in the degree of proteinuria, hypoalbuminemia, or in the rate of progression to chronic renal failure.

The dietary cholesterol-absorption inhibitors represent the newest class of cholesterol-lowering agents. However, these medications have not been extensively studied in children. They are assumed to act mainly on intestinal absorption; but these drugs are absorbed, enter the enterohepatic circulation, and may have systemic effects [11]. Additional studies will be needed to evaluate their long-term effectiveness in young patients and patients with kidney diseases.

Another approach to the management of hyperlipidemia in refractory NS is the use of LDL apheresis. A prospective uncontrolled trial of LDL apheresis and steroid treatment in 17 patients with FSGS revealed rapid improvement in hyperlipidemia and partial or complete remission of NS in 71 % of the patients [36]. In another study, 11 children with steroid- and cyclosporine-resistant NS due to FSGS were treated with LDL apheresis, and 63 % entered into either complete or partial remission [37]. These findings suggest that in addition to its ability to ameliorate the hyperlipidemia seen in NS, LDL apheresis may be useful in maintaining remission in pediatric FSGS patients.

In view of the available evidence, it seems logical to treat hyperlipidemia in patients with unremitting NS in order to prevent progression of atherosclerosis and chronic renal failure. However, slowing the progression of renal failure by lowering cholesterol has not yet been demonstrated in patients with NS, and the degree of the preventive effect of lowering cholesterol level in atherosclerosis prevention is presently not measurable exactly. Concerns about possible side effects of the medications and the absence of clearly defined therapeutic endpoints are clear limitations. Therefore, it is not possible to make evidence-based recommendations for treatment of hyperlipidemia in pediatric patients. Pharmacological therapy with statins in children with NS should be done cautiously until controlled studies are conducted in this population.

Dyslipidemias in Patients with Chronic Renal Insufficiency and End-Stage Renal Disease

Introduction

The association between CKD and dyslipidemia has long been recognized; however, compared to the adult population, data about dyslipidemia in children with CKD remain scarce. Findings in children largely parallel those in adults. Dyslipidemia in chronic renal insufficiency (CRI) manifests principally as increased triglyceride and decreased HDL with nearly normal total cholesterol. The degree of dyslipidemia is usually found to be parallel to the degree of renal impairment. The addition of hemodialysis (HD) does not seem to significantly alter the pattern of dyslipidemia found in CRI, while peritoneal dialysis (PD) usually results in elevation of the total cholesterol level with further increases in hypertriglyceridemia [38].

Epidemiology

In 1981, Papadopoulou et al. [39] showed for the first time that alterations in serum triglycerides and alpha lipoproteins (HDL) occur early in CRI and before the onset of uremia when the GFR falls below 40 mL/min/1.73 m^2 in pediatric patients. In these patients, the serum triglyceride levels become significantly elevated and alpha lipoproteins (HDL) markedly decreased as renal function deteriorates. These lipid abnormalities become further aggravated with the onset of hemodialysis. These findings were further supported by Zacchello et al. [40]. Recently, dyslipidemia profile of the largest number of patients ($n = 391$) with CKD was reported by Chronic Kidney Disease in Children (CKiD) investigators. One-third (32 %) of children had elevated triglyceride, 21 % had low HDL cholesterol, and 16 % had high non-HDL cholesterol. Overall, 45 % of the cohort had dyslipidemia, defined as one or more abnormal lipid measure; 45 % of those had combined dyslipidemia. Lower GFR was associated with higher triglyceride, lower HDL cholesterol, and higher non-HDL cholesterol. Compared to children with GFR >50 mL/min/1.73 m^2, children with GFR <30 mL/min/1.73 m^2 had an OR of 2.9 for any dyslipidemia (prevalence 65 %) and an OR of 8.58 for combined dyslipidemia (39 % prevalence). Compared to normal proteinuria, nephrotic proteinuria was strongly associated with dyslipidemia in these patients [41].

Dyslipidemia in pediatric HD patients were recognized earlier than CRI patients. Pennisi et al. [42] in 1976 reported that 93 % of the hemodialysis patients had elevated triglyceride levels and 13 % had elevated cholesterol. Then, further studies also showed elevated triglyceride levels and decreased HDL cholesterol in pediatric HD patients [7, 39, 40, 42, 43]. Papadopoulou et al. [39] showed the aggravation of these lipid abnormalities after onset of hemodialysis in CRI patients. Total cholesterol levels were found to be normal in majority of the hemodialysis patients. Elevated triglyceride and total cholesterol levels have been reported in 63–100 % and 30–100 % of pediatric PD patients, respectively [44–47]; some studies also revealed decreased HDL cholesterol levels [7, 47]. Muller et al. [48] compared the lipid profiles of patients with HD and PD and found that cholesterol and triglyceride levels were significantly higher in PD patients.

Pathogenesis

In CRI and end-stage renal disease (ESRD), lipoprotein synthesis does not appear to be significantly exaggerated, but studies consistently demonstrate impaired catabolism of triglyceride [38]. The diminished clearance of triglycerides, which can lead to hypertriglyceridemia, stems both from an alteration in the composition of triglycerides and from reductions in the activity of lipoprotein lipase and hepatic triglyceride lipase, which are involved in triglyceride removal. This results in accumulation of VLDL with impaired conversion to LDL, accompanied by low levels of circulating HDL. Therefore, uremic dyslipidemia is characterized by high triglyceride and low HDL cholesterol levels [49]. An important association is the consistent finding of increased concentrations of apoC-III, which has been implicated as a mediator of increased plasma triglyceride in several studies, in patients with CRI [50, 51].

Insulin resistance is a consistent finding of renal insufficiency [52]. The pattern of dyslipidemia associated with insulin resistance is similar to that found in patients with uremia [53]. Insulin regulates lipoprotein lipase in a tissue-specific manner, increasing its activity in adipose and decreasing it in muscle [54, 55]. Many individuals with uremia demonstrate a decreased insulin secretory response in addition to a post-receptor defect [56, 57]. Abnormalities of both insulin secretion and sensitivity may have significant roles in the development of disordered lipid metabolism in uremia.

The concentration of triglyceride-rich lipoproteins (TRL) (chylomicrons, VLDLs, and their remnants) is increased among individuals with CRI [58]. This relative hypertriglyceridemia also manifests within individual lipoprotein classes: the ratio of triglyceride to cholesteryl ester (CE) is higher in LDL and HDL and lower in VLDL and IDL [49, 59, 60]. A pathological increase in TRL is followed by the cholesterol ester transfer protein (CETP)-mediated transfer of the triglyceride from this expanded pool of substrate into HDL and LDL in exchange for CE [61]. Chylomicron and VLDL remnants have prolonged circulation and are found in increased levels in patients with CRI. HDL and its principal apolipoprotein, apoA-I, are found to be significantly decreased, probably as a consequence of elevated TRL, which induces transfer of excess triglyceride into HDL particles, increasing their susceptibility to serve as substrate for hepatic lipase [59, 62].

Patients with CRI usually demonstrate total cholesterol and LDL cholesterol that are similar to or slightly less than that of the general population, except for those on chronic PD, in whom these levels are usually elevated [58, 63]. Despite normal or low concentrations of LDL cholesterol, LDL particles are small and more dense than normal because of increased VLDL precursor and triglyceride/CE exchange followed by triglyceride lipolysis [64]. As small, dense LDL are prone to oxidation, and as oxidative stress is increased in CRI, levels of oxidized LDL are increased [65, 66].

Non-nephrotic proteinuria also affects lipoprotein physiology, and CRI is commonly associated with non-nephrotic proteinuria [49].

Peritoneal dialysis could aggravate dyslipidemia, since a high glucose load and peritoneal protein losses could stimulate hepatic production of VLDL. However, although most studies have observed an increase in lipoprotein lipids after the start of PD, reports have been inconsistent with respect to the influence of glucose load, nutrition, or protein losses on these abnormalities. Peritoneal losses of lipoproteins and apolipoproteins theoretically favor the loss of lower molecular weight lipoproteins, that is, HDL and apoA, which are protective against atherosclerosis [67].

Clinical Implications

Estimates of cardiovascular mortality rates in children and young adults who developed ESRD during childhood are 1,000 times greater than comparably aged healthy individuals [68]. For children on dialysis therapy, the anticipated lifespan is reduced by 40–60 years, and for transplant recipients, by 20–25 years compared with an age- and race-matched population [69, 70]. The most likely cause of this reduction in survival is an excessive burden of CV mortality, with 30–50 % of all deaths in this population attributed to CV causes that are related to both accelerated ischemic heart disease and premature development of dilated cardiomyopathy in young adult survivors of childhood-onset CKD [71]. Clinically evident CV lesions (symptomatic coronary artery disease, myocardial infarction, and cerebrovascular accident) luckily are rare in children and adolescents with CKD. However, there is increasing evidence showing significant subclinical CV abnormalities in this population [72]. In the 2006 American Heart Association guidelines for CV-risk reduction in high-risk pediatric patients, children with CKD were stratified for the first time as "high risk" for the development of CV disease, with associated "pathological and/or clinical evidence for manifest coronary disease before 30 years of age" [73]. As in adults, the risk factors believed to be responsible for accelerated CV disease in children with CKD can be divided into two primary groups: traditional risk factors for atherosclerotic disease (e.g., dyslipidemia, diabetes, hypertension, and smoking) and uremia-related risk factors that are unique to or far more prevalent in patients with CKD [72].

Treatment

Management of dyslipidemia is multifactorial. Therapeutic lifestyle changes (TLC) for children are similar to those recommended for adults. General nutritional guidelines on fat consumption, including lowering total, saturated, and trans fats and limiting cholesterol, should be carried out along with the proposals suitable for patients with CRI. Heart-healthy fats (margarines oils made from canola, corn, sunflower, soy, olives, peanuts) should be used. Obesity should be addressed, if present, and treatment of malnutrition related to CRI is essential, and increasing physical activity to reach and maintain a healthy body weight is recommended. Nutritional requirements to maintain growth should be provided. Studies in the general pediatric population have shown no adverse effects of dietary fat restriction on growth, development, or nutritional status; diet and lifestyle recommendations should be used with caution or not at all in children who are malnourished [74, 75]. Tube feeding can provide an appropriate energy intake with a balanced fat and carbohydrate profile that does not adversely affect serum lipids [76]. Correction of metabolic acidosis, vitamin D therapy, and correction of anemia with erythropoietin are essential because each of them is associated with improvements in lipid abnormalities [77–79]. Treatments known to reduce proteinuria may improve the lipid profile. Dietary fish oil supplementation (3–8 g/dL) was shown to reduce hypertriglyceridemia and improve atherogenic serum lipoprotein profiles in a small group of children with ESRD [80]. Dyslipidemia management should be undertaken in conjunction with all other available measures to reduce the overall risk of atherosclerotic CV disease. Modifiable, conventional risk factors (hypertension, cigarette smoking, obesity, glucose intolerance) should be assessed and managed according to existing guidelines. The phosphate binding agent sevelamer hydrochloride also acts as a bile acid sequestrant, and it has been shown to lower cholesterol levels in patients with CKD. A multicenter study that compared the efficacy and safety of sevelamer with calcium acetate in pediatric patients with CRI and ESRD showed that total cholesterol (−27 %) and LDL cholesterol (−34 %) levels decreased significantly with sevelamer treatment [81]. Similar results were shown by Gulati et al. [82] in pediatric patients with CKD stages 3 and 4.

The treatment of dyslipidemia in pediatric CKD is not well studied; there is limited information in the Kidney Disease Outcomes Quality Initiative (K/DOQI) guidelines, and it is recommended that prepubertal children be managed according to existing national guidelines for children in the general population and that pubertal and postpubertal children and adolescents in any stage of CKD or with a kidney transplant be managed according to the K/DOQI guidelines for adults [74]. According to K/DOQI guidelines, adolescents with CKD should be considered to be in the highest risk category for dyslipidemias. Evaluation of dyslipidemias should occur after presentation with CKD, after a change in kidney failure treatment modality, and annually. Adolescents with CKD should be evaluated for dyslipidemia with a fasting lipid profile for total cholesterol, LDL, HDL, and triglycerides. If LDL is 130–159 mg/dL, start TLC diet (if nutritional status is adequate), followed in 6 months by a statin if LDL ≥130 mg/dL. If LDL ≥160 mg/dL, start TLC plus a statin.

For prepubertal children, The National Cholesterol Expert Panel on Children (NCEP-C) recommendations exist for the management of dyslipidemia in younger children [83]. However, they are not specific for patients with CKD or kidney transplant recipients. The NCEP-C recommends diet therapy as the primary approach for treating dyslipidemia in children. If LDL levels are more than 130 mg/dL, a step I diet (less than 10 % of total calories from saturated fatty acids, no more than 30 % of calories from total fat, less than 300 mg/day of cholesterol) is prescribed, followed in 3 months by a step II diet (further reduction of the saturated fatty acid intake to less than 7 % of calories, the cholesterol intake to less than 200 mg/day) if the target levels are not achieved. Pharmacological treatment is recommended in children aged ≥10 years, after an adequate trial of diet therapy, if LDL cholesterol remains ≥190 mg/dL or if LDL is ≥160 mg/dL and there is a positive family history of CV disease or if two or more CV disease risk factors are present in the child. However, the American Heart Association expert panel released an updated scientific statement addressing high-risk pediatric patients that considered pediatric CKD patients to be in the highest risk group [73]. In children with CKD and a fasting LDL >100 mg/dL, TLC, such as reduced dietary saturated fat and cholesterol intake and moderate exercise, are first recommended for the initial 6 months. If target levels (<100 mg/dL) are not reached, initiation of statin therapy is indicated. According to American Academy of Pediatrics (AAP) 2008 guideline, for patients 8 years and older with an LDL concentration of ≥190 mg/dL (or ≥160 mg/dL with a family history of early heart disease or ≥2 additional risk factors present or ≥130 mg/dL if diabetes mellitus is present), pharmacological intervention should be considered [11]. The initial goal is to lower LDL concentration to <160 mg/dL.

However, targets as low as 130 mg/dL or even 110 mg/dL may be warranted when there is a strong family history of CV disease, especially with other risk factors, including obesity, diabetes mellitus, the metabolic syndrome, and other higher-risk situations [11].

It is difficult to develop an evidence-based approach for the specific age at which pharmacological treatment should be implemented. Statin use was limited in children. Long-term data on efficacy in pediatric patients are not available, and safety information on use of statins in children is not conclusive. The main indication was familial hyperlipidemia, and it was shown that they were efficacious and safe in this population [84]. In contrast to adults with CKD, there have been nearly no systematic studies on drug-induced lowering of serum lipids in children with CKD. A randomized, double-blind, placebo-controlled, cross-over clinical trial in children with hyperlipidemia secondary to kidney disorders showed that total cholesterol levels were significantly reduced by 23 %, LDL cholesterol levels by 34 %, and triglyceride levels by 21 % during the 3-month simvastatin treatment period. No differences were found across groups with respect to adverse events [85]. In another study, atorvastatin led to a decrease in total cholesterol and LDL levels in a small number of children with CKD stage 3–4 [86]. Thus, data on benefits of statin therapy in children with CKD are limited. Concerning the differences between the etiology of CKD in adults and children, adult data could not be directly interpreted in children [87]. Studies are needed to evaluate the benefits and adverse effects of statin and other treatment modalities in children with CKD.

Dyslipidemias in Patients with Renal Transplantation

Introduction

Together with improvements in the surgical techniques and immunosuppressive therapy, the success of pediatric renal transplantation increases and patient and organ survival get better. However, with the increase of long-term survivors, chronic complications are becoming more frequent. The expected lifespan is shortened compared with the age-matched population, mostly as a result of accelerated cardiovascular disease. The cardiovascular morbidity and mortality in renal transplant recipients are much lower than in dialysis patients, but still remain high. Heart disease is the second most common cause of death in children after infection, and is the leading cause of death in young adults who have undergone renal transplantation [68, 88, 89]. Post-transplant hyperlipidemia affects the majority of solid organ transplant recipients. Changes in serum lipid profiles reported after transplantation include an increase in total cholesterol, triglyceride, LDL cholesterol, and VLDL cholesterol and a variable effect on HDL cholesterol [90]. As a consequence, interest in monitoring and attempting to prevent and treat hyperlipidemia in the post-transplant period has increased dramatically.

Epidemiology

In the early reports, the incidence of hyperlipidemia in pediatric renal transplant recipients is reported to be 50 % on average, and as high as 66 %; increasing levels of cholesterol and triglyceride are also associated with higher corticosteroid dosages [91–95]. Alterations in lipid metabolism already exist prior to transplantation in patients with chronic renal failure. The pattern of hyperlipidemia is known to be different in uremic children according to the mode of renal replacement therapy before transplantation, and after transplantation the pattern of hyperlipidemia rapidly changes during the first few months. Muller et al. [48] showed that after transplantation, serum cholesterol tended to increase in HD and CRI patients, but to decrease in the PD group; similarly, triglyceride levels decrease in the PD and CRI patients and increase in the HD patients. Therefore, at 9 months post-transplant, the serum lipid levels in all children, with different pretransplant treatment modalities, were indiscernible and no longer influenced by prior renal replacement therapy. Thus, serum lipids converge to a common pattern of "post-transplant hyperlipidemia" in pediatric renal graft recipients.

The prevalence of dyslipidemia in the post-transplant period is thought to decrease over time and may reflect changes in immunosuppression. Sgambat et al. [96] evaluated the dyslipidemia profile of 38 pediatric patients who were at least 6 months post-transplant and receiving a lower dose of corticosteroids (0.1 mg/kg/day), tacrolimus, and mycophenolate mofetil. They found that 26 % had high total cholesterol, 24 % had high LDL cholesterol, 29 % had low HDL cholesterol, and 10 % had elevated triglyceride, although lower than the previous reports indicating the high prevalence of dyslipidemia even after immunosuppressive regimen change.

Oberholzer et al. [97] reported significantly less hyperlipidemia among children treated with an early steroid withdrawal protocol compared with those who continued on steroids after transplantation. Sarwal et al. [98] also reported no hyperlipidemia in ten pediatric recipients at 6 months post-transplant that were treated with complete steroid avoidance protocol. All children were treated with tacrolimus in both studies. On the other hand, steroid-minimization protocols were also associated with lower levels of HDL cholesterol.

Causes and Pathogenesis

There are many causes for the development of post-transplant dyslipidemia. Risk factors for the development of hyperlipidemia include degree of renal impairment, pretransplant hyperlipidemia, nephrotic syndrome that can occur after transplantation, use of antihypertensive agents such as thiazide diuretics and B-adrenergic blockers, genetic predisposition, lifestyle factors such as obesity, high-fat diet, and immunosuppressive agents [99, 100]. However, Siirtola et al. [101] recently showed that high serum cholesterol and triglyceride concentrations observed in renal transplant recipients were not explained by their diets, since comparable dietary intakes of total, saturated, and polyunsaturated fats and cholesterol were seen in their patients and controls.

The type of post-transplant treatment immunosuppressive regimen is one of the most important contributors to dyslipidemia prevalence. Of the immunosuppressive drugs, especially prednisone, cylosporin A (CSA) and sirolimus are more likely to be associated with dyslipidemia; however, tacrolimus and mycophenolate mofetil appear to have minimal to no dyslipidemic effects [102–104].

Corticosteroids, until recently, were used almost universally in the post-transplant period. A variety of mechanisms have been postulated for steroid-induced dyslipidemia. These include the induction of a hyperinsulinemic state that would increase the hepatic synthesis of TRL, inhibit the LDL receptor activity, reduce the activity of lipoprotein lipase and hepatic lipase, and an increase in the rate-limiting enzymes involved in lipogenesis (acetyl-CoA carboxylase and free fatty acid synthetase) [100]. On the other hand, corticosteroid therapy may raise the HDL level by increasing the apolipoprotein A-1 synthase and by decreasing the activity of CETP [105].

Possible mechanisms for CSA-induced hypercholesterolemia include impaired LDL clearance associated with interference at the LDL receptor, CSA-mediated impairment of steroid clearance and CSA-induced hepatic dysfunction. CSA also reduces bile acid synthesis by inhibiting hepatic 27-hydroxylation of cholesterol which is a potent suppresser of HMG-CoA reductase [106–109]. CSA is known to increase the rate of atherogenesis [110, 111]. The reasons for decreased incidence of hyperlipidemia observed on tacrolimus therapy when compared with CSA are not well understood. With the modern immunosuppression therapies, the incidence of acute rejection episodes decreases, together with the need for aggressive steroid therapy for the treatment of rejection.

Sirolimus increases serum triglycerides, LDL cholesterol, and HDL cholesterol levels in a dose-dependent manner. This defect in lipid metabolism is characterized by either a decrease in the catabolism of apoB100-containing lipoproteins or an increase in circulating free fatty acids leading to increased hepatic synthesis of triglycerides [112–114]. In pediatric renal transplant recipients, hyperlipidemia has been reported in a range of 10–61 % [104, 115–117]. Antiatherogenic effects of sirolimus via inhibiting vascular smooth muscle cell proliferation may balance the risk of hyperlipidemia [112].

Clinical Implications

Cardiovascular disease is one of the leading causes of death in pediatric kidney transplant recipients and accounts for over 15 % of all deaths [118]. Post-transplant CV disease has a multifactorial origin and is related to a combination of adverse factors that are prevalent in the post-transplant period to varying degrees. Silverstein et al. [119] assessed 45 children who received kidney transplants, all with stages 2–4 CKD at the time of study; two-thirds of patients had at least two risk factors for CVD, and one-third had at least three risk factors. A multicenter study of more than 200 kidney transplant recipients (aged 1–21 years) showed that 37 % met at least three (of a possible five) of the diagnostic criteria for metabolic syndrome at 1 year post-transplantation [120].

Dyslipidemia has been identified as a major contributor to CV mortality within this population. Very little direct data exist on the long-term clinical significance of lipid levels in children. Autopsy studies, such as the Pathobiological Determinants of Atherosclerosis in Youth (PDAY) study [121] and the Bogalusa Heart Study [122, 123], have demonstrated that the atherosclerotic process begins in childhood. PDAY study found that the development of fatty streaks (which are precursors of atherosclerotic plaques) in the coronary arteries and aorta was positively correlated with the elevated LDL cholesterol and low HDL cholesterol levels in young adults. In children, the extent of atherosclerotic lesions correlated significantly with serum total cholesterol, LDL cholesterol, and triglyceride concentrations. The Bogalusa Heart Study investigators followed a cohort of children who had their risk-factor status measured during assessments at school. As this population became older, some people died of accidental causes. The investigators obtained autopsies on these people in order to evaluate the presence and extent of atherosclerotic lesions. They reported that the extent of the arterial intimal surface covered with fatty streaks and fibrous plaques increased with age and the prevalence was almost 70 % in young adulthood. They also found that the extent to which the intimal surface was covered with atherosclerotic lesions was significantly associated with elevation of total cholesterol, LDL, and triglycerides concentrations, as well as a lower concentration of HDL. Another important discovery was that increased coverage of atherosclerotic lesions was positively correlated with the number of risk factors for CV disease present, such as dyslipidemia, obesity, and hypertension.

Dyslipidemia after transplantation has been associated with allograft injury, and therefore may contribute to the progression of chronic allograft nephropathy and subsequent graft loss [124, 125]. The prominence of the vascular lesions and certain similarities with the pathological features of atherosclerosis suggest that lipids may be involved in the pathogenesis of chronic rejection. In the series of Massy et al. [125], 706 consecutive renal transplants with long-term follow-up were included, increased post-transplant serum triglycerides, but not total cholesterol, were strong predictors of graft loss due to chronic rejection. This effect was independent of other risk factors for chronic rejection such as age, acute rejections, proteinuria, and hypoalbuminemia. Data in the pediatric population are also limited in this topic. Valavi et al. [126] performed a cross-sectional study in 62 renal transplant recipients, aged 5–18 years, with the mean follow-up time of 48 months and found that hypercholesterolemia and high LDL cholesterol levels have significant association with chronic allograft nephropathy.

Treatment

Adherence to standard practices of post-transplant care to ensure preservation of good renal function and education of patients regarding the benefits of maintaining a healthy lifestyle are extremely important. The first therapeutic step to be taken in all pediatric patients with post-transplant hyperlipidemia is dietary modification.

Despite the perception that dietary modification is not achievable for the majority of pediatric patients, it should be tried. In a study of Obarzanek et al. [127], 663 children, 8–10 years of age, with elevated LDL cholesterol without renal disease were randomized to a dietary intervention or usual care group, with a mean of 7.4 years follow-up, and it was shown that the intervention compared with the usual care group had lower LDL cholesterol. On the other hand, Delucchi et al. [128] offered the Step II American Heart Association diet (containing low fat and low saturated cholesterol content) to 22 children with hyperlipidemia after renal transplantation; only about half of the eligible children agreed to participate in the study. Moreover, none of the patients demonstrated 100 % compliance with the diet. No patient lost weight, nor was the mean body mass index affected, and while the total cholesterol and LDL cholesterol did decrease, the magnitude of the decline was small (11 % and 14 %, respectively, at 12 weeks). Recently, Filler et al. [129] showed that supplementation of omega-3 fatty acids may be effective in reducing total cholesterol in pediatric renal transplant recipients. Children with adequate graft function who have no other disabilities should be able to assume a normal exercise regimen.

Avoidance of medications implicated in causing lipid abnormalities, including substitution of tacrolimus for cyclosporine in the medication regimen, can be an alternative treatment option. Filler et al. [130] performed a multicenter, 6-month, randomized, prospective, open, parallel group study with an open extension phase in 18 centers from nine European countries. In total, 196 pediatric patients were randomly assigned to receive either tacrolimus or CSA administered concomitantly with azathioprine and corticosteroids. Tacrolimus was significantly more effective than CSA in preventing acute rejection in pediatric renal recipients. Renal function and graft survival were also superior with tacrolimus. Cholesterol remained significantly higher in the CSA group throughout follow-up. Another approach may be the use of calcineurin inhibitor (CNI) avoidance or withdrawal protocols. Most, if not all, of these CNI-free regimens are steroid-based and many have also employed the use of sirolimus as a substitute to the CNIs, which makes them more risky for the development of hyperlipidemia. However, by improving long-term graft function, a CNI-free regimen could reduce dyslipidemia.

Steroid withdrawal and minimization protocols seemed to be associated with a reduction in lipid abnormalities. Lau et al. [131] compared 16 children that were receiving maintenance steroids with 13 children on a steroid-minimization regimen, who were also receiving preemptive pravastatin treatment. At 1 month, children receiving maintenance steroids had higher cholesterol compared with the steroid minimization group. Statistically significant differences in total cholesterol were not seen at other time points. Similar findings were noted for the LDL cholesterol, LDL/HDL, and cholesterol/HDL ratios. At 1 month, the serum HDL cholesterol was substantially lower in the steroid-minimization group.

The National Kidney Foundation K/DOQI Working Group created guidelines for the management of dyslipidemia in kidney transplant recipients in 2004 [132]. The working group considered that adolescents be included in the guidelines and that children before the onset of puberty be managed according to existing national guidelines for children in the general population. The K/DOQI guidelines recommend that a fasting lipid profile (total cholesterol, LDL, HDL, triglycerides) be measured during the first 6 months post-transplant, at 1 year after transplant, and annually thereafter. A lipid profile should also be measured 2–3 months after stopping or starting an immunosuppressive medication known to affect lipid levels. Kidney transplant recipients with dyslipidemias should be evaluated for remediable, secondary causes. For adolescent kidney transplant recipients with fasting triglycerides ≥500 mg/dL that cannot be corrected by removing an underlying cause, treatment with TLC should be considered. For adolescent kidney transplant recipients with LDL ≥130 mg/dL, treatment should be considered to reduce LDL to <130 mg/dL. Secondary causes of dyslipidemias should be treated first. Thereafter, for LDL 130–159 mg/dL, TLC should be used first. If, after 6 months of TLC, LDL is ≥130 mg/dL, then consider pharmacological management. If LDL is ≥160 mg/dL, then consider starting atrovastatin at the same time as TLC. For adolescent kidney transplant recipients with LDL < 130 mg/dL, fasting triglycerides ≥200 mg/dL, and non-HDL cholesterol (total cholesterol minus HDL) ≥160 mg/dL, treatment should be considered to reduce non-HDL cholesterol to <160 mg/dL. Therefore, statins should be considered for therapy in adolescent kidney transplant recipients and elevated LDL, or in hypertriglyceridemic adolescent kidney transplant recipients and increased non-HDL cholesterol. For adolescents who do not achieve the desired target with a statin, addition of a bile acid sequestrant can be considered. For prepubertal children, the existing guidelines are already described in the CKD section [11, 83].

Statins is an option in patients who remain persistently dyslipidemic in spite of TLC and modification of their immunosuppressive regimen. There are only a limited number of studies describing the use of lipid-lowering agents in pediatric renal transplant patients. Penson et al. [133] showed for the first time that pravastatin therapy is effective and safe when used in 21 pediatric and adolescent cardiac transplant recipients. Patients receiving pravastatin experienced a mean 32 mg/dL decrease in total cholesterol and a mean 31 mg/dL decrease in LDL cholesterol, regardless of their immunosuppressive regimen. Krmar et al. [134] used low-dose atorvastatin in eight children and young adult renal transplant recipients who had inadequately controlled hypercholesterolemia; at the end of the study, the total serum cholesterol was lowered by 32 % and the LDL cholesterol by about 42 %. Argent et al. [135], in a prospective study, showed that atorvastatin safely reduced total cholesterol, LDL cholesterol, and serum triglyceride by approximately 40 %, 60 %, and 45 %, respectively, in nine children with renal transplants who had persistent hyperlipidemia. Butani et al. [136] demonstrated that the preemptive use of pravastatin in seven pediatric renal transplant recipients appears to be effective in significantly reducing serum cholesterol. At 1 month only 43 % of the pravastatin group had hypercholesterolemia compared with 67 % of the controls; by 12 months this difference was even more significant (0 % in the pravastatin group vs. 45 % in the control group). The same group further evaluated the efficacy of the preemptive use of pravastatin in the post-transplant period in 17 children who were receiving maintenance steroids, and demonstrated it to effectively reduce total cholesterol, triglyceride, and LDL cholesterol after transplantation. The general linear model analysis showed that with time, there was a significant decline in the total cholesterol, serum triglyceride, LDL, and also HDL cholesterol. Compared with the controls, the mean serum cholesterol was lower at all time points post-transplant in the treated patients. However, despite treatment, the prevalence of hypercholesterolemia increased from 31 % pretransplant to 53 % at 1 month, but declined thereafter to 6 % at 3 and 6 months and 0 % at 1 year. Multivariable regression analyses showed the prednisone dose, pre-transplant cholesterol, and age to be the most important risk factors for the development of dyslipidemia. This group remarkably has been using a fixed dose of pravastatin preemptively in pediatric renal allograft recipients since 1999 [137]. Sgambat et al. [96] also showed a significant reduction in total cholesterol, LDL, VLDL, and triglyceride levels after 3–6 months of atrovastatin treatment compared with pretreatment value in five children. No difference in HDL was observed. There are various potential side effects associated with statins such as myopathy, rhabdomyolysis, and elevation of liver enzymes. In addition, there appears to be interaction between statins and cyclosporine, based upon their similar metabolism via the P450 cytochrome pathway [100]. Thus, drug levels should be monitored carefully.

It is not possible to make evidence-based recommendations for treatment of hyperlipidemia in pediatric renal transplant patients. The prevalence of dyslipidemia in the post-transplant period seems to decrease over time, together with the improvements in the immunosuppression regimen. Pharmacological therapy with statins in children with renal transplantation must be done carefully until controlled studies are conducted in this population.

References

1. Nephrotic syndrome in children: prediction of histopathology from clinical and laboratory characteristics at time of diagnosis. A report of the International Study of Kidney Disease in Children. Kidney Int. 1978;13:159–65.
2. McKinney PA, Feltbower RG, Brocklebank JT, Fitzpatrick MM. Time trends and ethnic patterns of childhood nephrotic syndrome in Yorkshire, UK. Pediatr Nephrol. 2001;16:1040–4.
3. White RH, Glasgow EF, Mills RJ. Clinicopathological study of nephrotic syndrome in childhood. Lancet. 1970;1:1353–9.
4. Niaudet P. Steroid resistant idiopathic nephrotic syndrome in children. In: Avner ED, Harmon WE, Niaudet P, editors. Pediatric nephrology. Philadelphia, PA: Lippincott Williams & Wilkins; 2004. p. 557–73.
5. Gbadegesin R, Smoyer WE. Nephrotic syndrome. In: Geary DF, Schaefer F, editors. Comprehensive pediatric nephrology. 1st ed. Philadelphia, PA: Mosby, Elsevier; 2008. p. 204–18.
6. Querfeld U. Should hyperlipidemia in children with the nephrotic syndrome be treated? Pediatr Nephrol. 1999;13:77–84.
7. Querfeld U, Lang M, Friedrich JB, Kohl B, Fiehn W, Schörer K. Lipoprotein(a) serum levels and apolipoprotein(a) phenotypes in children with chronic renal disease. Pediatr Res. 1993;34:772–6.
8. American Academy of Pediatrics. National Cholesterol Education Program: report of the expert panel on blood cholesterol levels in children and adolescents. Pediatrics. 1992;89:525–84.

9. Kavey RE, Daniels SR, Lauer RM, Atkins DL, Hayman LL, Taubert K. American Heart Association guidelines for primary prevention of atherosclerotic cardiovascular disease beginning in childhood. Circulation. 2003;107(11):1562–6; copublished in J Pediatr. 2003;142:368–72.
10. Tamir I, Heiss G, Glueck CJ, Christensen B, Kwiterovich P, Rifkind B. Lipid and lipoprotein distributions in white children ages 6–19 yrs: the lipid research clinics program prevalence study. J Chronic Dis. 1981;34:27–39.
11. Daniels SR, Greer FR. Lipid screening and cardiovascular health in childhood. Pediatrics. 2008;122:198–208.
12. Baxter JH, Goodman HC, Havel RJ. Serum lipid and lipoprotein alterations in nephrosis. J Clin Invest. 1960;39:455–65.
13. Valentini RP, Smoyer WE. Nephrotic syndrome. In: Kher KK, Schnaper HW, Makker SP, editors. Clinical pediatric nephrology. 2nd ed. London: Informa; 2007. p. 155–94.
14. Tsukahara H, Haruki S, Hiraoka M, Hori C, Sudo M. Persistent hypercholesterolaemia in frequently relapsing steroid-responsive nephrotic syndrome. J Paediatr Child Health. 1997;33:253–5.
15. Merouani A, Levy E, Mongeau JG, Robitaille P, Lambert M, Delvin EE. Hyperlipidemic profiles during remission in childhood idiopathic nephrotic syndrome. Clin Biochem. 2003;36:571–4.
16. Berlyne G, Mallick N. Ischemic heart disease as a complication of nephrotic syndrome. Lancet. 1969;II:339–40.
17. Hopp L, Gilboa N, Kurland G, Weichler N, Orchard TJ. Acute myocardial infarction in a young boy with nephrotic syndrome: a case report and review of the literature. Pediatr Nephrol. 1994;8:290–4.
18. Kallen RJ, Brynes RK, Aronson AJ, Lichtig C, Spargo BH. Premature coronary atherosclerosis in a 5-year-old with corticosteroid-refractory nephrotic syndrome. Am J Dis Child. 1977;131:976–80.
19. Silva JM, Oliveira EA, Marino VSP, Oliveira JS, Torres RM, Ribeiro AL, et al. Premature acute myocardial infarction in a child with nephrotic syndrome. Pediatr Nephrol. 2002;17:169–72.
20. Antikainen M, Sariola H, Rapola J, Taskinen MR, Holthöfer H, Holmberg C. Pathology of renal arteries of dyslipidemic children with congenital nephrosis. APMIS. 1994;102:129–34.
21. Portman R, Hawkins E, Verani R. Premature atherosclerosis in pediatric renal patients: report of the Southwest Pediatric Nephrology Study Group. Pediatr Res. 1991;29:2075A (Abstract).
22. Lechner BL, Bockenhauer D, Iragorri S, Kennedy TL, Siegel NJ. The risk of cardiovascular disease in adults who have had childhood nephrotic syndrome. Pediatr Nephrol. 2004;19:744–8.
23. Moorhead JF, El-Nahas M, Chan MK, Varghese Z. Lipid nephrotoxicity in chronic progressive glomerular and tubulointerstitial disease. Lancet. 1982;II:1309–12.
24. Diamond J. Hyperlipidemia of nephrosis: pathophysiologic role in progressive glomerular disease. Am J Med. 1989;87:25–9.
25. Keane WF, Mulcahy WS, Kasiske BL, Kim Y, O'Donnell MP. Hyperlipidemia and progressive renal disease. Kidney Int. 1991;39:41–8.
26. Keane WF, Kasiske BL, O'Donnell P, Kim Y. The role of altered lipid metabolism in the progression of renal disease: experimental evidence. Am J Kidney Dis. 1991;17:38–42.
27. O'Donnell MP, Kasiske BL, Kim Y, Schmitz PG, Keane WF. Lovastatin retards the progression of established glomerular disease in obese Zucker rats. Am J Kidney Dis. 1993;22:83–9.
28. Muntner P, Coresh J, Smith JC, Eckfeldt J, Klag MJ. Plasma lipids and risk of developing renal dysfunction: the atherosclerosis risk in communities study. Kidney Int. 2000;58:293–301.
29. Cerkauskiene R, Kaminskas A, Kaltenis P, Vitkus D. Influence of omega-3 fatty acids on lipid metabolism in children with steroid sensitive nephrotic syndrome. Medicina (Kaunas). 2003;39:82–7.

30. Kwiterovich PO. Clinical and laboratory assessment of cardiovascular risk in children: guidelines for screening, evaluation, and treatment. J Clin Lipidol. 2008;2:248–66.
31. Büyükçelik M, Anarat A, Bayazıt AK, Noyan A, Ozel A, Anarat R, et al. The effect of gemfibrozil on hyperlipidemia in children with persistent nephrotic syndrome. Turk J Pediatr. 2002;44:40–4.
32. Yamashita S, Matsuzawa Y. Where are we with probucol: a new life for an old drug? Atherosclerosis. 2009;207:16–23.
33. Querfeld U, Kohl B, Fiehn W, Minor T, Michalk D, Schörer K, et al. Probucol for treatment of hyperlipidemia in persistent childhood nephrotic syndrome. Pediatr Nephrol. 1999;13:7–12.
34. Coleman JE, Watson AR. Hyperlipidemia, diet and simvastatin therapy in steroid resistant nephrotic syndrome of childhood. Pediatr Nephrol. 1996;10:171–4.
35. Sanjad SA, Al-Abbad A, Al-Shorafa S. Management of hyperlipidemia in children with refractory nephrotic syndrome: the effect of statin therapy. J Pediatr. 1997;130:470–4.
36. Muso E, Mune M, Fujii Y, Imai E, Ueda N, Hatta K, et al. Low density lipoprotein apheresis therapy for steroid-resistant nephrotic syndrome. Kansai-FGS-Apheresis Treatment (K-FLAT) Study Group. Kidney Int. 1999;71(Suppl):122–5.
37. Hattori M, Chikamoto H, Akioka Y, Nakakura H, Ogino D, Matsunaga A, et al. A combined low-density lipoprotein apheresis and prednisone therapy for steroid-resistant primary focal segmental glomerulosclerosis in children. Am J Kidney Dis. 2003;42:1121–30.
38. Saland JM, Ginsberg H, Fisher EA. Dyslipidemia in pediatric renal disease: epidemiology, pathophysiology, and management. Curr Opin Pediatr. 2002;14:197–204.
39. Papadopoulou ZL, Sandler P, Tina LU, Jose PA, Calcagno PL. Hyperlipidemia in children with chronic renal insufficiency. Pediatr Res. 1981;15:887–91.
40. Zacchello G, Pagnan A, Sidran MP, Ziron L, Braggion M, Pavanello L, et al. Further definition of lipid-lipoprotein abnormalities in children with various degrees of chronic renal insufficiency. Pediatr Res. 1987;21:462–5.
41. Saland JM, Pierce CB, Mitsnefes MM, Flynn JT, Goebel J, Kupferman JC, et al. Dyslipidemia in children with chronic kidney disease: a report of the chronic kidney disease in children (CKiD) study. Kidney Int. 2010;78:1154–63.
42. Pennisi AJ, Heuser ET, Mickey MR, Lipsey A, Malekzadeh M, Fine RN. Hyperlipidemia in pediatric haemodialysis and renal transplant patients. Am J Dis Child. 1976;130:957–61.
43. El Bishti M, Counahan R, Jarrett RJ, Stimmler L, Wass V, Chantler C. Hyperlipidaemia in children on regular haemodialysis. Arch Dis Child. 1977;52:932–6.
44. Querfeld U, Salusky IB, Nelson P, Foley J, Fine RN. Hyperlipidemia in pediatric patients undergoing peritoneal dialysis. Pediatr Nephrol. 1988;2:447–52.
45. Querfeld U, LeBoeuf RC, Salusky IB, Nelson P, Laidlaw S, Fine RN. Lipoproteins in children treated with continuous peritoneal dialysis. Pediatr Res. 1991;29:155–9.
46. Scolnik D, Balfe JW. Initial hypoalbuminemia and hyperlipidemia persist during chronic peritoneal dialysis in children. Perit Dial Int. 1993;13:136–9.
47. Kosan C, Sever L, Arisoy N, Caliskan S, Kasapcopur O. Carnitine supplementation improves apolipoprotein B levels in pediatric peritoneal dialysis patients. Pediatr Nephrol. 2003;18: 1184–8.
48. Muller T, Koeppe S, Arbeiter K, Luckner D, Salzer U, Balzar E, et al. Serum lipid pattern unifies following renal transplantation in children. Pediatr Nephrol. 2003;18:939–42.
49. Saland JM, Ginsberg HN. Lipoprotein metabolism in chronic renal insufficiency. Pediatr Nephrol. 2007;22:1095–112.
50. Moberly JB, Attman PO, Samuelsson O, Johansson AC, Knight-Gibson C, Alaupovic P. Apolipoprotein C-III, hypertriglyceridemia and triglyceride-rich lipoproteins in uremia. Miner Electrolyte Metab. 1999;25:258–62.
51. Monzani G, Bergesio F, Ciuti R, Rosati A, Frizzi V, Serruto A, et al. Lipoprotein abnormalities in chronic renal failure and dialysis patients. Blood Purif. 1996;14:262–72.
52. Hager SR. Insulin resistance of uremia. Am J Kidney Dis. 1989;14:272–6.
53. Howard BV. Insulin resistance and lipid metabolism. Am J Cardiol. 1999;84:28–32.

54. Lithell H, Boberg J, Hellsing K, Lundqvist G, Vessby B. Lipoprotein-lipase activity in human skeletal muscle and adipose tissue in the fasting and the fed states. Atherosclerosis. 1978;30:89–94.
55. Farese Jr RV, Yost TJ, Eckel RH. Tissue-specific regulation of lipoprotein lipase activity by insulin/glucose in normal-weight humans. Metabolism. 1991;40:214–6.
56. Mak RH. Insulin secretion and growth failure in uremia. Pediatr Res. 1995;38:379–83.
57. Alvestrand A, Mujagic M, Wajngot A, Efendic S. Glucose intolerance in uremic patients: the relative contributions of impaired beta-cell function and insulin resistance. Clin Nephrol. 1989;31:175–83.
58. Kimak E, Ksiazek A, Solski J. Disturbed lipoprotein composition in non-dialyzed, hemodialysis, continuous ambulatory peritoneal dialysis and post-transplant patients with chronic renal failure. Clin Chem Lab Med. 2006;44:64–9.
59. Grutzmacher P, Marz W, Peschke B, Gross W, Schoeppe W. Lipoproteins and apolipoproteins during the progression of chronic renal disease. Nephron. 1988;50:103–11.
60. Horkko S, Huttunen K, Laara E, Kervinen K, Kesaniemi YA. Effects of three treatment modes on plasma lipids and lipoproteins in uraemic patients. Ann Med. 1994;26:271–82.
61. Horowitz BS, Goldberg IJ, Merab J, Vanni TM, Ramakrishnan R, Ginsberg HN. Increased plasma and renal clearance of an exchangeable pool of apolipoprotein A-I in subjects with low levels of high density lipoprotein cholesterol. J Clin Invest. 1993;91:1743–52.
62. Bergesio F, Monzani G, Ciuti R, Serruto A, Benucci A, Frizzi V, Salvadori M. Lipids and apolipoproteins change during the progression of chronic renal failure. Clin Nephrol. 1992;38:264–70.
63. Kasiske BL. Hyperlipidemia in patients with chronic renal disease. Am J Kidney Dis. 1998;32:142–56.
64. Berneis KK, Krauss RM. Metabolic origins and clinical significance of LDL heterogeneity. J Lipid Res. 2002;43:1363–79.
65. Massy ZA, Nguyen-Khoa T. Oxidative stress and chronic renal failure: markers and management. J Nephrol. 2002;15:336–41.
66. Oberg BP, McMenamin E, Lucas FL, McMonagle E, Morrow J, Ikizler TA, et al. Increased prevalence of oxidant stress and inflammation in patients with moderate to severe chronic kidney disease. Kidney Int. 2004;65:1009–16.
67. Querfeld U. Cardiovascular considerations of pediatric ESRD. In: Warady BA, Schaefer FS, Fine RN, Alexander SR, editors. Pediatric dialysis. Dordrecht: Kluwer Academic; 2004. p. 353–67.
68. Parekh RS, Carrol CE, Wolfe RA, Port FK. Cardiovascular mortality in children and young adults with end-stage kidney disease. J Pediatr. 2002;141:191–7.
69. National Kidney Foundation Task Force on Cardiovascular Disease. Controlling the epidemic of cardiovascular disease in chronic renal disease: what do we know? What do we need to know? Special report from the National Kidney Foundation task force on cardiovascular disease. Am J Kidney Dis. 1998;32:1–121.
70. U.S. Renal Data System: USRDS Annual Report. Bethesda: The National Institute of Diabetes and Digestive and Kidney Diseases. 2003. http://www.usrds.org
71. Mitsnefes MM. Cardiovascular complications of pediatric chronic kidney disease. Pediatr Nephrol. 2008;23:27–39.
72. Wilson AC, Mitsnefes MM. Cardiovascular disease in CKD in children: update on risk factors, risk assessment, and management. Am J Kidney Dis. 2009;54:345–60.
73. Kavey RE, Allada V, Daniels SR, Hayman LL, McCrindle BW, Newburger JW, et al. Cardiovascular risk reduction in high-risk pediatric patients: a scientific statement from the American Heart Association expert panel on population and prevention science: the councils on cardiovascular disease in the young, epidemiology and prevention, nutrition, physical activity and metabolism, high blood pressure research, cardiovascular nursing, and the kidney in heart disease; and the Interdisciplinary Working Group on quality of care and outcomes research: endorsed by the American Academy of Pediatrics. Circulation. 2006;114: 2710–38.

74. National Kidney Foundation: K/DOQI. Clinical practice guidelines for managing dyslipidemias in chronic kidney disease. Am J Kidney Dis. 2003;41 Suppl 3:61–70.
75. Secker D, Mak R. Nutritional challenges in pediatric chronic kidney disease. In: Geary DF, Schaefer F, editors. Comprehensive pediatric nephrology. 1st ed. Philadelphia, PA: Mosby, Elsevier; 2008. p. 743–59.
76. Kari JA, Shaw V, Vallance DT, Rees L. Effect of enteral feeding on lipid subfractions in children with chronic kidney failure. Pediatr Nephrol. 1998;12:401–4.
77. Mak RH. Metabolic effects of erythropoietin in patients on peritoneal dialysis. Pediatr Nephrol. 1998;12:660–5.
78. Mak RH. 1,25-Dihydroxyvitamin D3 corrects insulin and lipid abnormalities in uremia. Kidney Int. 1998;53:1353–7.
79. Mak RH. Effect of metabolic acidosis on hyperlipidemia in uremia. Pediatr Nephrol. 1999;13:891–3.
80. Goren A, Stankiewicz H, Goldstein R, Drukker A. Fish oil treatment of hyperlipidemia in children and adolescents receiving renal replacement therapy. Pediatrics. 1991;88:265–8.
81. Pieper AK, Haffner D, Hoppe B, Dittrich K, Offner G, Bonzel KE, et al. A randomized crossover trial comparing sevelamer with calcium acetate in children with CKD. Am J Kidney Dis. 2006;47:625–35.
82. Gulati A, Sridhar V, Bose T, Hari P, Bagga A. Short-term efficacy of sevelamer versus calcium acetate in patients with chronic kidney disease stage 3–4. Int Urol Nephrol. 2010;42:1055–62.
83. National Cholesterol Education Program. Report of the expert panel on blood cholesterol levels in children and adolescants. Pediatrics. 1992;89:495–584.
84. Avis HJ, Vissers MN, Stein EA, Wijburg FA, Trip MD, Kastelein JJ, et al. A systematic review and meta-analysis of statin therapy in children with familial hypercholesterolemia. Arterioscler Thromb Vasc Biol. 2007;27:1803–10.
85. Garcia-de-la-Puenta S, Arredondo-Garcia JL, Gutierrez-Castrellon P, Bojorquez-Ochoa A, Maya ER, Perez-Martinez MDP. Efficacy of simvastatin in children with hyperlipidemia secondary to kidney disorders. Pediatr Nephrol. 2009;24:1205–10.
86. Mackie FE, Rosenberg AR, Harmer JA, Kainer G, Celermajer DS. HMG CoA reductase inhibition and endothelial function in children with chronic kidney disease (CKD)—a pilot study. Acta Paediatr. 2010;99:457–9.
87. Tullus K. Dyslipidemia in children with CKD: should we treat with statins. Pediatr Nephrol. 2012;27:357–62.
88. McDonald SP, Craig JC. Long-term survival of children with end-stage renal disease. N Engl J Med. 2004;350:2654–62.
89. United States Renal Data System. Experts from the USRDS 2001 annual report. Am J Kidney Dis. 2001;38 Suppl 3:147–58.
90. Kobashigawa JA, Kasiske BL. Hyperlipidemia in solid organ transplantation. Transplantation. 1997;63:331–8.
91. Pennisi AJ, Fiedler J, Lipsey A, Mickey R, Malekzadeh MH, Fine NR. Hyperlipidemia in pediatric renal allograft recipients. J Pediatr. 1975;87:249–51.
92. Saldanha LF, Hurst KS, Amend Jr WJ, Lazarus JM, Lowrie EG, Ingelfinger J, et al. Hyperlipidemia after renal transplantation in children. Am J Dis Child. 1976;130:951–3.
93. Goldstein S, Duhamel G, Laudat MH, Berthelier M, Hervy C, Tete MJ, et al. Plasma lipids, lipoproteins and apolipoproteins AI, AII, and B in renal transplanted children: what risk for accelerated atherosclerosis? Nephron. 1984;38:87–92.
94. Sharma AK, Myers TA, Hunninghake DB, Matas AJ, Kashtan CE. Hyperlipidemia in long-term survivors of pediatric renal transplantation. Clin Transplant. 1994;8:252–7.
95. Silverstein DM, Palmer J, Polinsky MS, Braas C, Conley SB, Baluarte HJ. Risk factors for hyperlipidemia in long-term pediatric renal transplant recipients. Pediatr Nephrol. 2000;14:105–10.
96. Sgambat K, He J, McCarter R, Moudgil A. Lipoprotein profile changes in children after renal transplantation in the modern immunosuppression era. Pediatr Transplant. 2008;12: 796–803.

97. Oberholzer J, John E, Lumpaopong A, Testa G, Sankary HN, Briars L, et al. Early discontinuation of steroids is safe and effective in pediatric kidney transplant recipients. Pediatr Transplant. 2005;9:456–63.
98. Sarwal MM, Yorgin PD, Alexander S, Millan MT, Belson A, Belanger N, et al. Promising early outcomes with a novel, complete steroid avoidance immunosuppression protocol in pediatric renal transplantation. Transplantation. 2001;72:13–21.
99. Massy ZA, Kasiske BL. Post-transplant hyperlipidemia: mechanisms and management. J Am Soc Nephrol. 1996;7:971–7.
100. Butani L. Dyslipidemia after renal transplantation: a cause for concern? Pediatr Transplant. 2008;12:724–8.
101. Siirtola A, Virtanen SM, Ala-Houhala M, Koivisto AM, Solakivi T, Lehtimäki T, et al. Diet does not explain the high prevalence of dyslipidaemia in paediatric renal transplant recipients. Pediatr Nephrol. 2008;23:297–305.
102. Perrea DN, Moulakakis KG, Poulakou MV, Vlachos IS, Nikiteas N, Kostakis A. Correlation between lipid abnormalities and immunosuppressive therapy in renal transplant recipients with stable renal function. Int Urol Nephrol. 2008;40:521–7.
103. Mathis AS, Dave N, Knipp GT, Friedman GS. Drug-related dyslipidemia after renal transplantation. Am J Health Syst Pharm. 2004;61:565–85.
104. Kasap B. Sirolimus in pediatric renal transplantation. Pediatr Transplant. 2011;15:673–85.
105. Moulin P, Appel GB, Ginsberg HN, Tall AR. Increased concentration of plasma cholesteryl ester transfer protein in nephrotic syndrome: role in dyslipidemia. J Lipid Res. 1992;33:1817–22.
106. Bittar AE, Ratcliffe PJ, Richardson AJ, Raine AE, Jones L, Yudkin PL, et al. The prevalence of hyperlipidemia in renal transplant recipients. Associations with immunosuppressive and antihypertensive therapy. Transplantation. 1990;50:987–92.
107. Ost L. Impairment of prednisolone metabolism by cyclosporine treatment in renal graft recipients. Transplantation. 1987;44:533–5.
108. Lopez-Miranda J, Vilella E, Perez-Jimenez F, Espino A, Jiménez-Perepérez JA, Masana L, et al. Low-density lipoprotein metabolism in rats treated with cyclosporine. Metabolism. 1993;42:678–83.
109. Gueguen Y, Ferrari L, Souidi M, Batt AM, Lutton C, Siest G, et al. Compared effect of immunosuppressive drugs cyclosporine A and rapamycin on cholesterol homeostasis key enzymes CYP27A1 and HMGCoA reductase. Basic Clin Pharmacol Toxicol. 2007;100:392–7.
110. Apanay DC, Neylan JF, Ragab MS, Sgoutas DS. Cyclosporine increases the oxidizability of low-density lipoproteins in renal transplant recipients. Transplantation. 1994;58:663–9.
111. Emeson EE, Shen ML. Accelerated atherosclerosis in hyperlipidemic C57BL/6 mice treated with cyclosporin A. Am J Pathol. 1993;142:1906–15.
112. Augustine JJ, Bodziak KA, Hricik DE. Use of sirolimus in solid organ transplantation. Drugs. 2007;67:369–91.
113. Hoogeveen RC, Ballantyne CM, Pownall HJ, Opekun AR, Hachey DL, Jaffe JS, et al. Effect of sirolimus on the metabolism of apoBl00-containing lipoproteins in renal transplant patients. Transplantation. 2001;72:1244–50.
114. Morrisett JD, Abdel-Fattah G, Hoogeveen R, Mitchell E, Ballantyne CM, Pownall HJ, et al. Effects of sirolimus on plasma lipids, lipoprotein levels, and fatty acid metabolism in renal transplant patients. J Lipid Res. 2002;43:1170–80.
115. Hymes LC, Warshaw BL. Sirolimus in pediatric patients: results in the first 6 months post-renal transplant. Pediatr Transplant. 2005;9:520–2.
116. Powell HR, Kara T, Jones CL. Early experience with conversion to sirolimus in a pediatric renal transplant population. Pediatr Nephrol. 2007;22:1773–7.
117. Hymes LC, Warshaw BL, Amaral SG, Greenbaum LA. Tacrolimus withdrawal and conversion to sirolimus at three months post-pediatric renal transplantation. Pediatr Transplant. 2008;12:773–7.
118. Smith JM, Stablein DM, Munoz R, Hebert D, McDonald RA. Contributions of the transplant registry: the 2006 annual report of the North American Pediatric Renal Trials and Collaborative Studies (NAPRTCS). Pediatr Transplant. 2007;11:366–73.

119. Silverstein DM, Mitchell M, LeBlanc P, Boudreaux JP. Assessment of risk factors for cardiovascular disease in pediatric renal transplant patients. Pediatr Transplant. 2007;11:721–9.
120. Wilson AC, Greenbaum LA, Barletta GM, Chand D, Lin JJ, Patel HP, et al. High prevalence of the metabolic syndrome and associated left ventricular hypertrophy in pediatric renal transplant recipients. Pediatr Transplant. 2010;14:52–60.
121. McGill Jr HC, McMahan CA. Determinants of atherosclerosis in the young. Pathobiological determinants of atherosclerosis in youth (PDAY) research group. Am J Cardiol. 1998;82:30–6.
122. Newman III WP, Freedman DS, Voors AW, Gard PD, Srinivasan SR, Cresanta JL, et al. Relation of serum lipoprotein levels and systolic blood pressure to early atherosclerosis: the Bogalusa Heart Study. N Engl J Med. 1986;314:138–44.
123. Berenson GS, Srinivasan SR, Bao W, Newman III WP, Tracy RE, Wattigney WA. Association between multiple cardiovascular risk factors and the early development of atherosclerosis. Bogalusa Heart Study. N Engl J Med. 1998;338:1650–6.
124. Guijarro C, Massy ZA, Kasiske BL. Clinical correlation between renal allograft failure and hyperlipidemia. Kidney Int Suppl. 1995;52:56–9.
125. Massy ZA, Guijarro C, Wiederkehr MR, Ma JZ, Kasiske BL. Chronic renal allograft rejection: immunologic and nonimmunologic risk factors. Kidney Int. 1996;49:518–24.
126. Valavi E, Otukesh H, Fereshtehnejad SM, Sharifian M. Clinical correlation between dyslipidemia and pediatric chronic allograft nephropathy. Pediatr Transplant. 2008;12:748–54.
127. Obarzanek E, Kimm SY, Barton BA, Van Horn LL, Kwiterovich Jr PO, Simons-Morton DG, et al. Long-term safety and efficacy of a cholesterol-lowering diet in children with elevated low-density lipoprotein cholesterol: seven-year results of the dietary intervention study in children (DISC). Pediatrics. 2001;107:256–64.
128. Delucchi A, Marin V, Trabucco G, Azocar P, Salas E, Gutierrez E, et al. Dyslipidemia and dietary modification in Chilean renal pediatric transplantation. Transplant Proc. 2001;33: 1297–301.
129. Filler G, Weiglein G, Gharib MT, Casier S. Ω3 fatty acids may reduce hyperlipidemia in pediatric renal transplant recipients. Pediatr Transplant. 2012;16:835–9.
130. Filler G, Webb NJ, Milford DV, Watson AR, Gellermann J, Tyden G, et al. Four-year data after pediatric renal transplantation: a randomized trial of tacrolimus vs. cyclosporin microemulsion. Pediatr Transplant. 2005;9:498–503.
131. Lau KK, Tancredi DJ, Perez RV, Butani L. Unusual pattern of dyslipidemia in children receiving steroid minimization immunosuppression after renal transplantation. Clin J Am Soc Nephrol. 2010;5:1506–12.
132. Kasiske B, Cosio FG, Beto J, Bolton K, Chavers BM, Grimm Jr R, et al. Clinical practice guidelines for managing dyslipidemias in kidney transplant patients: a report from the managing dyslipidemias in Chronic Kidney Disease Work Group of the National Kidney Foundation kidney disease outcomes quality initiative. Am J Transplant. 2004;4 Suppl 7:13–53.
133. Penson MG, Fricker FJ, Thompson JR, Harker K, Williams BJ, Kahler DA, et al. Safety and efficacy of pravastatin therapy for the prevention of hyperlipidemia in pediatric and adolescent cardiac transplant recipients. J Heart Lung Transplant. 2001;20:611–8.
134. Krmar RT, Ferraris JR, Ramirez JA, Sorroche P, Legal S, Cayssials A. Use of atorvastatin in hyperlipidemic hypertensive renal transplant recipients. Pediatr Nephrol. 2002;17:540–3.
135. Argent E, Kainer G, Aitken M, Rosenberg AR, Mackie FE. Atorvastatin treatment for hyperlipidemia in pediatric renal transplant recipients. Pediatr Transplant. 2003;7:38–42.
136. Butani L, Pai MV, Makker SP. Pilot study describing the use of pravastatin in pediatric renal transplant recipients. Pediatr Transplant. 2003;7:179–84.
137. Butani L. Prospective monitoring of lipid profiles in children receiving pravastatin preemptively after renal transplantation. Pediatr Transplant. 2005;9:746–53.

Chapter 14
Dyslipidemias in the Geriatric Chronic Kidney Disease Patients

Zeynel Abidin Ozturk and Zekeriya Ulger

Increased life expectancy is one of the most important successes of medicine in this century, and older people comprise the most rapidly growing age segment. As the growing older adult population constitutes a larger proportion of the general population, the incidence of chronic diseases such as cardiovascular diseases (CVDs), diabetes mellitus (DM), and chronic kidney disease (CKD) as well as dyslipidemia has increased over the past several decades. Metabolic changes that occur with progressive renal failure and aging predispose patients to lipid abnormalities with increased atherogenic potential. As the incidence of kidney dysfunction increases with aging and as the risk for poor cardiovascular outcome increases in this population, understanding and treating abnormalities in lipid metabolism become central in the geriatric CKD patients.

Dyslipidemia in the Elderly

Epidemiological studies show that a substantial proportion of older adults are dyslipidemic, including persons 80 years and older; however, controversy persists regarding the relative importance of specific dyslipidemias in this population. It has been established that in older adults, dyslipidemia often coexists with diabetes mellitus (DM), hypertension, and obesity, making its management crucial in attempting to decrease cardiovascular risk. The absolute risk associated with dyslipidemia rises substantially with advancing age [1].

Z.A. Ozturk, M.D.
Division of Geriatrics, Department of Internal Medicine, School of Medicine, Gaziantep University, Üniversite Bulvarı, Şehitkamil, Gaziantep 27310, Turkey
e-mail: zaodr79@yahoo.com

Z. Ulger, M.D. (✉)
Division of Geriatrics, Department of Internal Medicine, School of Medicine, Gazi University Hospital, Besevler, Ankara 06500, Turkey
e-mail: zekeriyaulger@yahoo.com

A. Covic et al. (eds.), *Dyslipidemias in Kidney Disease*, DOI 10.1007/978-1-4939-0515-7_14,

Coronary artery disease (CAD) is estimated to remain the leading cause of death in developed countries over the next three decades due to increasing prevalence of older population. Dyslipidemia is an important risk factor for CAD in the elderly, and this association has been shown in many studies [2–8]. The World Health Organization predicts that more than half of the CAD cases in the world are associated with dyslipidemia. It has been firmly established that the risk of CAD increases with high levels of low-density lipoprotein cholesterol (LDL-C) and, inversely, the risk also increases with low levels of high-density lipoprotein cholesterol (HDL-C) [9, 10]. Both the Framingham Heart Study and Multiple Risk Factor Intervention Trial confirmed this correlation [2, 11]. Systolic Hypertension in the Elderly Program, which is including 4,736 elderly persons with a 4.4 years follow-up, demonstrated that the incidence of CAD events was increased by 30–35 % when non-HDL or LDL cholesterol levels increased by 1.03 mmol/L (40 mg/dL) [6].

On the other hand, some studies have observed that lower cholesterol levels also are associated with increased cardiovascular risk, especially in patients who have no additional risk factors for CAD. Some reports have observed a U- or J-shaped curve in the elderly in which lower cholesterol levels are paradoxically associated with an increase in cardiovascular risk. In a longitudinal study of 4,066 elderly men and women, for example, death from CAD increased at serum cholesterol levels below 160 mg/dL (4.1 mmol/L). If, however, adjustments were made for CAD risk factors and for serum iron and albumin (to account for comorbid disease and frailty), the increase in risk at lower cholesterol values disappeared [12].

Lipid Metabolism in the Elderly

Aging is associated with undesirable changes in body composition that expose older adults to a host of metabolic complications. It is well known that body fat increases with age and is preferentially accumulated in the abdominal region, thereby increasing the risk of CVD and DM in older adults [1, 13].

The lipid levels are similar in both genders before puberty [14]. LDL-C increases more rapidly with age after adolescence in men compared with women [15, 16]. The LDL-C levels reach a plateau in males by age 50–60 years, whereas in females, between the ages of 60 and 70 years. The mechanisms that result in this rise are not simple. The hepatic synthesis of very-low-density lipoprotein (VLDL) and its conversion to LDL increases with male aging. In addition, a decrease in lipid metabolism due to reduced functional LDL-C receptors in the hepatic cells and the alternations in the function of LDL-C receptors due to aging contribute to pathogenesis [17].

Serum HDL-C levels do not vary much in women throughout their lifetime, whereas HDL-C concentrations decrease in males during puberty and remain lower than in women after that time [18]. Testosterone plays an important role in HDL metabolism. Testosterone stimulates the expression of genes encoding for hepatic lipase and scavenger receptor B1 [19–21]. Via this mechanism, catabolism of HDL-C increases and results in lower HDL levels in males compared with females of the same age. HDL-C levels are higher in the elderly men than in the middle-aged men due to reduced androgen levels with aging [22]. However, inflammatory diseases, hormonal and metabolic changes can cause no increase in HDL levels in the elderly [23].

Studies have established that with aging, there is both an increase in the release of free fatty acids (FFA) from adipocytes and a decrease in the mass of metabolically active tissue combined with a decrease in the oxidative capacity of tissues. The net effect of these cellular changes is increased blood levels of FFA, which increase the risk of CVD, and result in hyperinsulinemia with insulin resistance and increased nonoxidative disposal of FFA as VLDL. These metabolic changes produce an atherogenic lipid profile [24–26].

In women triglyceride levels increase throughout their lifespan, whereas in men triglyceride levels peak between 40 and 50 years old and later decrease [27].

Before menopause, women have lower total cholesterol levels than those of men of the same age. After menopause, with reducing levels of estrogen, their LDL-C increase and HDL-C decrease [18]. These changes in lipid metabolism play an important role in the increased incidence of CVD in older adults.

Pseudocapillarization is a novel mechanism for age-related dyslipidemia [28]. Morphological changes occur in the liver sinusoidal endothelial cell with aging. These changes include reduction of fenestrations that have been called pseudocapillarization. Fenestrations provide transfer of lipoproteins, and their loss alters hepatic lipoprotein metabolism.

Treatment of Dyslipidemia in the Elderly

The primary target for treatment of dyslipidemia is LDL-C, and statins are the well-known and most used therapy for management of dyslipidemic patients. Many kinds of studies, including primary and secondary prevention trials, demonstrated the benefit of dyslipidemia treatment. National Cholesterol Education Program Adult Treatment Panel III recommends no age restriction for treatment of elderly persons with lipid-lowering drug therapy if they have CAD or higher risk factors for CAD [29]. This guideline also recommends similar LDL targets in the elderly individuals compared with younger patients.

Primary Prevention Trials

The Air Force/Texas Coronary Atherosclerosis Prevention Study was one of the earliest trials demonstrating the importance of statin usage in the elderly. Twenty-two percent of all patients were older than 65 years old [30]. There was a significant risk reduction in the incidence of first acute major coronary events such as myocardial infarction, unstable angina, and coronary revascularization regardless of age.

The Prospective Study of Pravastatin in Elderly Individuals at Risk of Vascular Disease randomized 5,804 men and women ages 70–82 years to placebo or pravastatin [31]. The patients had a history of or risk factors for vascular disease. Pravastatin treatment demonstrated a significant reduction with a combined endpoint of coronary death, nonfatal myocardial infarction, and fatal or nonfatal stroke after 3 years follow-up.

The Anglo-Scandinavian Cardiac Outcomes Trial Lipid-Lowering Arm randomized 10,305 hypertensive patients with cardiovascular risk factors but no history of CVDs [32]. In this study, 23 % of all patients were over 70 years of age. The results demonstrated benefit of atorvastatin therapy regardless of age at entry.

The Collaborative Atorvastatin Diabetes Study compared benefit of statin usage in 1,229 diabetic patients aged 65–75 years with 1,709 younger patients [33, 34]. Atorvastatin 10 mg/day reduced first major cardiovascular events by 38 % in older patients and by 37 % in younger patients.

The Cardiovascular Health Study showed that both all-cause mortality and cardiovascular events significantly decreased in the elderly patients with no known coronary heart diseases [35].

Justification for the use of statins in prevention: an intervention trial evaluating rosuvastatin followed up 17,802 healthy men and women with elevated high-sensitivity C-reactive protein between ages 60 and 71 for 1.9 years [36]. The results showed 44 % relative risk reduction in combined primary endpoint of myocardial infarction, stroke, arterial revascularization, cardiovascular death, or hospitalization for unstable angina.

Secondary Prevention Trials

The Scandinavian Simvastatin Survival Study included 1,021 patients older than 65 years of age who had angina or a prior myocardial infarction [37]. A reduction by 29 % in major cardiovascular events and 27 % in all-cause mortality was noted in the statin-using group in comparison to a placebo-control group. Older patients had twice as much absolute risk reduction compared with younger patients.

The Cholesterol and Recurrent Events (CARE) trial included 1,283 patients between the ages of 65 and 75 and showed that use of pravastatin resulted in 27 % reduction in major cardiovascular events in patients with known CAD and average cholesterol levels [38, 39]. It was estimated that for every 1,000 older patients treated, 207 cardiovascular events would be prevented compared with 150 cardiovascular events in 1,000 younger patients.

The Long-term Intervention with Pravastatin in Ischemic Disease Study included 3,514 patients between the ages of 65 and 75 years with a history of unstable angina or myocardial infarction [40, 41]. Statin therapy significantly reduced total mortality, CAS-related deaths, stroke, and coronary revascularization in the elderly patients compared to younger patients, and the absolute benefit was greater in the elderly.

The Heart Protection Study (HPS) included 20,536 patients up to the age of 80 years with documented CAD or a risk-factor profile that conveyed CAD risk equivalence [42]. Among all patients, 10,697 were over 65 years of age, and patients were randomly assigned to simvastatin or placebo. After the 5-year treatment period, all-cause mortality, coronary events, and stroke were significantly reduced in the statin group, regardless of age and initial serum lipids.

Trials Including Intensive Lipid-Lowering Therapy

To compare efficacy and safety of high-dose atorvastatin (80 mg/day) versus low (10 mg/day) in patients with CHD and a LDL level less than 130 mg/dL, the Treating to New Targets Study was performed [43]. High-dose statin appeared to reduce more major cardiovascular and neurological events without a significant increase in adverse effects.

The Study Assessing Goals in the Elderly trial randomized 893 patients with stable CAD who were between 65 and 85 years to atorvastatin 80 mg/day or pravastatin 40 mg/day [44]. In both groups a similar, significant reduction in the duration of myocardial ischemia was observed. However, there was a trend toward a reduction in major cardiovascular events in the high-dose atorvastatin group.

The Myocardial Ischemia Reduction with Acute Cholesterol Lowering trial randomized 3,086 patients between the ages of 18 and 80 to placebo or high-dose atorvastatin and resulted in a significant reduction in death, nonfatal MI, or recurrent myocardial ischemia [45, 46].

Undertreatment of Hyperlipidemia in the Elderly

Although randomized, controlled, multicenter trials demonstrated that elderly patients with highest cardiovascular risks derive the highest benefits from hypolipidemic treatment, this group of patients lastly receives appropriate therapy. There is also an inverse relationship between absolute coronary risk, advancing age, and statin prescription.

A retrospective analysis including 1.4 million elderly people demonstrated that 19 % of patients with CAD or diabetes mellitus used statins [47]. The percentage of patients receiving statin treatment was 37.3 % in low and 23.4 % in high cardiovascular risk patients. The likelihood of statin prescription decreased 6 % for each year of increasing patient age.

Potential reasons for hypolipidemic undertreatment in the elderly were determined by researchers [48]. The main reason given was lack of an indication in the elderly. Many physicians believe that cholesterol level could be less predictive of CHD or there is an inverse relationship between serum cholesterol level and mortality in the elderly patients. Drug side effects, cost effectiveness, and patient noncompliance are other important reasons for underprescription.

Dyslipidemia and Chronic Kidney Disease

Dyslipidemia and CKD are significant public health concerns in the world among elderly people. Human and animal studies support that dyslipidemia plays a role in progression and initiation of renal diseases. In addition, CKD causes development of alternations in lipid metabolism that result in increased cardiovascular morbidity and mortality. The contribution of dyslipidemia in renal diseases was first reported by Virchow in the middle of nineteenth century [49]. In an experimental study, Peric-Golia et al. demonstrated that feeding rats with a high cholesterol diet causes more focal glomerulosclerosis (FGS) at age 1 year than controls fed with a standard diet [50]. There was also a positive correlation between serum cholesterol level and FGS. Another study by Kasiske et al. showed that obese Zucker rats have significant glomerulosclerosis and albuminuria and after treatment by lipid-lowering agents glomerular injury was reduced [51]. There was an association between hypertriglyceridemia and podocyte injury, proteinuria and interstitial injury without mesangial changes in a rat model study [52].

The results of human studies were similar to animal data. Correlation between triglyceride-rich apoB-containing lipoproteins and rate of decrease in renal functions was demonstrated by Samuelsson et al. [53]. Patients with lecithin-cholesterol acyltransferase deficiency have hyperlipidemia, and this causes deposits of LDL-C in glomerules with developing renal failure from glomerulosclerosis [54, 55]. In The Atherosclerosis Risk in Communities Study, participants were followed up to 2.9 years and high triglycerides with low HDL-C but LDL-C predicted an increased risk of renal dysfunction [56]. In addition, hypertriglyceridemia was a strong parameter in the initiation of mild renal insufficiency. The results of the Physicians Health Study and the Framingham Offspring Study suggested that a low HDL-C and high LDL/HDL cholesterol ratio were risk factors for an increase in serum creatinine [57–59].

Structural features of glomerules are similar to arteries that are involved in atherosclerosis. Lipid-laden macrophages, which are thought to be important in initiation of atherosclerosis, are found in both atherosclerotic lesions and glomerules of FGS [60]. Atchley et al. demonstrated that oxidatively modified lipoproteins are found in diabetic patients with nephropathy and suggested they may contribute to pathogenesis of glomerulosclerosis [61].

Treatment of Dyslipidemia in Geriatric CKD Patients

Numerous changes in lipoprotein metabolism and serum lipids occur with increasing age and with renal dysfunction. Therefore, the benefit of lipid-lowering treatment in the elderly patients with renal dysfunction is an important era of research. Unfortunately, there is no big randomized clinical study about outcomes of dyslipidemia treatment specifically in this particular age group. The data on this issue are generally derived from the subgroup analysis of several landmark secondary prevention trials.

According to these data, lipid-lowering agents among elderly patients with CKD seem to have a benefit, but the data remain limited. Although improved cardiovascular outcomes have been suggested in CKD, similar findings of treatment benefit have not been evident in patients with end-stage renal disease (ESRD) [62]. Moreover, it should always be considered that elderly patients with CKD are at greater risk of adverse drug reactions; therefore, the lowest possible dose of medications should be used for the treatment of dyslipidemia [63].

In the treatment of dyslipidemia, lifestyle modifications should be considered first, because we very well know that the treatment of dyslipidemia requires two approaches: therapeutic lifestyle changes and medications. Most patients need both approaches simultaneously to achieve target LDL cholesterol levels. Lifestyle changes include regular exercise and a reduced intake of saturated fat (<7 % of total calories) and cholesterol (<200 mg/day). Dietary calories should be derived predominantly from foods rich in complex carbohydrates, such as whole grains, fruit, and vegetables [64]. However, while consuming these foods, the patient should be careful not to exceed the limits of a kidney failure diet. Therapeutic lifestyle changes can achieve an almost 30 % reduction in LDL cholesterol level in highly motivated individuals [27].

Although it was not a study specific to the older age group, the HPS is one of the largest studies from which we gained information about the endpoints of statin treatment in patients with CKD [65]. HPS enrollment included 20,000 British men and women age 40–80 years who were at increased risk of death from CVD due to diabetes, CAD, or other atherosclerotic disease. This 5-year study evaluated the benefit of lowering cholesterol with simvastatin 40 mg/day. The primary outcomes were total mortality and fatal and nonfatal vascular events [65, 66]. A subgroup analysis of 1,329 CKD patients in the HPS, including patients with a creatinine level from 1.3 to 2.3 mg/dL over 5 years' duration, showed a relative risk reduction of 28 % (95 % CI, 0.75–0.85; $p=0.05$) with simvastatin use of 40 mg/day [62]. The proportional reduction in the rate of major vascular events with allocation to simvastatin also seemed to be about one-quarter, irrespective of the age of the participants. Indeed, even among the 1,263 individuals aged 75–80 years at entry, and so aged about 80–85 years by the end of the study, the reduction in the event rate was substantial and definite (142 [23.1 %] versus 209 [32.3 %]; $p=0.0002$) [66].

In a large group of renal transplant recipients with mild to moderate increases in LDL cholesterol levels, the ALERT (Assessment of Lescol in Renal Transplant Trial) examined the effect of fluvastatin 40–80 mg/day versus placebo. In this randomized double-blind placebo-controlled study, the mean age was 48 ± 10 years in the fluvastatin group and 49 ± 10 years in the placebo group [67]. Findings show no detrimental effect on renal function with the long-term use of fluvastatin in this high-risk post-transplant patient population already on multiple medications, including immunosuppressive agents. After 4 years of fluvastatin treatment, there was a statistically significant risk correlation for major cardiac adverse events, cardiac death, and non-CV death [63].

In a 4-year, randomized, double-blind, placebo-controlled study of 1,255 patients with diabetes who required long-term hemodialysis (The Deutsche Diabetes Dialyse

Studie; the 4D study), no significant effects on the composite primary endpoint of cardiovascular events were obtained. The 4D study is the only large study evaluating with a mean age over the geriatric age limit the effect of statin therapy in CKD patients. The mean age was 65.7 ± 8.3 years, while 42.2 % of the patients were 65–74 years of age and 14.6 % were 75–83 years of age [68, 69]. Similarly, in a 3.8-year, randomized, double-blind, placebo-controlled study of 2,776 patients requiring long-term hemodialysis (the AURORA study), a reduction in cardiovascular events was not demonstrated from the use of rosuvastatin therapy. Mean age was 64.1 ± 8.6 years in the rosuvastatin group and 64.3 ± 8.7 in the placebo group in this study [70].

From the Prevention of Renal and Vascular End-Stage Disease Intervention Trial (PREVEND IT), extended follow-up data to investigate the long-term effects of fosinopril 20 mg and pravastatin 40 mg on cardiovascular outcomes in subjects with microalbuminuria were obtained [71]. Pravastatin 40 mg/day resulted in a nonsignificant 13 % reduction ($p = 0.649$) in the primary endpoint of cardiovascular mortality and hospitalization for cardiovascular morbidity [65]. But again, the age of participants was not in the geriatric age group in PREVEND IT (52.1 ± 11.9 years in pravastatin group, 50.5 ± 11.7 years in placebo group) [71].

Cholesterol and Recurrent Events trial (CARE Study) was conducted to determine whether pravastatin reduced rates of loss of renal function in patients (21–75 years of age) with moderate chronic renal insufficiency [72]. After a median follow-up period of 58.9 months, the incidence of the death from coronary disease or symptomatic nonfatal myocardial infarction was 28 % lower in participants receiving pravastatin 40 mg than in those receiving placebo [62]. The mean age was 63.2 ± 7.7 years in the statin group and 63.7 ± 7.4 years in the placebo group [72].

Study of Heart and Renal Protection (SHARP) evaluated the efficacy and safety of the combination of simvastatin plus ezetimibe on major atherosclerotic events in patients with a serum or plasma creatinine of at least 1.7 mg/dL in men or 1.5 mg/dL in women but no history of myocardial infarction. In this randomized, double-blind, placebo-controlled study with a median follow-up of 4.9 years, a 17 % proportional reduction in major atherosclerotic events with simvastatin–ezetimibe therapy was observed. However, in the subset of patients requiring dialysis, the incidence of major atherosclerotic events was not significantly different than the placebo group [73].

Fibric acid derivatives and gemfibrozil are frequently used agents in lowering triglyceride levels in the elderly patients with severe hypertriglyceridemia who have failed the diet treatment. They are associated with increased risk of rhabdomyolysis in patients with renal insufficiency; therefore, they need to be monitored carefully because the risk may exceed the potential benefit [62, 74]. Nicotinic acid, although very advantageous due to the effect of increased HDL, should be used cautiously in older adults, because of adverse effects on glycemic control [75].

Dyslipidemia has a significant and important role in the progression and initiation of renal diseases. On the other hand, CKD causes alternations in lipid metabolism that result in increased cardiovascular morbidity and mortality. Structural features of glomerules are also similar to arteries that are involved in atherosclerosis. There is no big randomized clinical study about outcomes of dyslipidemia treatment specifically in geriatric patients with CKD. The data about this topic are related to subgroup analysis of several landmark secondary prevention trials that demonstrated that improved cardiovascular outcomes have been suggested in CKD, but not in patients with ESRD. It is remarkable that elderly patients with CKD are at greater risk of adverse drug reactions, so the lowest possible dose of medications should be applied for dyslipidemia treatment. Further prospective studies including large numbers of elderly patients with CKD are required for comments on this issue.

References

1. Shanmugasundaram M, Rough SJ, Alpert JS. Dyslipidemia in the elderly: should it be treated? Clin Cardiol. 2010;33(1):4–9.
2. Castelli WP, Wilson PW, Levy D, Anderson K. Cardiovascular risk factors in the elderly. Am J Cardiol. 1989;63(16):12H–9.
3. Benfante R, Reed D. Is elevated serum cholesterol level a risk factor for coronary heart disease in the elderly? JAMA. 1990;263(3):393–6.
4. Agner E, Hansen PF. Fasting serum cholesterol and triglycerides in a ten-year prospective study in old age. Acta Med Scand. 1983;214(1):33–41.
5. Rubin SM, Sidney S, Black DM, Browner WS, Hulley SB, Cummings SR. High blood cholesterol in elderly men and the excess risk for coronary heart disease. Ann Intern Med. 1990;113(12):916–20.
6. Frost PH, Davis BR, Burlando AJ, Curb JD, Guthrie GP, Isaacsohn JL, et al. Serum lipids and incidence of coronary heart disease. Findings from the Systolic Hypertension in the Elderly Program (SHEP). Circulation. 1996;94(10):2381–8.
7. Houterman S, Verschuren WM, Hofman A, Witteman JC. Serum cholesterol is a risk factor for myocardial infarction in elderly men and women: the Rotterdam Study. J Intern Med. 1999;246(1):25–33.
8. Manolio TA, Pearson TA, Wenger NK, Barrett-Connor E, Payne GH, Harlan WR. Cholesterol and heart disease in older persons and women. Review of an NHLBI workshop. Ann Epidemiol. 1992;2(1–2):161–76.
9. Miller GJ, Miller NE. Plasma-high-density-lipoprotein concentration and development of ischaemic heart-disease. Lancet. 1975;1(7897):16–9.
10. Gordon T, Castelli WP, Hjortland MC, Kannel WB, Dawber TR. High density lipoprotein as a protective factor against coronary heart disease. The Framingham Study. Am J Med. 1977; 62(5):707–14.
11. Stamler J, Vaccaro O, Neaton JD, Wentworth D. Diabetes, other risk factors, and 12-yr cardiovascular mortality for men screened in the Multiple Risk Factor Intervention Trial. Diabetes Care. 1993;16(2):434–44.
12. Corti MC, Guralnik JM, Salive ME, Harris T, Ferrucci L, Glynn RJ, et al. Clarifying the direct relation between total cholesterol levels and death from coronary heart disease in older persons. Ann Intern Med. 1997;126(10):753–60.
13. Poehlman ET, Toth MJ, Bunyard LB, Gardner AW, Donaldson KE, Colman E, et al. Physiological predictors of increasing total and central adiposity in aging men and women. Arch Intern Med. 1995;155(22):2443–8.
14. Bagatell CJ, Bremner WJ. Androgen and progestagen effects on plasma lipids. Prog Cardiovasc Dis. 1995;38(3):255–71.
15. Ferrara A, Barrett-Connor E, Shan J. Total, LDL, and HDL cholesterol decrease with age in older men and women. The Rancho Bernardo Study 1984-1994. Circulation. 1997;96(1):37–43.
16. Ericsson S, Eriksson M, Vitols S, Einarsson K, Berglund L, Angelin B. Influence of age on the metabolism of plasma low density lipoproteins in healthy males. J Clin Invest. 1991;87(2):591–6.

17. Li Y, Sugiyama E, Yokoyama S, Jiang L, Tanaka N, Aoyama T. Molecular mechanism of age-specific hepatic lipid accumulation in PPARalpha (+/-):LDLR (+/-) mice, an obese mouse model. Lipids. 2008;43(4):301–12.
18. Kreisberg RA, Kasim S. Cholesterol metabolism and aging. Am J Med. 1987;82(1B):54–60.
19. Florentin M, Liberopoulos EN, Wierzbicki AS, Mikhailidis DP. Multiple actions of high-density lipoprotein. Curr Opin Cardiol. 2008;23(4):370–8.
20. Herbst KL, Amory JK, Brunzell JD, Chansky HA, Bremner WJ. Testosterone administration to men increases hepatic lipase activity and decreases HDL and LDL size in 3 wk. Am J Physiol Endocrinol Metab. 2003;284(6):E1112–8.
21. Nakagawa A, Nagaosa K, Hirose T, Tsuda K, Hasegawa K, Shiratsuchi A, et al. Expression and function of class B scavenger receptor type I on both apical and basolateral sides of the plasma membrane of polarized testicular Sertoli cells of the rat. Dev Growth Differ. 2004; 46(3):283–98.
22. Schleich F, Legros JJ. Effects of androgen substitution on lipid profile in the adult and aging hypogonadal male. Eur J Endocrinol. 2004;151(4):415–24.
23. Walter M. Interrelationships among HDL metabolism, aging, and atherosclerosis. Arterioscler Thromb Vasc Biol. 2009;29(9):1244–50.
24. Sial S, Coggan AR, Carroll R, Goodwin J, Klein S. Fat and carbohydrate metabolism during exercise in elderly and young subjects. Am J Physiol. 1996;271(6 Pt 1):E983–9.
25. Wolfe RR, Klein S, Carraro F, Weber JM. Role of triglyceride-fatty acid cycle in controlling fat metabolism in humans during and after exercise. Am J Physiol. 1990;258(2 Pt 1):E382–9.
26. Boden G, Chen X, Ruiz J, White JV, Rossetti L. Mechanisms of fatty acid-induced inhibition of glucose uptake. J Clin Invest. 1994;93(6):2438–46.
27. Gobal FA, Mehta JL. Management of dyslipidemia in the elderly population. Ther Adv Cardiovasc Dis. 2010;4(6):375–83.
28. Le Couteur DG, Cogger VC, McCuskey RS, De Cabo R, Smedsrød B, Sorensen KK, et al. Age-related changes in the liver sinusoidal endothelium: a mechanism for dyslipidemia. Ann N Y Acad Sci. 2007;1114:79–87.
29. Expert Panel on Detection Evaluation, and Treatment of High Blood Cholesterol in Adults. Executive Summary of The Third Report of The National Cholesterol Education Program (NCEP) Expert Panel on Detection, Evaluation, and Treatment of High Blood Cholesterol in Adults (Adult Treatment Panel III). JAMA. 2001;285(19):2486–97.
30. Downs JR, Clearfield M, Weis S, Whitney E, Shapiro DR, Beere PA, et al. Primary prevention of acute coronary events with lovastatin in men and women with average cholesterol levels: results of AFCAPS/TexCAPS. Air Force/Texas Coronary Atherosclerosis Prevention Study. JAMA. 1998;279(20):1615–22.
31. Shepherd J, Blauw GJ, Murphy MB, Bollen EL, Buckley BM, Cobbe SM, et al. Pravastatin in elderly individuals at risk of vascular disease (PROSPER): a randomised controlled trial. Lancet. 2002;360(9346):1623–30.
32. Sever PS, Dahlöf B, Poulter NR, Wedel H, Beevers G, Caulfield M, et al. Prevention of coronary and stroke events with atorvastatin in hypertensive patients who have average or lower-than-average cholesterol concentrations, in the Anglo-Scandinavian Cardiac Outcomes Trial-Lipid Lowering Arm (ASCOT-LLA): a multicentre randomised controlled trial. Lancet. 2003;361(9364):1149–58.
33. Colhoun HM, Betteridge DJ, Durrington PN, Hitman GA, Neil HA, Livingstone SJ, et al. Primary prevention of cardiovascular disease with atorvastatin in type 2 diabetes in the Collaborative Atorvastatin Diabetes Study (CARDS): multicentre randomised placebo-controlled trial. Lancet. 2004;364(9435):685–96.
34. Neil HA, DeMicco DA, Luo D, Betteridge DJ, Colhoun HM, Durrington PN, et al. Analysis of efficacy and safety in patients aged 65-75 years at randomization: Collaborative Atorvastatin Diabetes Study (CARDS). Diabetes Care. 2006;29(11):2378–84.
35. Lemaitre RN, Psaty BM, Heckbert SR, Kronmal RA, Newman AB, Burke GL. Therapy with hydroxymethylglutaryl coenzyme a reductase inhibitors (statins) and associated risk of incident cardiovascular events in older adults: evidence from the Cardiovascular Health Study. Arch Intern Med. 2002;162(12):1395–400.

36. Ridker PM, Danielson E, Fonseca FA, Genest J, Gotto AM, Kastelein JJ, et al. Rosuvastatin to prevent vascular events in men and women with elevated C-reactive protein. N Engl J Med. 2008;359(21):2195–207.
37. Miettinen TA, Pyörälä K, Olsson AG, Musliner TA, Cook TJ, Faergeman O, et al. Cholesterol-lowering therapy in women and elderly patients with myocardial infarction or angina pectoris: findings from the Scandinavian Simvastatin Survival Study (4S). Circulation. 1997;96(12): 4211–8.
38. Lewis SJ, Moye LA, Sacks FM, Johnstone DE, Timmis G, Mitchell J, et al. Effect of pravastatin on cardiovascular events in older patients with myocardial infarction and cholesterol levels in the average range. Results of the Cholesterol and Recurrent Events (CARE) trial. Ann Intern Med. 1998;129(9):681–9.
39. Sacks FM, Pfeffer MA, Moye LA, Rouleau JL, Rutherford JD, Cole TG, et al. The effect of pravastatin on coronary events after myocardial infarction in patients with average cholesterol levels. Cholesterol and Recurrent Events Trial investigators. N Engl J Med. 1996;335(14): 1001–9.
40. Hunt D, Young P, Simes J, Hague W, Mann S, Owensby D, et al. Benefits of pravastatin on cardiovascular events and mortality in older patients with coronary heart disease are equal to or exceed those seen in younger patients: results from the LIPID trial. Ann Intern Med. 2001; 134(10):931–40.
41. Prevention of cardiovascular events and death with pravastatin in patients with coronary heart disease and a broad range of initial cholesterol levels. The Long-Term Intervention with Pravastatin in Ischaemic Disease (LIPID) Study Group. N Engl J Med. 1998;339(19): 1349–57.
42. Group HPSC. MRC/BHF Heart Protection Study of antioxidant vitamin supplementation in 20,536 high-risk individuals: a randomised placebo-controlled trial. Lancet. 2002;360(9326): 23–33.
43. Wenger NK, Lewis SJ, Herrington DM, Bittner V, Welty FK. Investigators TtNTSSCa. Outcomes of using high- or low-dose atorvastatin in patients 65 years of age or older with stable coronary heart disease. Ann Intern Med. 2007;147(1):1–9.
44. Deedwania P, Stone PH, Bairey Merz CN, Cosin-Aguilar J, Koylan N, Luo D, et al. Effects of intensive versus moderate lipid-lowering therapy on myocardial ischemia in older patients with coronary heart disease: results of the Study Assessing Goals in the Elderly (SAGE). Circulation. 2007;115(6):700–7.
45. Schwartz GG, Olsson AG, Ezekowitz MD, Ganz P, Oliver MF, Waters D, et al. Effects of atorvastatin on early recurrent ischemic events in acute coronary syndromes: the MIRACL study: a randomized controlled trial. JAMA. 2001;285(13):1711–8.
46. Olsson AG, Schwartz GG, Szarek M, Luo D, Jamieson MJ. Effects of high-dose atorvastatin in patients > or =65 years of age with acute coronary syndrome (from the myocardial ischemia reduction with aggressive cholesterol lowering [MIRACL] study). Am J Cardiol. 2007; 99(5):632–5.
47. Ko DT, Mamdani M, Alter DA. Lipid-lowering therapy with statins in high-risk elderly patients: the treatment-risk paradox. JAMA. 2004;291(15):1864–70.
48. Cournot M, Cambou JP, Quentzel S, Danchin N. Key factors associated with the under-prescription of statins in elderly coronary heart disease patients: results from the ELIAGE and ELICOEUR surveys. Int J Cardiol. 2006;111(1):12–8.
49. Saito K, Kihara K. Role of C-reactive protein as a biomarker for renal cell carcinoma. Expert Rev Anticancer Ther. 2010;10(12):1979–89.
50. Peric-Golia L, Peric-Golia M. Aortic and renal lesions in hypercholesterolemic adult, male, virgin Sprague-Dawley rats. Atherosclerosis. 1983;46(1):57–65.
51. Kasiske BL, O'Donnell MP, Cleary MP, Keane WF. Treatment of hyperlipidemia reduces glomerular injury in obese Zucker rats. Kidney Int. 1988;33(3):667–72.
52. Joles JA, Kunter U, Janssen U, Kriz W, Rabelink TJ, Koomans HA, et al. Early mechanisms of renal injury in hypercholesterolemic or hypertriglyceridemic rats. J Am Soc Nephrol. 2000;11(4):669–83.

53. Samuelsson O, Mulec H, Knight-Gibson C, Attman PO, Kron B, Larsson R, et al. Lipoprotein abnormalities are associated with increased rate of progression of human chronic renal insufficiency. Nephrol Dial Transplant. 1997;12(9):1908–15.
54. Lambert G, Sakai N, Vaisman BL, Neufeld EB, Marteyn B, Chan CC, et al. Analysis of glomerulosclerosis and atherosclerosis in lecithin cholesterol acyltransferase-deficient mice. J Biol Chem. 2001;276(18):15090–8.
55. Ohta Y, Yamamoto S, Tsuchida H, Murano S, Saitoh Y, Tohjo S, et al. Nephropathy of familial lecithin-cholesterol acyltransferase deficiency: report of a case. Am J Kidney Dis. 1986; 7(1):41–6.
56. Muntner P, Coresh J, Smith JC, Eckfeldt J, Klag MJ. Plasma lipids and risk of developing renal dysfunction: the atherosclerosis risk in communities study. Kidney Int. 2000;58(1):293–301.
57. Cases A, Coll E. Dyslipidemia and the progression of renal disease in chronic renal failure patients. Kidney Int Suppl. 2005;99:S87–93.
58. Fox CS, Larson MG, Leip EP, Culleton B, Wilson PW, Levy D. Predictors of new-onset kidney disease in a community-based population. JAMA. 2004;291(7):844–50.
59. Schaeffner ES, Kurth T, Curhan GC, Glynn RJ, Rexrode KM, Baigent C, et al. Cholesterol and the risk of renal dysfunction in apparently healthy men. J Am Soc Nephrol. 2003;14(8): 2084–91.
60. Abrass CK. Cellular lipid metabolism and the role of lipids in progressive renal disease. Am J Nephrol. 2004;24(1):46–53.
61. Atchley DH, Lopes-Virella MF, Zheng D, Kenny D, Virella G. Oxidized LDL-anti-oxidized LDL immune complexes and diabetic nephropathy. Diabetologia. 2002;45(11):1562–71.
62. Choudhury D, Tuncel M, Levi M. Disorders of lipid metabolism and chronic kidney disease in the elderly. Semin Nephrol. 2009;29(6):610–20.
63. Olyaei A, Greer E, Delos Santos R, Rueda J. The efficacy and safety of the 3-hydroxy-3-methylglutaryl-CoA reductase inhibitors in chronic kidney disease, dialysis, and transplant patients. Clin J Am Soc Nephrol. 2011;6(3):664–78.
64. Adult Treatment Panel III. Third report of the National Cholesterol Education Program (NCEP) Expert Panel on detection, evaluation, and treatment of high blood cholesterol in adults. Circulation. 2002;106:3143–421.
65. Harper CR, Jacobson TA. Managing dyslipidemia in chronic kidney disease. J Am Coll Cardiol. 2008;51(25):2375–84.
66. Heart Protection Study Collaborative Group. MRC/BHF Heart Protection Study of cholesterol lowering with simvastatin in 20,536 high-risk individuals: a randomised placebo-controlled trial. Lancet. 2002;360:7–22.
67. Jardine AG, Holdaas H, Fellstrom B, Cole E, Nyberg G, Grönhagen-Riska C, et al. Fluvastatin prevents cardiac death and myocardial infarction in renal transplant recipients: post-hoc subgroup analyses of the ALERT study. Am J Transplant. 2004;4:988–95.
68. Wanner C, Krane V, März W, Olschewski M, Mann JF, Ruf G, et al. Atorvastatin in patients with type 2 diabetes mellitus undergoing hemodialysis. N Engl J Med. 2005;353:238–48.
69. Wanner C, Krane V, März W, Olschewski M, Asmus HG, Krämer W, et al. Randomized controlled trial on the efficacy and safety of atorvastatin in patients with type 2 diabetes on hemodialysis (4D study): demographic and baseline characteristics. Kidney Blood Press Res. 2004;27(4):259–66.
70. Fellström BC, Jardine AG, Schmieder RE, Holdaas H, Bannister K, Beutler J, et al. Rosuvastatin and cardiovascular events in patients undergoing hemodialysis. N Engl J Med. 2009;360:1395–407.
71. Brouwers FP, Asselbergs FW, Hillege HL, de Boer RA, Gansevoort RT, van Veldhuisen DJ, van Gilst WH. Long-term effects of fosinopril and pravastatin on cardiovascular events in subjects with microalbuminuria: ten years of follow-up of Prevention of Renal and Vascular End stage Disease Intervention Trial (PREVEND IT). Am Heart J. 2011;161(6):1171–8.
72. Tonelli M, Moyé L, Sacks FM, Cole T, Curhan GC, Cholesterol and Recurrent Events Trial Investigators. Effect of pravastatin on loss of renal function in people with moderate chronic renal insufficiency and cardiovascular disease. J Am Soc Nephrol. 2003;14(6):1605–13.

73. Baigent C, Landray MJ, Reith C, Emberson J, Wheeler DC, Tomson C, et al. The effects of lowering LDL cholesterol with simvastatin plus ezetimibe in patients with chronic kidney disease (Study of Heart and Renal Protection): a randomised placebo-controlled trial. Lancet. 2011;377(9784):2181–92.
74. Pierides AM, Alvarez-Ude F, Kerr DN. Clofibrate-induced muscle damage in patients with chronic renal failure. Lancet. 1975;2:1279–82.
75. Sendur MA, Gurlek A. Treatment of hyperlipidemia in the elderly. Akad Geriatri. 2009;1:59–66.

Chapter 15
Apheresis Methods in Hyperlipidemias

Serdar Sivgin

Introduction

Familial hypercholesterolemia (FH) is an autosomal dominant disease that is carried on chromosome 19p. This would cause reduction in the synthesis of the low-density lipoprotein (LDL) receptor. This will lead to reduced catabolism of low-density lipoprotein cholesterol (LDL-C). Heterozygote FH occurs in 1 in 500 births, while the frequency of homozygotes FH (HFH) is 1:million [1]. More than 700 mutations can cause defects in LDL receptors, which are located mainly in the liver [2, 3].

The main function of LDL receptors is removing the LDL particles from the plasma by endocytosis. Many studies established that the receptor-negative mutations differ in various populations, leading to a variety of symptoms and severity in different countries [4–7]. The end result of all of these defects is a failure to clear LDL-C from the circulation.

Patients who are heterozygous for an abnormal low-density lipoprotein receptors (LDL-R) gene have lower LDL-C levels and a less severe course than the patients who are homozygous or who are double heterozygotes, inheriting two different mutations [8].

Other factors that could affect the clinical course of the disorder include the presence of other inherited abnormalities in lipid metabolism (e.g., type III hyperlipidemia, lipoprotein lipase deficiency), metabolic factors (e.g., variation in thyroid hormone and estrogen levels, factors influencing coagulation), and environmental factors (e.g., diet, behavioral factors such as smoking) [9]. Heterozygote patients for an LDL-R mutation have twofold increase in LDL-C (350–550 mg/dL), soft-tissue

S. Sivgin, M.D. (✉)
Department of Hematology and Stem Cell Transplantation, Hematology Oncology Hospital, Erciyes University, Talas Street, Kayseri, Talas 38039, Turkey
e-mail: drssivgin@gmail.com

A. Covic et al. (eds.), *Dyslipidemias in Kidney Disease*, DOI 10.1007/978-1-4939-0515-7_15,

Table 15.1 Symptoms and clinical characteristics of FH

Gene type	Characteristic
Heterozygotes	Twofold increase in LDL cholesterol (350–550 mg/dL)
	Premature coronary artery disease (age <30)
	Development of aortic stenosis
	Dietary and medical management probability
	Xanthomas before age 20
Homozygotes	Fourfold increase in LDL cholesterol (650–1,000 mg/dL)
	Premature coronary artery disease (age <20) and death (age <30)
	Aortic stenosis (always)
	No response to dietary and medical management
	Xanthomas before age 10

Table created with data from [8, 9]
LDL low-density lipoprotein

deposition of cholesterol (tendon xanthoma) appearing by the second decade of life, premature coronary artery disease appearing in the third decade of life, and frequent development of aortic stenosis [8]. Unfortunately; heterozygote patients may respond to dietary and medical management [9].

Homozygotes for an LDL-R mutation, as well as double heterozygotes, demonstrate a fourfold increase in LDL-C (650–1,000 mg/dL), soft-tissue deposition of cholesterol (tendon xanthoma and cutaneous xanthoma) appearing during the first decade of life, premature coronary artery disease appearing in the second decade of life with death in the third decade, and the common development of aortic stenosis [10, 11]. Homozygotes for FH do not respond to dietary and medical management [8, 9]. The general characteristics and clinical features of the patients with FH are summarized in Table 15.1.

The goal in the treatment of FH is the reduction of LDL-C. For the initial treatment goals, inhibition of endogenous cholesterol production with hydroxymethylglutaryl coenzyme A (HMG-CoA) reductase inhibitors, prevention of dietary cholesterol adsorption using ezetimibe, disruption of enterohepatic circulation of cholesterol using bile acid-binding agents, and reduction in cholesterol intake could be mentioned [9]. As indicated, all homozygotes and double heterozygotes and some heterozygotes will not respond to these therapies. This is in contrast to other inherited forms of hypercholesterolemia in which medical management is usually effective [12]. This resistance to medical management has led to the use of more invasive therapies in these patients. Among the treatments that have been used distal ileal bypass, portacaval shunting, and liver transplantation could be mentioned [12]. However, these treatments are associated with a high morbidity rate [13–15].

Dietary interventions in some countries aim to reduce fat, saturated fatty acids, and cholesterol intake and to consider carbohydrates to compensate for the low energy caused by low-fat diet. Along with the positive effects of the diet, some problems, including lower intake of fat-soluble vitamins and lower levels of high-density lipoprotein (HDL) as well as an increase in triglycerides caused by high

Table 15.2 Guidelines for the methods of therapeutic apheresis applications defined by the committee of ASFA

Type of disease	Apheresis modality	Category	Category	Recommendations 2010 (grade)
FH, homozygous	Selective removal methods TPE	I	I, II	1A, 1C
FH, heterozygous LDL >300 mg/dL	Selective removal methods TPE	II	II	1A, 1C
FH, heterozygous with CDH	Selective removal methods TPE	II	II	–
FH during pregnancy	Selective removal methods TPE	II	II	–
CHD and elevated Lp(a)	Selective removal methods TPE	–	–	–
Hypertriglyceridemic pancreatitis	–	III	III	2C

Table created with data from [11, 27]

carbohydrate intake, may occur. Use of bile acid sequestrants such as cholestyramine showed that they only have minor effects on lowering cholesterol levels [16].

The other category of drugs that have been used effectively in adults with hypercholesterolemia are HMG-CoA reductase inhibitors [17, 18]. Various meta-analysis studies have confirmed the role of statins on the clinical results of hyperlipidemias. Based on such findings, they finally concluded that statin monotherapy is safe, well tolerated, and efficacious. However, long-term safety still remains unknown [19, 20].

As a less frequent method for FH, liver transplantation has become a treatment of choice for affected patients that are nonresponsive to routine pharmacologic treatments [21, 22]. The transplanted liver retains the specific qualities of the donor, so liver transplantation can transfer a rich source of functioning LDL receptors to the recipient, which may lead to a cure of the hypercholesterolemia and resolution of the symptoms. However, the success of this type of treatment depends on the total functional receptors transplanted and, hence, on the graft size [23].

In patients with FH, an inherited abnormality in LDL-R, plasma exchange slows aortic and coronary artery atherosclerosis [24, 25] and prolongs survival [26] in individuals who are homozygous for the LDL-R mutation. Plasma exchange, however, also removes HDL, which is protective against atherosclerosis. To prevent removal of the beneficial HDL, selective removal techniques were developed to remove LDL-C while sparing other plasma proteins.

The American Society for Apheresis (ASFA) has determined the indications for therapeutic apheresis in the treatment of hyperlipidemias (Table 15.2). Besides this, the FDA approved the major indications [27] for patients with FH who have failed to respond to pharmacological and dietary strategies as follows:

- Functional homozygotes with an LDL-C >500 mg/dL.
- Functional heterozygotes with no known cardiovascular disease but an LDL-C >300 mg/dL.
- Functional heterozygotes with known cardiovascular disease but an LDL-C >200 mg/dL.

Epidemiology and Management of Hyperlipidemias (LDL Apheresis)

Plasma exchange (plasmapheresis, PE) has been used as a safe and effective technique of extracorporeal blood purification not only for the treatment of renal diseases, but also for many other indications in neurological and toxicological disorders (Table 15.3). The method was considered highly effective in anti-glomerular basement membrane glomerulonephritis, hemolytic–uremic syndrome, and recurrence of glomerulopathies in transplanted kidney. However, the method has some disadvantages, such as the risk for transmission of some viral infections that could be carried with the fresh frozen plasma used as the supplement fluid during process. During the last decade, many researchers focused on more selective and effective techniques that could be used in renal diseases. Despite significant progress in the diagnostic techniques and new medications for the diagnosis and treatment of coronary heart disease (CHD), it still remains one of the major causes of death worldwide. Plasmapheresis has been used as a safe and effective technique of extracorporeal blood purification not only for the treatment of renal diseases, but also for many other indications in neurological and toxicological disorders. The method was considered highly effective in anti-glomerular basement membrane glomerulonephritis, hemolytic–uremic syndrome, recurrence of glomerulopathies in transplanted kidney. However, the method has some disadvantages, such as the risk for transmission of some viral infections that could be carried with the fresh frozen plasma used as the supplement fluid during process.

During the last decade, many researchers focused on more selective and effective techniques that could be used in renal diseases. Despite significant progress in the diagnostic techniques and new medications for the diagnosis and treatment of CHD, it still remains one of the major causes of death worldwide.

Table 15.3 The methods of extracorporeal LDL apheresis

Year	Author	Method of therapeutic apheresis	Advantages	Disadvantages
1967	De Gennes et al.	Plasmapheresis	Quick and well-tolerated	Not selective, infection risk and bleeding
1980	Agishi et al.	Cascade filtration	Semi-selective	Infection risk, less effective
1983	Borberg et al.	Immunoadsorption	Selective and effective	Expensive
1983	Wieland and Seidel	Heparin-induced extracorporeal LDL precipitation (HELP)	Selective and effective	Expensive
1985	Antwiller et al.	Dextransulfate-induced LDL precipitation	Selective and effective	Expensive, low availability
1987	Mabuchi et al.	Dextransulfate LDL adsorption (Liposorber)	Selective and effective	Expensive
1993	Bosch et al.	LDL hemoperfusion (DALI)	Selective and effective	Not defined
2003	Otto et al.	LDL hemoperfusion (Liposorber D)	Selective and effective	Not defined

Adapted from [10]. Courtesy of Dr. Rolf Bambauer

The effective reduction in serum cholesterol levels has been achieved with the administration of HMG-CoA reductase inhibitors, which could be combined with other lipid-lowering agents. The available treatment alternatives are fenofibrate, β-pyridylcarbinol, nicotinic acid, probucol, colestyramin, colestipol, D-thyroxine, and β-fibrates.

Among older treatment choices, the combination of niacin and bile acid sequestrants should be mentioned. This was the best therapy available before the statins were used for FH [28]. However, this study was performed with 10 g of bile acid sequestrant three times a day and the administration of 3–7 g of immediate-release niacin and was very difficult to accomplish.

In current treatment options, statins have been tested extensively in children with FH. Lovastatin, simvastatin, atorvastatin, and rosuvastatin have all been studied in adolescents [29–32]. In the study, patients achieved reduction in plasma LDL levels of 27 %, 41 %, 40 %, and 50 %, respectively. Statins have been used effectively, and their effectiveness could be improved by appropriate dietary regulations.

Serum cholesterol levels higher than 200 mg/dL represent an increased coronary risk. It should be noted that the risk is double in case of serum cholesterol levels between 200 and 250 mg/dL and fourfold at values of 250–300 mg/dL [33]. Additional risk factors include familial disposition, adiposity, diabetes mellitus, smoking, reduced HDL, increased Lipoprotein (a) (Lp(a)), and fibrinogen.

Almost all forms of treatment-resistant hypercholesterolemia might be treated effectively after the development of semiselective extracorporeal reducing strategies for hyperlipidemia [34–37].

The major treatment principle for various forms of FH includes dietetic regulations and medical therapy. The goal of the treatment was to reduce the LDL levels below 200 mg/dL. In case of treatment resistance to first-step alternatives or the presence of side effects, LDL-apheresis should be planned for the patients. The diagnosis of FH should be supported by corresponding examinations, and it is preferred to choose the patients who are nonsmokers. All patients should be monitored for cardiological risk status with findings in ECG under exercise, thallium sintigraphy, or coronary angiography. These attempts aim to reduce progression or to achieve the regression of the coronary heart condition.

In general, the basic concept of LDL-apheresis seems to reduce the LDL-C in treatment-resistant FH. However, this method has been considered effective in patients with nephrotic syndrome (NS). The current data established the potency of LDL-apheresis not only by reducing the plasma lipids, but also by its positive effect on the progress of different nephropathies. There are some disorders in which the effectiveness of LDL-apheresis in renal patients seems to be proven by current data. These disorders are lupus nephritis, primary focal glomerulosclerosis (FGS), and recurrence of FGS in transplanted kidney. The method of LDL-apheresis in lupus nephritis should be planned for patients who do not respond to other treatment strategies and who do not have renal involvement. LDL-apheresis method could be a good alternative method for patients with NS who are resistant to immunosuppressive therapy, such as minimal change disease [38]. Besides the lowering effect on plasma lipids, LDL-apheresis might improve renal function in diabetic nephropathy [39].

Table 15.4 The effectiveness of LDL apheresis techniques (the values represent the reduction in percent of original concentration)

Variables	Cascade filtration	Immunoadsorption	HELP	LDL adsorption	LDL hemoperfusion (DALI)	LDL hemoperfusion (Liposorber)
Cholesterol	35–50	30	50	45	60	55
LDL	30–45	35	45	35–40	60–75	60–75
HDL	35–50	20	10–20	–	16–29	5–13
Lp(a)	60–70	60	46	60	60–75	60–75
Triglycerides	60	60	60	70	40	66
Fibrinogen	50	10–20	50	30	16	20–40
Ig M	35	10–20	–	–	21	14
Ig A	55	10–20	–	–	–	–
Factor VIII	–	10–20	10–20	20	–	–
C3	–	–	50	–	–	–
C4	–	–	50	–	–	–
Plasminogen	–	–	50	–	–	–

Adapted from [10]. Courtesy of Dr. Rolf Bambauer

The effectiveness of LDL-apheresis techniques is summarized in Table 15.4. In today's medical practice, the following LDL-apheresis strategies are the most effective and common treatment options worldwide.

Immunoadsorption

As an effective method for LDL-apheresis, immunoadsorption (IA) technique depends upon the perfusion of plasma through sepharosis columns covered with LDL antibodies (Fig. 15.1). In this way, the LDL molecules are easily adsorbed onto the antibodies of the columns in the system. This method was first described in some studies [40, 41] in the 1980s as LDL-apheresis containing anti-LDL sepharose columns. This method is mostly based on the affinity chromatography forming antigen-antibody complex. The source of antibodies against the protein part in human LDL-C molecules (apolipoprotein B 100) are mostly derived from sheep, and these molecules are covalently bound to sepharose particles.

The working procedure is that when one column is used for adsorption, the non-working part should be generated with neutral solutions of saline buffer, glycine buffer, and again with neutral buffer. This cycle should be completed after the column has been saturated with the absorbed lipoproteins (600–800 mL of plasma).

The immunoadsorption columns should be used for at least 40 treatment sessions. During the procedure, the operated plasma is mixed with the cellular part of the blood and then returned to the patient. This operational procedure takes approximately 3 h with a computerized apheresis monitor. At the end of the treatment, the columns should be rinsed and filled with sterilized solution after the same procedure.

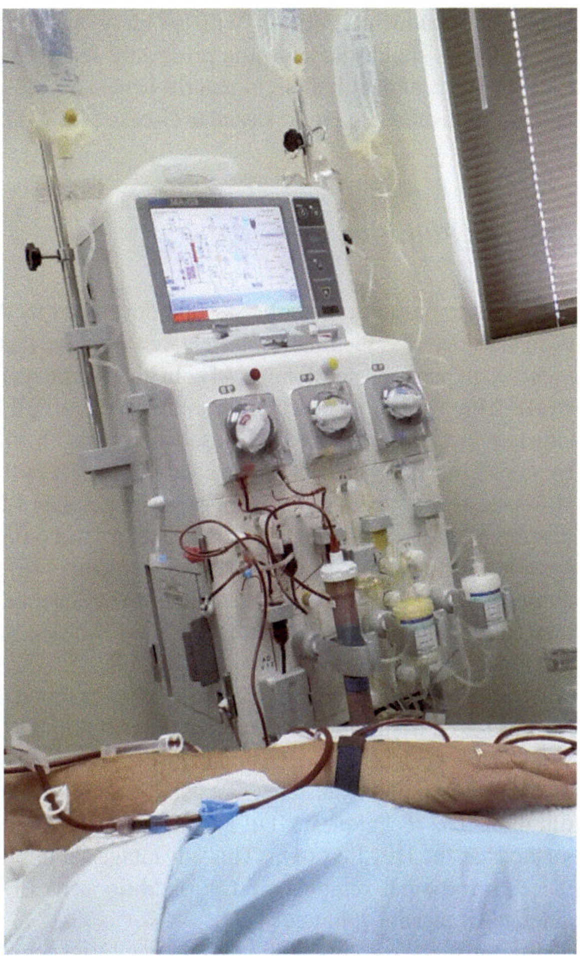

Fig. 15.1 A photo of the patient and LDL-apheresis device with medical equipment used for LDL-apheresis procedures (immunoadsorption)

Factors such as selectivity, effectiveness, and high regenerating ability of the columns are among the advantages of the method. The disadvantage of the method is that the treatment is very expensive. It is a great deal that the implementation of the system is viable on a long-term basis due to the high cost of the columns, which means 40 times at least per each patient. An LDL-C level that could reduce 30–40 % of the pretreatment level could be achieved with a perfusion volume of 4–6 L for each session. The other parameters that are expected to decline with this method are serum proteins, immunoglobulins, HDL, and fibrinogen by 15–20 %. The levels return to their original ranges within 24 h following the procedure.

Here we should mention two different systems that are currently available worldwide, the LDL Therasorb system (Miltenyi Biotec, Germany), and the LDL and Lp(a)-Excorim system (Fresenius, Germany). These two systems could be considered as safe and effective methods for clinical use, even for patients requiring long-term treatment. Patients with primary and secondary dyslipoproteinemia and Lp(a) IA should undergo the procedure for the extracorporeal elimination of LDL-C. IA treatment had significantly beneficial effects on serum LDL levels in patients with atherosclerotic vascular disease [42, 43].

Cascade Filtration

The cascade filtration method was first developed by Agishi et al. in Japan. It has been considered as the first semiselective technique that could be used for the treatment of hypercholesterolemia [44]. In this technique, the secondary membrane works with a cutoff of nearly one million daltons. We know that an LDL-C molecule has a weight of 2,300,000 Da, so it is retained by this membrane. It should also be noted that all other molecules larger than 1,000,000 Da are also retained. However, some molecules in the plasma smaller than 1,000,000 Da pass through the membrane and then are returned to the patient. It should be mentioned that the lipid-lowering techniques cascade filtration, membrane differential filtration (MDF), or double filtration plasmapheresis are accepted as having advantages compared to the conventional plasmapheresis method. Nevertheless, adsorption or precipitation techniques seem superior these methods [45].

Towards the development of some synthetic secondary membranes like the lipid-filter EC-50 (Asahi, Japan), improved outcomes in the treatment of hypercholesterolemia have been achieved via higher effectiveness and selectivity for the separation of the blood components. This cascade filtration system can be considered as lipid filtration. The techniques MDF and lipid filtration are used as safe and effective methods as the HELP-system. This advantage should be mentioned with respect to the extracorporeal removal of Lp(a), fibrinogen, LDL-C by processing similar amounts of plasma volumes [46].

Recently, for patients with diabetes mellitus, peripheral arterial occlusive disease, coronary artery disease, cerebrovascular stroke, and age-related macular degeneration, a new technique has been developed for impaired microcirculation. This method has been named rheopheresis, which should be used as a special form of cascade filtration, which aims to reduce blood viscosity. Some studies established that the treatment results of rheopheresis could have promising results in patients with diabetic retinopathy and age-related macular degeneration [47, 48].

Dextran Sulfate Low-Density Lipoprotein (Liposorber)

This technique works with dextran sulfate on the basis of its high affinity and low toxicity for LDL adsorbent. Low-molecular dextran sulfate (MW 4,500) can selectively absorb all molecules containing apolipoprotein B. The mechanism is that dextran sulfate is covalently bound to cellulose particles. As a result of direct

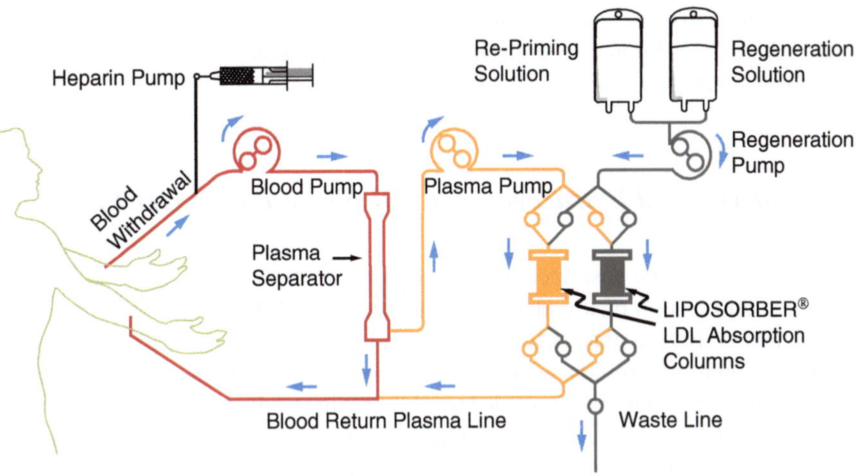

Fig. 15.2 The schematic configuration of the principles of the LDL-apheresis method (Liposorber)

interaction between dextran sulfate and apolipoprotein B-containing lipoproteins (such as LDL and VLDL) that are positively charged, a binding operation is usually achieved (Fig. 15.2). It should be emphasized that the dextran sulfate structurally mimics the structure of LDL receptor and acts as a type of pseudoreceptor [49, 50]. All compounds containing apolipoprotein B-like cholesterol, VLDL, triglycerides, and LDL are absorbed within the penetrating of plasma through columns after the primary separation is completed. Later, the plasma is directed to the patient without cholesterol. In recent years, this technique has found large clinical use by physicians due to its high effectiveness in the elimination of serum cholesterol [51, 52].

The advantage of the Liposorber system is that the technique is highly selective for the elimination of all apolipoprotein B-containing lipoproteins. The high effectiveness of the system should not be omitted even in patients with life-threatening hypercholesterolemia.

The Liposorber LA-15 (Kaneka, Japan) system could be considered a safe and effective treatment modality in patients with severe hypercholesterolemia that was not responsive to diet and maximum drug use. There are some data regarding the effectiveness of LDL-apheresis on coronary arterial lesions that the method could not only prevent the development of CHD but also slow the regression in patients with hypercholesterolemia [53]. Among the side effects for the method are hypotension, hypoglycemia, nausea, and light allergic reactions. Low-molecular dextran sulfate could be considered to have less allergenic potential than the forms of dextran that have a higher molecular weight to 80,000. The effectiveness of Liposorber has been experienced in various clinical studies. The data showed that the majority of the patients (75 %) achieved reduction of coronary atherosclerosis risk. In these studies, side effects were observed at very low percentage, such as 0.5–4 % [54, 55].

The effectiveness and safety of the Liposorber system in children has been established with some studies [56]. The experience of these authors led them to recommend early therapeutic intervention with extracorporeal treatment with LDL-apheresis in children severely affected by homozygous or double heterozygous familial hypercholesterolemia.

Heparin-Induced Extracorporeal LDL Precipitation (HELP)

This method was first described and experienced in 1982 for the purpose of extracorporeal elimination of low-density lipoproteins, or HELP [57]. The principle of the method is that the plasma is mixed with a ratio of 1:1 using acetate acetic acid buffer and then the primary separation is performed. This aims to keep the pH of this mixture at 5.1. It is recommended to add heparin at a dose of 100,000 U/L to the buffer. LDL-C precipitates in the acidic environment interfere with heparin and fibrinogen in order to form insoluble particles. This operation is performed following the forming of mixture with the acetate acetic acid buffer and heparin. Later, the precipitates are removed from the plasma with the action of a polycarbonate membrane. The operation continues with the removal of free heparin through a heparin absorber (DEAE cellulose). The technical part of the system seems quite confusing, but it is a very effective and reliable lipid-lowering strategy. The other parameters in the blood such as HDL reach their original levels within 24 h following operation. Here it should be mentioned that the amount of plasma should be limited to 3 L, as the fibrinogen concentration increases gradually [58].

Because the treatment uses only disposable materials, the device does not need disinfection.

Besides this, no piped water supply or reverse osmosis is required for the progress of the operation. During the operation, the levels of various components in the blood such as C3, C4, fibrinogen, and plasminogen decline by 50 %. The system also reduces the levels of cholesterol, LDL, and triglycerides, so it could be suggested that the technique is not specific. High fibrinogen levels decline during the HELP operation, so excess amounts of plasma units could lead to bleeding complications. The effectiveness of the system on cholesterol levels is shown in Table 15.4. The risk of cardiovascular events might be prevented in an earlier period by using antihyperlipidemic agents in patients who undergo regular extracorporeal LDL-elimination.

The mechanism of action of the LDL apheresis procedure depends on reducing the shear-stress of the flowing blood that puts stress on plaques, which form the viscosity of the plasma. This leads to a significant reduction in the resistance of peripheral arteries of lower extremities. In addition to the high safety profile and effectiveness of the system, serious complications have rarely been observed [59]. Some studies have strongly established that the HELP method has lowered the incidence of cardiovascular complications in patients with high serum cholesterol [60, 61]. Another significant result of LDL-apheresis is that oxidized LDL could be removed effectively. We should mention that oxidized LDL promotes plaque stabilization that could lead to atherothrombotic events.

Fibrinogen is one of the major molecules that has an effect on the formation of blood viscosity. The removal of fibrinogen with some other molecules results in significant improvement in the microcirculatory status of the body by which numerous studies have published evidence-based data [62]. In familial hypercholesterolemia, ischemic heart disease, and heart transplantation, the HELP method had successful results as established in some studies [63, 64].

Lipoprotein (a) Apheresis

Today the current data show that Lp(a) has seriously negative effects on the development of atherothrombotic complications due to its structural similarity to plasminogen [65]. The major similar part of Lp(a) is with LDL and also apo-B that represents such as a lipid molecule. There are many studies regarding the data that elevated levels of plasma Lp(a) are associated with an increased risk of CHD [66]. Lp(a) is considered to have both atherogenic and thrombogenic activity due to its structural potential [67]. Many drug therapies have failed to maintain reductions in the plasma Lp(a) levels, so these strategies have limited effectiveness.

LDL-apheresis methods seem to be the most effective strategy for reducing the elevated levels of plasma Lp(a). For approximately 20 years, some special antibodies for immunoadsorption with sepharose bound anti-Lp(a) have been used for the treatment of patients with high Lp(a) levels [68, 69]. For the treatment strategy, two columns are required. During the process, both columns are filled with 400 mL of sorbent solution that has been tested for sterility. The columns are reusable for anti-Lp(a) immunoadsorption. In the time intervals between treatment sessions, the device columns should be stored at 4 °C. For each patient, two personal columns are reserved to keep the procedure on [70]. In the pathogenesis of CHD and arteriosclerosis, high Lp(a) levels are considered as a significant risk factor. Diet or drugs do not have beneficial effect on reducing the elevated levels of Lp(a). The current available device that could remove Lp(a) specifically from plasma is Lipopak, Pocard (Moscow, Russia).

Low-Density Lipoprotein Hemoperfusion (DALI System)

The first definition and clinical administration of this system was performed in 1993 as low-density lipoprotein hemoperfusion (direct adsorption of lipoproteins [DALI]) [71]. In the DALI system, an absorber is used for perfusion (Fig. 15.3). These absorbers contain 480 mL of polyacrylate-coated polyacrylamide. The columns have a capacity of more than 1.5–2.0 L blood volumes for effective adsorption. The major molecules that the operation targets are LDL, triglycerides, cholesterol, and Lp(a). In this method, regeneration is not required because the columns are usually used for only one treatment session [72]. The principle in this method is performed by

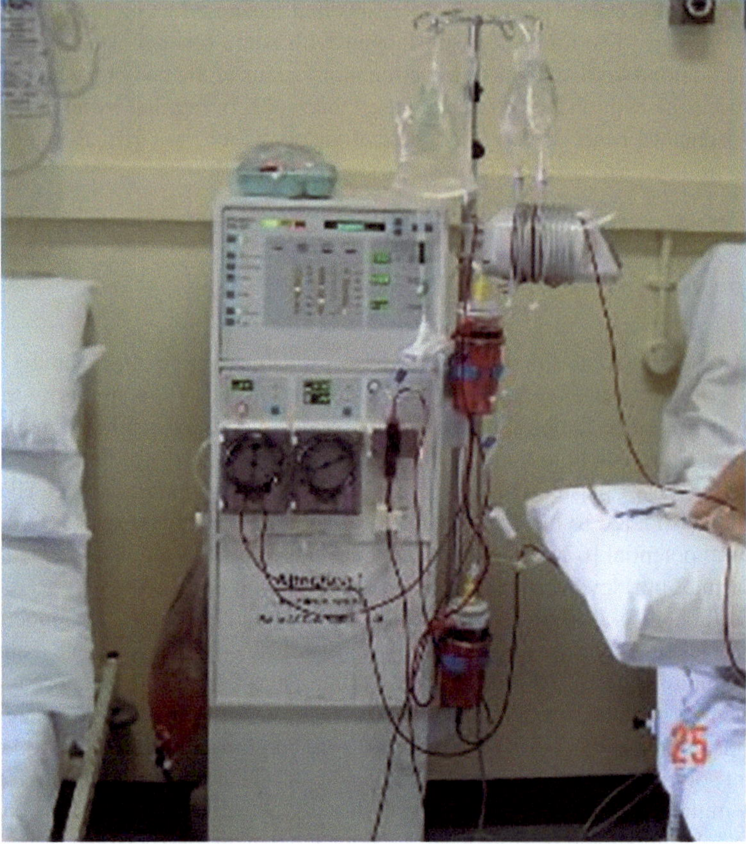

Fig. 15.3 The DALI machine that is used for lipid apheresis in patients with FH

adsorption onto polyacrylate-coated polyacrylamide beads in order to reduce the elevated levels of Lp(a) molecules, LDL, and other lipoproteins.

The adsorption of LDL and Lp(a) and other lipoproteins occurs by polyacrylate ligands that bind covalently to the polyacrylamide surface. The main part of the system, polyacrylate, consists of polyanions, which are negatively charged with carboxylate groups like LDL-receptor [73]. As the polyanions interact with cationic groups in apoprotein B, the lipoproteins are moved through the beads. We should mention that by flowing, the whole blood affects only a minor interaction between the blood cells and small outer surface of the beads [74]. The small-size lipoproteins have advantages for penetrating through the inner sponge-like body of the beads by the pores. HDL molecules have disadvantages due to the fact that the apo AI-coated HDL is not attracted to the ligand. As a result, it is not affected by the adsorber and cannot be eliminated by the system. Heparin could be used for anticoagulation in the system and then anticoagulation could be maintained by continuous acid citrate dextrose (ACD-A) solution infusion into the blood. For adequate anticoagulation in extracorporeal device, the volume of ACD is calculated as approximately 5 % of whole blood for the majority of the patients. The DALI system can eliminate calcium and magnesium as well as lipoproteins.

This property requires one to maintain the presence of mentioned electrolytes in the columns with a volume of 5 L of priming solution. This operation could prevent hypocalcemia and hypomagnesia during the apheresis period. The DALI system might be performed with three different adsorber sizes. These are DALI 500, DALI 750, and DALI 1000 mL adsorbers. During the operation, the blood pressure in both afferent and efferent blood lines are measured for the monitorization of the system [10]. The DALI system can be considered as a safe, effective, and selective therapy for apheresis in hyperlipidemias. Some microparticles may release from the columns, so the columns should be rinsed carefully to avoid the risk. A second filter might be added after the column in order to reduce the possibility of microparticle release. This filter is recommended to maximize the safety of the system. There are some data regarding the safety and effectiveness of the DALI system that could be suggested to reduce LDL and Lp(a) at 60 % at the end of a treatment period lasting 100 min. The patients had rare side effects that could negatively effect the operation survey [75].

Conclusion

It should be noted that all the aforementioned techniques could be considered as safe and effective methods of lipid reduction. The goal of the treatment should be to lower the plasma LDL-C levels to 50–60 % of the original levels by performing weekly or biweekly apheresis sessions. The primary aim in reducing cholesterol concentration is to prevent the development and progression of atherosclerosis. The evolution of the techniques used in medicine will enable one to achieve more satisfying outcomes related to the hyperlipidemic status of the patients.

References

1. Goldstein JL, Hobbs HH, Brown MS. Familial hypercholesterolemia. In: Scriver CR, Beaudet AL, Sly WS, Valle D, editors. The metabolic and molecular basis of inherited disease. New York: McGraw-Hill; 1995. p. 1981–2030.
2. Austin MA, Hutter CM, Zimmern RL, Humphries SE. Familial hypercholesterolemia and coronary heart disease: a HuGE association review. Am J Epidemiol. 2004;160(5):421–9.
3. Shafiq N, Singh M, Kaur S, Khosla P, Malhotra S. Dietary treatment for familial hypercholesterolaemia. Cochrane Database Syst Rev. 2010;(1):CD001918.
4. Bertolini S, Cassanelli S, Garuti R, Ghisellini M, Simone ML, Rolleri M, et al. Analysis of LDL receptor gene mutations in Italian patients with homozygous familial hypercholesterolemia. Arterioscler Thromb Vasc Biol. 1999;19(2):408–18.
5. Bujo H, Takahashi K, Saito Y, Maruyama T, Yamashita S, Matsuzawa Y, et al. Clinical features of familial hypercholesterolemia in Japan in a database from 1996–1998 by the research committee of the ministry of health, labour and welfare of Japan. J Atheroscler Thromb. 2004;11(3):146–51.

6. Cao S, Wang L, Qin Y, Lin J, Wu B, Liu S, et al. Analysis of low-density lipoprotein receptor gene mutations in a Chinese patient with clinically homozygous familial hypercholesterolemia. Chin Med J (Engl). 2003;116(10):1535–8.
7. Chiou KR, Charng MJ. Detection of mutations and large rearrangements of the low-density lipoprotein receptor gene in Taiwanese patients with familial hypercholesterolemia. Am J Cardiol. 2010;105(12):1752–8.
8. Ueda M. Familial hypercholesterolemia. Mol Genet Metab. 2005;86:423–6.
9. Bhatnagar D. Diagnosis and screening for familial hypercholesterolaemia: finding the patients, finding the genes. Ann Clin Biochem. 2006;43:441–56.
10. Bambauer R, Bambauer C, Lehmann B, Latza R, Schiel R. LDL-apheresis: technical and clinical aspects. ScientificWorldJournal. 2012;2012:314283.
11. Szczepiorkowski M, Bandarenko N, Kim HC, Linenberger ML, Marques MB, Sarode R, et al. Guidelines on the use of therapeutic apheresis in clinical practice-evidence-based approach from the apheresis applications committee of the American Society for Apheresis. J Clin Apher. 2007;22:106–75.
12. Soutar AK, Naoumova RP. Mechanisms of disease: genetic causes of familial hypercholesterolemia. Nat Clin Pract Cardiovasc Med. 2007;4:214–25.
13. Grundy SM, Vega GI, Bilheimer DM. Influence of combined therapy with mevinolin and interruption of bile-acid reabsorption on low density lipoprotein in heterozygous familial hypercholesterolemia. Ann Intern Med. 1985;103:339–43.
14. Stein EA, Mieny C, Spitz L. Portocaval shunt in four patients with homozygous hypercholesterolima. Lancet. 1975;1:832–5.
15. Buchwald H, Varco RL, Matts IP, et al. Effect of partial heart bypass surgery on mortality and morbidity from coronary heart disease in patients with hypercholesterolemia. Report of the Program on the Surgical Control of the Hyperlipidemias. N Engl J Med. 1990;323:946–55.
16. Tonstad S, Knudtzon J, Sivertsen M, Refsum H, Ose L. Efficacy and safety of cholestyramine therapy in peripubertal and prepubertal children with familial hypercholesterolemia. J Pediatr. 1996;129(1):42–9.
17. Alonso R, Mata N, Mata P. Benefits and risks assessment of simvastatin in familial hypercholesterolaemia. Expert Opin Drug Saf. 2005;4(2):171–81.
18. Avellone G, Di Garbo V, Abruzzese G, Campisi D, De Simone R, Raneli G, et al. One-year atorvastatin treatment in hypercholesterolemic patients with or without carotid artery disease. Int Angiol. 2006;25(1):26–34.
19. Avis HJ, Vissers MN, Stein EA, Wijburg FA, Trip MD, Kastelein JJ, et al. A systematic review and metaanalysis of statin therapy in children with familial hypercholesterolemia. Arterioscler Thromb Vasc Biol. 2007;27(8):1803–10.
20. Arambepola C, Farmer AJ, Perera R, Neil HA. Statin treatment for children and adolescents with heterozygous familial hypercholesterolaemia: a systematic review and meta-analysis. Atherosclerosis. 2007;195(2):339–47.
21. Moghadasian MH, Frohlich JJ, Saleem M, Hong JM, Qayumi K, Scudamore CH. Surgical management of dyslipidemia: clinical and experimental evidence. J Invest Surg. 2001;14(2):71–8.
22. Bilheimer DW, Goldstein JL, Grundy SM, Starzl TE, Brown MS. Liver transplantation to provide low-density-lipoprotein receptors and lower plasma cholesterol in a child with homozygous familial hypercholesterolemia. N Engl J Med. 1984;311(26):1658–64.
23. Lopez-Santamaria M, Migliazza L, Gamez M, Murcia J, Diaz-Gonzalez M, Camarena C, et al. Liver transplantation in patients with homozygotic familial hypercholesterolemia previously treated by end-to-side portocaval shunt and ileal bypass. J Pediatr Surg. 2000;35(4):630–3.
24. Thompson GR, Myant NB, Kilpatrick D, Oakley CM, Raphael MJ, Steiner RE. Assessment of long-term plasma exchange for familial hypercholesterolaemia. Br Heart J. 1980;43:680–8.
25. Tatami R, Inoue N, Itoh H, Kishino B, Koga N, Nakashima Y, et al. Regression of coronary atherosclerosis by combined LDL apheresis and lipid-lowering drug therapy in patients with familial hypercholesterolemia: a multicenter study. Atherosclerosis. 1992;95:1–13.
26. Thompson GR, Miller JP, Breslow JL. Improved survival of patients with homozygous familial hypercholesterolaemia treated by plasma exchange. Br Med J. 1985;291:1671–3.

27. Szczepiorkowski ZM, Winters JL, Bandarenko N, Kim HC, Linenberger ML, Marques MB, et al. Guidelines on the use of therapeutic apheresis in clinical practice—evidence-based approach from the Apheresis Applications Committee of the American Society for Apheresis. J Clin Apher. 2010;25:83–177.
28. Kuo PT, Kostis JB, Moreyra AE, Hayes JA. Familial type II hyperlipoproteinemia with coronary heart disease: effect of diet-colestipol-nicotinic acid treatment. Chest. 1981;79:286–91.
29. Clauss SB, Holmes KW, Hopkins P, Stein E, Cho M, Tate A, et al. Efficacy and safety of lovastatin therapy in adolescent girls with heterozygous familial hypercholesterolemia. Pediatrics. 2005;116:682–8.
30. de Jongh S, Ose L, Szamosi T, Gagné C, Lambert M, Scott R, et al. Efficacy and safety of statin therapy in children with familial hypercholesterolemia: a randomized double-blind, placebo-controlled trial with simvastatin. Circulation. 2002;106:2231.
31. McCrindle BW, Ose L, Marais AD. Efficacy and safety of atorvastatin in children and adolescents with familial hypercholesterolemia or severe hyperlipidemia: a multicenter, randomized, placebo-controlled trial. J Pediatr. 2003;143:74–80.
32. Avis HJ, Hutten BA, Gagne C, Langslet G, McCrindle BW, Wiegman A, et al. Efficacy and safety of rosuvastatin therapy for children with familial hypercholesterolemia. J Am Coll Cardiol. 2010;55:1121–6.
33. European Atherosclerosis Society (Study Group). Strategies for prevention of coronary heart disease: a policy statement of the European atherosclerosis society. Eur Heart J. 1987;8:77–88.
34. Berger ML, Wilson HM, Liss CL. A comparison of the tolerability and efficacy of lovastatin 20 and fluvastatin 20 mg in the treatment of primary hypercholesterolemia. J Cardiovasc Pharmacol Ther. 1996;2:101–6.
35. Illingworth DR, Stein EA, Knopp RH, Hunninghake DB, Davidson MH, Dujovne CA, et al. A randomized multicenter trial comparing the efficacy of simvastatin and fluvastatin. J Cardiovasc Pharmacol Ther. 1996;1:23–9.
36. Duell PE, Connor WE, Illingworth DR. Rhabdomyolysis after taking atorvastatin with gemfibrozil. Am J Cardiol. 1998;81:368–9.
37. Treasure CB, Klein JL, Weintraub WS, Talley JD, Stillabower ME, Kosinski AS, et al. Beneficial effects of cholesterol-lowering therapy on the coronary endothelium in patients with coronary artery disease. N Engl J Med. 1995;332:481–7.
38. Muso E, Mune M, Fujii Y, Imai E, Ueda N, Hatta K, et al. Significant rapid relief from steroid-resistant nephrotic syndrome by LDL-apheresis compared with steroid monotherapy. Nephron. 2001;89:408–15.
39. Nakao T, Yoshino M, Matsumoto H, Okada T, Han M, Hidaka H, et al. Low-density lipoprotein apheresis retards the progression of hyperlipidemic overt diabetic nephropathy. Kidney Int. 1999;56 Suppl 71:206–9.
40. Borberg H, Stoffel W, Oette K. The development of specific plasma immunoadsorption. Plasma Ther Transfus Technol. 1983;4:459–66.
41. Stoffel W, Demant T. Selective removal of apolipoprotein B-containing serum lipoproteins from blood plasma. Proc Natl Acad Sci U S A. 1981;78:611–5.
42. Bambauer R, Schiel R, Latza R. Current topics on low-density lipoprotein apheresis. Ther Apher. 2001;5:293–300.
43. Borberg H. Results of an open, longitudinal multicenter LDL-apheresis trial. Transfus Sci. 1999;20:83–94.
44. Agishi T, Kaneko J, Hasuo Y, Hayasaka Y, Sanaka T, Ota K, et al. Double filtration plasmapheresis with no or minimal amount of blood derivate for substitution. In: Sieberth HG, editor. Plasma exchange. Stuttgart, Germany: Schattauer; 1980. p. 53.
45. Yamamoto A, Kawaguchi A, Harada-Shiba M, Tsushima M, Kojima SI. Apheresis technology for prevention and regression of atherosclerosis: an overview. Ther Apher. 1997;1:233–41.
46. Klingel R, Mausfeld P, Fassbender C, Goehlen B. Lipidfiltration—safe and effective methodology to perform lipid-apheresis. Transfus Apher Sci. 2004;30:245–54.
47. Klingel R, Fassbenderm C, Fassbender T, Erdtracht B, Berrouschot J. Rheopheresis: rheologic, functional, and structural aspects. Ther Apher. 2000;4:348–57.

48. Klingel R, Erdtracht B, Gauss V, Piazolo A, Mausfeld-Lafdhiya P, Diehm C. Rheopheresis in patients with critical limb ischemia—results of an open label prospective pilot trial. Ther Apher Dial. 2005;9:473–81.
49. Agishi T, Wood W, Gordon B. LDL apheresis using the Liposorber LA-15 system in coronary and peripheral vascular disease associated with severe hypercholesterolemia. Curr Ther Res. 1994;55:879–904.
50. Knisel W, Muller M, Besenthal I, di Nicuolo A, Rebstock M, Risler T, et al. Application of a new LDL apheresis system using two dextran sulfate cellulose columns in combination with an automatic column-regenerating unit and a blood cell separator. J Clin Apher. 1991;6:11–5.
51. Kojima S, Harada-Shiba M, Toyoto Y, Kimura G, Tsushima M, Kuramochi M, et al. Changes in coagulation factors by passage through a dextran sulfate cellulose column during low-density lipoprotein apheresis. Int J Artif Organs. 1992;15:185–90.
52. Burgstaler EA, Pineda AA. Plasma exchange versus an affinity column for cholesterol reduction. J Clin Apher. 1992;7:69–74.
53. Bambauer R, Schiel R, Latza R. Low-density lipoprotein apheresis: an overview. Ther Apher. 2003;7:382–90.
54. Gordon BR, Kelsey SF, Bilheimer DW, Brown DC, Dau PC, Gotto Jr AM, et al. Treatment of refractory familial hypercholesterolemia by low-density lipoprotein apheresis using an automated dextran sulfate cellulose adsorption system. For the Lipsorber Study Group. Am J Cardiol. 1992;70:1010–3.
55. Richter WO, Donner MG, Schwandt P. Three low density lipoprotein apheresis techniques in treatment of patients with familial hypercholesterolemia: a long-term evaluation. Ther Apher. 1999;3:203–8.
56. Stefanutti C, Notarbartolo A, Collridi V, Nigri A, Vivenzio A, Bertolini S, et al. LDL apheresis in a homozygous familial hypercholesterolemic child aged 4.5. Artif Organs. 1997;21:1126–7.
57. Seidel D, Wieland H. Ein neues verfahren zur selektiven messung und extrakorporalen elimination von low-densitylipoproteinen. J Clin Chem Clin Biochem. 1982;20:684–8.
58. Stefanutti C, Morozzi C, Perrone G, Di Giacomo S, Vivenzio A, D'Alessandri G. The lipid- and lipoprotein- [LDL-Lp(a)] apheresis techniques. Updating. G Chir. 2012;33:444–9.
59. Seidel D, Armstrong VW, Schuff-Werner P. The HELP-apheresis multicenter study, an angiography assessed trial on the role of LDL-apheresis in the secondary prevention of coronary heart-disease. Eur J Clin Invest. 1991;21:375–83.
60. Xue J, Dong Q, Han X, You H, Gu Y, Lin S. Effects of HELP therapy on acute ischemic stroke and vascular endothelial cell function. Ther Apher Dial. 2007;11:171–6.
61. Thiery J, Seidel D. Safety and effectiveness of long-term LDL-apheresis in patients at high risk. Curr Opin Lipidol. 1998;9:521–6.
62. Eisenhauer T, Schuff-Werner P, Armstrong VW, Talartschik J, Scheler F, Seidel D. Long-term experience with the HELP system for treatment of severe familial hypercholesterolemia. ASAIO Trans. 1987;33:395–7.
63. Jaeger BR, Meiser B, Nagel D, Uberfuhr P, Thiery J, Brandl U, et al. Aggressive lowering of fibrinogen and cholesterol in prevention of graft vessel disease after heart transplantation. Circulation. 1997;96:154–8.
64. Jaeger BR, Marx P, Pfefferkorn T, Hamann G, Seidel D. Heparin-mediated extracorporeal LDL/fibrinogen precipitation—HELP—in coronary and cerebral ischemia. Acta Neurochir. 1999;73:81–4.
65. Ullrich H, Mansouri-Taleghani B, Lackner KJ, Schalke B, Bogdahn U, Schmitz G. Chronic inflammatory demyelinating polyradiculoneuropathy: superiority of protein A immunoadsorption over plasma exchange treatment. Transfus Sci. 1998;19:33–8.
66. Kostner GM, Krempler F. Lipoprotein (a). Curr Opin Lipidol. 1992;3:279–84.
67. Jauhiainen M, Koskinen P, Ehnholm C, Frick MH, Mänttäri M, Manninen V, et al. Lipoprotein (a) and coronary heart disease risk: a nested case–control study of the Helsinki heart study participants. Atherosclerosis. 1991;89:59–67.

68. Ullrich H, Lackner KJ, Schmitz G. Lipoprotein(a) apheresis in severe coronary heart disease: an immunoadsorption method. Artif Organs. 1998;22:135–9.
69. Pokrovsky SN, Adamova IY, Afanasieva OY, Benevolenskaya GF. Immunosorbent for selective removal of lipoprotein (a) from human plasma: in vitro study. Artif Organs. 1991;15:136–46.
70. Pokrovsky SN, Sussekov AV, Afanasieva OI, Adamova IY, Lyakishev AA, Kukharchuk VV. Extracorporeal immunoadsorption for the specific removal of lipoprotein (a) (Lp(a) apheresis): preliminary clinical data. Chem Phys Lipids. 1994;67:323–30.
71. Bosch T, Thiery J, Gurland HJ, Seidel D. Long-term efficiency, biocompatibility, and clinical safety of combined simultaneous LDL apheresis and hemodialysis in patients with hypercholesterolemia and endstage renal failure. Nephrol Dial Transplant. 1993;8:1350–8.
72. Bosch T, Lnnertz A, Schmidt B, Fink E, Keller C, Toepfer M, et al. Dali apheresis in hyperlipidemic patients: biocompatibility, efficacy, and selectivity of direct adsorption of lipoprotein from whole blood. Artif Organs. 2000;24:81–90.
73. Bosch T, Schmidt B, Kleophas W, Otto V, Samtleben W. LDL-hemoperfusion—a new procedure for LDL apheresis: biocompatibility results from a first pilot study in hypercholesterolemic atherosclerosis patients. Artif Organs. 1993;21:1060–5.
74. Drager LJ, Julius U, Kraezle K, Schaper J, Toepfer M, Zygan K, et al. Dali-the first human blood low-density lipoprotein and lipoprotein (a) systemin a clinical use: procedure and clinical results. Eur J Clin Invest. 1998;28:994–1002.
75. Bosch T, Gahr S, Belchner U, Schaefer C, Lennertz A, Rammo J, DALI Study Group. Direct adsorption of low-density lipoprotein by DALI-LDL-apheresis: results of a prospective long-term multicenter follow-up covering 12,291 sessions. Ther Apher Dial. 2006;10:210–8.

Chapter 16
Review of Current Guidelines: National Cholesterol Education Program and Kidney Disease Outcomes Quality Initiative as They Apply to CKD with Dyslipidemias

Baris Afsar

Introduction

The number of patients with chronic kidney disease (CKD) is increasing. Unfortunately, the survival of CKD patients remains poor. Among other factors, cardiovascular disease (CVD) is the leading cause of death in CKD patients. Both traditional and nontraditional factors play a role for this increased cardiovascular mortality. Among traditional risk factors, diabetes, hypertension, and dyslipidemia are the leading causes. Anemia, inflammation, oxidative stress, disorders of calcium phosphorus metabolism, arterial stiffness, and malnutrition can be stated as nontraditional risk factors [1–3]. Thus, it is of no question that CKD patients can be considered as high-risk patients. In previous reports such as adult treatment panel (ATP) III, there was no specific interest regarding the dyslipidemia in CKD patients. Thus, in response to recommendations of the National Kidney Foundation (NKF) Task Force on CVD, the NKF Kidney Disease Outcomes Quality Initiative (K/DOQI) convened a work group to develop guidelines for the management of dyslipidemias, one of the risk factors for CVD in CKD. This section will give detailed information about these guidelines first and the interpretation of these guidelines based on the recently conducted randomized prospective studies thereafter.

B. Afsar, M.D. (✉)
Konya Numune State Hospital, Department of Nephrology, Konya, Selcuklu 42250, Turkey
e-mail: afsarbrs@yahoo.com

A. Covic et al. (eds.), *Dyslipidemias in Kidney Disease*, DOI 10.1007/978-1-4939-0515-7_16,

Adult Treatment Panel III Guidelines

The Executive Summary of the Third Report of the National Cholesterol Education Program (NCEP) Expert Panel on Detection, Evaluation, and Treatment of High Blood Cholesterol in Adults (ATP III) was published in May 2001 [4]. ATP III provides evidence-based recommendations on the management of high blood cholesterol and related disorders. For development of its recommendations, ATP III places primary emphasis on large, randomized, controlled clinical trials (RCTs). The classification of dyslipidemias according to ATP III was given in Table 16.1.

According to ATP III guidelines, management of all lipid disorders begins with therapeutic lifestyle changes (TLCs), given the fact that TLC has the potential to reduce cardiovascular risk through several mechanisms beyond lowering of low-density lipoprotein (LDL) cholesterol. Among TLCs, diet (saturated fat <7 % of calories, cholesterol <200 mg/day, and increased viscous [soluble] fiber [10–25 g/day] and plant sterols [2 g/day] as therapeutic options to enhance LDL lowering), weight management, and increased physical activity are strongly recommended.

ATP III reports have identified low-density lipoprotein cholesterol (LDL-C) as the primary target of cholesterol-lowering therapy. Lipoprotein levels must be obtained after 9–12 h of fasting.

According to the ATP III algorithm, persons are categorized into three risk categories:

1. Established coronary heart disease (CHD) and CHD risk equivalents
2. Multiple (2+) risk factors
3. Zero to one (0–1) risk factor

Table 16.1 Dyslipidemias as defined in the Adult Treatment Panel III guidelines

	Level (mg/dL)[a]
Total cholesterol	
• Desirable	<200
• Borderline high	200–239
• High	≥240
Low-density lipoprotein (LDL) cholesterol	
• Optimal	<100
• Near optimal	100–129
• Borderline	130–159
• High	160–189
• Very high	≥190
Triglyceride	
• Normal	<150
• Borderline high	150–199
• High	200–499
• Very high	≥500
High-density lipoprotein (HDL) cholesterol	
• Low	<40

[a]To convert mg/dL to mmol/L, multiply triglycerides by 0.01129 and cholesterols by 0.02586

CHD risk equivalents include non-coronary forms of clinical atherosclerotic disease and diabetes. Major risk factors other than LDL cholesterol include cigarette smoking, hypertension (BP >140/90 mmHg or on antihypertensive medication), low high-density lipoprotein cholesterol (HDL-C) (<40 mg/dL), family history of premature CHD (CHD in male first-degree relative <55 years; CHD in female first-degree relative <65 years), age (men >45 years; women >55 years). HDL-C >60 mg/dL counts as a "negative" risk factor, and its presence removes one risk factor from the total count. All persons with CHD or CHD risk equivalents should be accepted as high risk. The goal for LDL-lowering therapy in high-risk patients is an LDL-C level <100 mg/dL. If treatment LDL-C is <100 mg/dL, no further LDL-lowering therapy was recommended. For all high-risk patients with LDL-C levels ≥100 mg/dL, LDL-lowering dietary therapy should be initiated first. When baseline LDL-C is ≥130 mg/dL, an LDL-lowering drug should be started simultaneously with dietary therapy. However, LDL-lowering drugs were not mandated if the baseline LDL-C level is in the range of 100–129 mg/dL; in this range, ATP III suggested several therapeutic options. Dietary therapy should be intensified, whereas adding or intensifying an LDL-lowering drug was said to be optional. Alternatively, if the patient has elevated triglycerides or low HDL-C, a drug that targets these abnormalities may be added.

For patients with 2+ risk factors the LDL-C should be <130 mg/dL. ATP III further recommended that Framingham risk scoring be carried out in individuals with 2+ risk factors so as to triage them into three levels of 10-year risk for hard CHD events (myocardial infarction + CHD death), namely >20 % risk, 10–20 % risk, and <10 % risk. Persons with a 10-year risk >20 % were elevated to the high-risk category; in these patients, the LDL-C goal is <100 mg/dL. For others with 2+ risk factors, a 10-year risk ≤20 %, the LDL-C goal is <130 mg/dL. If the 10-year risk is 10–20 %, drug therapy should be considered if the LDL-C level is above the goal level (≥130 mg/dL) after a trial of dietary therapy. When 10-year risk is <10 %, an LDL-lowering drug can be considered if the LDL-C level is ≥160 mg/dL on maximal dietary therapy. Finally, for persons with 0–1 risk factor, the goal is to lower LDL-C concentrations to 160 mg/dL. If the LDL-C is ≥190 mg/dL after an adequate trial of dietary therapy, consideration should be given to adding a cholesterol-lowering drug. When serum LDL-C ranges from 160 to 189 mg/dL, introduction of a cholesterol-lowering drug is a therapeutic option in appropriate circumstances, such as when a severe risk factor is present [5]. In the ATP III guidelines, no specific comment was made on patients with CKD, and CKD patients are not managed differently from other patients. The ATP III only notes that nephrotic syndrome is a cause of secondary dyslipidemia, and suggests consideration be given to the use of cholesterol-lowering drugs if hyperlipidemia persists despite specific treatment for kidney disease. The ATP III also notes that various dyslipidemias have been reported in persons with kidney failure. However, the ATP III suggests that a cautious approach be taken, since these persons are prone to drug side effects, e.g., they are at increased risk for myopathy from both fibrates and statins. Indeed, fibrates are contraindicated in Stage 5 CKD patients in ATP III reports.

Kidney Disease Outcomes Quality Initiative Guidelines for Dyslipidemia

One may ask why we need a specific guideline regarding the dyslipidemias in CKD. There are several answers to this question. Firstly, both the ATP III guidelines [4] and its older component in children (NCEP-C) [6], without excluding or including patients with CKD, make few specific recommendations for the evaluation and treatment of dyslipidemias in CKD. Secondly, the CKD patients were entirely different from other patients with their own traditional and nontraditional risk factors. Thirdly, CKD should be accepted as a CHD risk equivalent. Fourthly, the K/DOQI work group concluded that the NCEP guidelines are applicable to patients with stages 1–4 CKD. Therefore, these K/DOQI guidelines target adults and adolescents with Stage 5 CKD and kidney transplant recipients [7]. Lastly, there is also a debate about whether dyslipidemia is a true risk factor for CVD in CKD patients. While some studies showed that dyslipidemia was indeed associated with increased risk of incident atherosclerotic CVD and with increased risk of death after CVD events [8], others reported the opposite association in CKD patients [9, 10]—a discrepancy that was explained with the context of reverse epidemiology [11, 12].

For all these reasons, the K/DOQI established a specific guideline regarding the dyslipidemias in CKD patients. The differences of the K/DOQI guidelines from those of the ATP III are given in Table 16.2.

The K/DOQI Clinical Practice Guidelines for Managing Dyslipidemias in Chronic Kidney Disease may be divided into three parts. First part explains the target population, scope, intended users, and methods. Second part was about the assessment of dyslipidemias and the third part was about the treatment of dyslipidemias. The data regarding these three parts are given below.

Table 16.2 Features that differ between K/DOQI guidelines and ATP III guidelines

K/DOQI guidelines	ATP III guidelines
CKD patients should be considered as CHD risk equivalent	No specific mention of CKD patients
Evaluation of dyslipidemias should be made annually	Evaluation of dyslipidemias should occur every 5 years
Drug therapy should be used for LDL 100–129 mg/dL after 3 months of TCL (initial drug therapy should be statin)	Drug therapy is optional for LDL 100–129 mg/dL (initial drug therapy can be statin, bile acid sequestrant, or nicotinic acid)
Recommendations were made for patients <20 years old	No recommendations were made for patients <20 years old
Fibrates may be used under special conditions. Gemfibrozil may be the drug of choice	Fibrates are contraindicated in Stage 5 CKD

TLC therapeutic lifestyle changes

Target Population, Scope, Intended Users, and Methods

Due to the reasons explained above, an expert committee performed seminal work and the K/DOQI guidelines were published regarding the management of dyslipidemias in all stages of CKD and renal transplant patients. One of the most important issues reported by the work group was the acceptance of CKD as a CHD risk equivalent. The work group also underscored the importance of other risk factors for the development of atherosclerotic cardiovascular disease (ACVD) and pointed out that dyslipidemia management should be undertaken in conjunction with all other available measures to reduce the overall risk of ACVD. It was also suggested that modifiable, conventional risk factors (including hypertension, cigarette smoking, glucose intolerance or diabetes control, and obesity) should be assessed at initial presentation and at least yearly thereafter. These guidelines are intended for use by physicians, nurses, nurse practitioners, pharmacists, dietitians, and other health-care professionals who care for patients with CKD. The guidelines were developed using a scientifically rigorous process, and the rationale and evidentiary basis for each guideline are clearly explained. All the members of the working group are experts in the management of CKD and dyslipidemias. The experts worked independently from any organizational affiliations and had final responsibility for determining guideline content. The guidelines underwent widespread critical review before being finalized.

Assessment of Dyslipidemias

The principal reason to evaluate dyslipidemias in patients with CKD is to detect abnormalities that may be treated to reduce the incidence of ACVD. However, there may be other reasons to evaluate and treat dyslipidemias in CKD. A number of observational studies have reported that various dyslipidemias are associated with decreased kidney function in the general population and in patients with CKD. Besides, the prevalence of dyslipidemias in patients with CKD is high. Factors such as proteinuria, glomerular filtration rate changes, and treatment of CKD may all alter lipoprotein levels. Lipoprotein levels may change during the first 3 months of hemodialysis, peritoneal dialysis, and kidney transplantation. On the other hand, waiting 3 months to measure the first lipid profile may needlessly delay effective treatment for patients who present with dyslipidemia. Therefore, it is prudent to evaluate dyslipidemias more often than is recommended in the general population. Another potential concern is the effect of dialysis procedure on lipid levels. There is some evidence that the hemodialysis procedure acutely alters plasma lipid levels due to hemoconcentration and/or effects of the dialysis membrane or heparin on lipoprotein metabolism [13].

Based on all these data, the working group suggests that

- All adults and adolescents with CKD should be evaluated for dyslipidemias (moderate evidence).
- For adults and adolescents with CKD, the assessment of dyslipidemias should include a complete fasting lipid profile with total cholesterol, LDL-C, HDL-C, and triglycerides (moderate evidence).
- For adults and adolescents with Stage 5 CKD, dyslipidemias should be evaluated upon presentation (when the patient is stable), at 2–3 months after a change in treatment or other conditions known to cause dyslipidemias; and at least annually thereafter (moderate evidence).
- For adults and adolescents with Stage 5 CKD, a complete lipid profile should be measured after an overnight fast whenever possible (moderate evidence).
- Hemodialysis patients should have lipid profiles measured either before dialysis, or on days not receiving dialysis (moderate evidence).
- Stage 5 CKD patients with dyslipidemias should be evaluated for remediable, secondary causes (moderate evidence).

Treating Dyslipidemias

The rationale for treating dyslipidemias is similar to the ATP III guidelines focus on lowering LDL-C levels. One important remark was the acceptance of CKD as a CHD risk equivalent. However, for the rare adult patient with markedly elevated serum triglyceride levels, triglyceride reduction is the principal focus of treatment in order to prevent pancreatitis. Based on these data, the working group suggests that

- For adults with Stage 5 CKD and fasting triglycerides ≥500 mg/dL that cannot be corrected by removing an underlying cause, treatment with TLCs and a triglyceride-lowering agent should be considered (weak evidence).
- For adults with Stage 5 CKD and LDL ≥100 mg/dL (≥2.59 mmol/L), treatment should be considered to reduce LDL to <100 mg/dL (<2.59 mmol/L) (moderate evidence).
- For adults with Stage 5 CKD and LDL <100 mg/dL (<2.59 mmol/L), fasting triglycerides ≥200 mg/dL and non-HDL cholesterol (total cholesterol minus HDL) ≥130 mg/dL (≥3.36 mmol/L), treatment should be considered to reduce non-HDL cholesterol to <130 mg/dL (<3.36 mmol/L) (weak evidence).
- For adolescents with Stage 5 CKD and LDL ≥130 mg/dL, treatment should be considered to reduce LDL to <130 mg/dL (<3.36 mmol/L) (weak evidence).
- For adolescents with Stage 5 CKD and LDL <130 mg/dL (<3.36 mmol/L), fasting triglycerides ≥200 mg/dL and non-HDL cholesterol (total cholesterol minus HDL) ≥160 mg/dL treatment should be considered to reduce non-HDL cholesterol to <160 mg/dL (weak evidence).

Until these guidelines were published by the working group, there were very few randomized controlled studies examining the effect of lipid-lowering therapy in CKD patients. However, after the report of the working group, several prospective studies were published regarding the use of lipid-lowering agents and cardiovascular outcomes in CKD patients including peritoneal and hemodialysis patients. Since these studies are very important in the field of treatment of dyslipidemias in CKD patients, they should be mentioned.

Studies of Dyslipidemia Treatment in Chronic Kidney Disease Patients Not on Dialysis

Few studies have been designed primarily to investigate the effects of statins (HMG-CoA [3-hydroxy-3-methylglutaryl coenzyme A] reductase inhibitor) on cardiovascular outcomes in patients with CKD who are not undergoing dialysis therapy. The pravastatin pooling project examined the effects of statin therapy on the risk of major cardiovascular events based on other large trials. The relative risk reduction in major cardiovascular events observed among patients with an estimated GFRs (eGFRs) of ≥30 mL/min/1.73 m^2 and <60 mL/min/1.73 m^2 was similar to that observed in patients with a GFR ≥60 mL/min/1.73 m^2 (23 % and 22 %, respectively) [14]. A meta-analysis of randomized, placebo-controlled trials that included >6,500 patients with CKD demonstrated that statins significantly reduced both serum lipid concentrations and the incidence of cardiovascular endpoints, without evidence of increased adverse effects [15]. These studies were primarily designed to assess cardiovascular outcomes in patients with cardiac disease or at high risk of developing cardiac disease and lacked predefined kidney function outcomes; consequently, the renal findings derived from post hoc analyses might be misleading [14]. Thus, to diminish these drawbacks; various trials randomly assigned participants to statin therapy vs. control [16–19], and one trial randomly assigned participants to high-dose vs. low-dose statin and reported relevant outcomes for patients with CKD [20]. These later studies varied in respect to definitions, patient characteristics, and methods. Mean baseline LDL cholesterol levels ranged from 96.3 to 140 mg/dL. Study duration ranged from 3.9 to 5.4 years. As a cumulative result of these studies, it was concluded that statins did not decrease all-cause mortality or stroke in participants with diabetes and CKD [21]. Besides, high-dose statin therapy did not decrease all-cause mortality, stroke, or the risk of major cardiovascular events compared to lower-dose statin therapy in participants with diabetes and CKD. However, statin therapy increased regression of microalbuminuria to normoalbuminuria, but did not attenuate the decrease in eGFR in patients with baseline albuminuria [17].

However, the aforementioned studies were carried out in diabetic CKD patients. To be more comprehensive, Navaneethan et al. evaluated the benefits of statins in patients with non-dialysis-dependent CKD, with or without cardiovascular comorbidities, including randomized controlled trials and comparing statins with placebo. The meta-analysis involved more than 18,500 patients and showed that statins reduced the relative risk of all cause mortality by 19 %, the relative risk of cardiovascular mortality by 20 %, and the relative risk of nonfatal cardiovascular events by 25 % [22]. Thus, it was concluded that statin therapy is effective in reducing CVD, especially in early stages of CKD [23–26]. Based on these data, a recent review suggests more specifically that it is better for CKD patients with stages 1–3 to use statins, whereas the beneficial role of statins beyond Stage 3 CKD is less clear [14].

Apart from statins, there are also studies investigating the effects of fibrates in CKD patients. In a randomized study by Tonelli et al. that included 2,531 men (1,046 of them had chronic renal insufficiency defined as by creatinine clearance ≤75 mL/min using the Cockcroft–Gault equation) to investigate the effects of gemfibrozil in secondary prevention of cardiovascular events. After a median follow-up of a 5.3 years, gemfibrozil treatment significantly reduced the risk of the composite outcome of fatal CHD, nonfatal myocardial infarction, and stroke compared to placebo [27]. In another study by Davis et al., the effect of fenofibrate therapy on renal function was investigated in 9,795 type 2 diabetic patients. Patients were randomly assigned to fenofibrate ($n=4.895$) or placebo ($n=4.900$) for 5 years, following 6 weeks of fenofibrate run-in. Although in the run-in period plasma creatinine increased, it quickly reversed on placebo assignment. However, eGFR had fallen less from baseline on fenofibrate than on placebo ($p<0.001$). Fenofibrate reduced urine albumin concentrations and, hence, albumin/creatinine ratio by 24 % vs. 11 % ($p<0.001$; mean difference 14 % [95 % confidence interval (CI) 9–18]; $p<0.001$), with 14 % less progression and 18 % more albuminuria regression ($p<0.001$) than in participants on placebo. End-stage renal event frequency was similar ($n=21$ vs. 26, $p=0.48$). The authors concluded that fenofibrate reduced albuminuria and slowed eGFR loss over 5 years, despite initially and reversibly increasing plasma creatinine. Fenofibrate may delay albuminuria and GFR impairment in type 2 diabetes patients [28].

Studies of Dyslipidemia Treatment in Chronic Kidney Disease Patients on Dialysis

The Deutsche Diabetes Dialyse Studie (4D) study randomly assigned participants with end-stage renal disease (ESRD) and diabetes to statin therapy vs. placebo [29]. In the 4D study, Wanner et al. recruited 1,255 diabetic patients with ESRD; 619 were in intervention group (atorvastatin 20 mg/dL) and 636 served as controls. The primary endpoint was a composite of death from cardiac causes, nonfatal myocardial infarction, and stroke. Secondary endpoints included death from all causes and all cardiac and cerebrovascular events combined. After a median of 4 years follow-up; 469 patients (37 %) reached the primary endpoint, of whom 226 were assigned to atorvastatin and 243 to placebo (relative risk, 0.92; 95 % CI, 0.77–1.10; $p=0.37$). Atorvastatin had no significant effect on the individual components of the primary endpoint, except that the relative risk of fatal stroke among those receiving the drug was 2.03 (95 % CI, 1.05–3.93; $p=0.04$). Atorvastatin reduced the rate of all cardiac events combined (relative risk, 0.82; 95 % CI, 0.68–0.99; $p=0.03$, nominally significant) but not all cerebrovascular events combined (relative risk, 1.12; 95 % CI, 0.81–1.55; $p=0.49$) or total mortality (relative risk, 0.93; 95 % CI, 0.79–1.08; $p=0.33$). The authors concluded that atorvastatin had no statistically significant effect on the composite primary endpoint of cardiovascular death, nonfatal myocardial infarction, and stroke in patients with diabetes receiving hemodialysis [29]. The authors speculated regarding the lack of effectiveness of the lipid lowering by atorvastatin. A possible reason for the unexpected results with regard to the primary endpoint might be related to the low LDL cholesterol concentrations at baseline. Indeed post hoc analysis of 4D study demonstrated that atorvastatin significantly reduced the rate of adverse outcomes in patients with a baseline LDL cholesterol level in the highest quartile (≥3.76 mmol/L) but not in any of the other three quartiles [30]. Secondly, the pathogenesis of vascular events in patients with diabetes mellitus who are receiving hemodialysis may, at least in part, be different from that in patients without ESRD. Additionally, patients with diabetic ESRD may also be different with respect to disease characteristics than other ESRD patients without diabetes. Thus, it could be possible that the absence of a significant effect on mortality from cardiac causes and cardiac endpoints may be the presence of additional pathogenetic pathways in diabetes. Reverse epidemiology and protein energy malnutrition may be another explanation. Another potential reason may be the low dose of atorvastatin. Lastly, the effect of lipid-lowering therapy may not be observed since the disease has already progressed and the lipid-lowering therapy may work in earlier stages of renal disease. Thus, the benefit of atorvastatin is limited when intervention with statins is postponed until patients have reached ESRD.

Another randomized, double-blind prospective trial with rosuvastatin in ESRD was recently published. The AURORA trial (A Study to Evaluate the Use of Rosuvastatin in Subjects on Regular Hemodialysis: An Assessment of Survival and Cardiovascular Events) involved 2,776 patients, 50–80 years of age, who were undergoing maintenance hemodialysis. Patients were randomly assigned to receive rosuvastatin, 10 mg daily, or placebo. The combined primary endpoint was death from cardiovascular causes, nonfatal myocardial infarction, or nonfatal stroke. Secondary endpoints included death from all causes and individual cardiac and vascular events. During a median follow-up period of 3.8 years, 396 patients in the rosuvastatin group and 408 patients in the placebo group reached the primary endpoint (9.2 and 9.5 events per 100 patient-years, respectively; hazard ratio for the combined endpoint in the rosuvastatin group vs. the placebo group, 0.96; 95 % CI, 0.84–1.11; $p=0.59$). Rosuvastatin had no effect on individual components of the primary endpoint. There was also no significant effect on all-cause mortality (13.5 vs. 14.0 events per 100 patient-years; hazard ratio, 0.96; 95 % CI, 0.86–1.07; $p=0.51$). Interestingly, an increased incidence of fatal hemorrhagic stroke was noted in patients with diabetes mellitus in the rosuvastatin group, compared to patients with diabetes mellitus in the placebo group ($p=0.03$). Of note, a total of 1,296 patients died during the follow-up period, and approximately half of these were deaths from cardiovascular causes. The authors concluded that undergoing hemodialysis, the initiation of treatment with rosuvastatin lowered the LDL cholesterol level but had no significant effect on the composite primary endpoint of death from cardiovascular causes, nonfatal myocardial infarction, or nonfatal stroke [31]. The lack of potential benefit in the AURORA trial was explained by several mechanisms, including lack of sufficient statistical power, high dropout rate, and exclusion of patients using statins during the 6 months before enrollment [32].

Lastly, it is worth mentioning the study Heart and Renal Protection (SHARP) trial [33]. This randomized double-blind trial included 9,270 patients both with CKD and ESRD on hemodialysis and peritoneal dialysis (3,023 on dialysis and 6,247 not) with no known history of myocardial infarction or coronary revascularization. Patients were randomly assigned to simvastatin 20 mg plus ezetimibe 10 mg daily (4,650 patients) vs. matching placebo (4,620 patients). The key pre-specified outcome was first major atherosclerotic event (nonfatal myocardial infarction or coronary death, non-hemorrhagic stroke, or any arterial revascularization procedure). All analyses were by intention to treat. After 4.9 years follow-up, there was a 17 % proportional reduction in major atherosclerotic events in simvastatin plus ezetimibe vs. placebo; (rate ratio [RR] 0.83, 95 % CI 0.74–0.94; log-rank $p=0.0021$) and there were significant reductions in non-hemorrhagic stroke (131 [2.8 %] vs. 174 [3.8 %]; RR 0.75, 95 % CI 0.60–0.94; $p=0.01$) and arterial revascularization procedures (284 [6.1 %] vs. 352 [7.6 %]; RR 0.79, 95 % CI 0.68–0.93; $p=0.0036$) in the simvastatin plus ezetimibe group. Of note, the authors were aware that SHARP did not have sufficient power to assess the effects on major atherosclerotic events separately in dialysis and non-dialysis patients, but there was not good statistical evidence that the proportional effects in dialysis patients differed to those seen in patients not on dialysis. On subgroup analysis, however, the investigators did not observe a clinically or statistically significant reduction in either mortality or the cardiovascular event rate in the dialysis population given active treatment compared with those on placebo (15 % vs. 16.5 %, respectively). Consequently, the results of the SHARP study for patients on dialysis were similar to those from the AURORA and 4D studies. However, the results of the SHARP trial must be interpreted with caution. Compliance with statin therapy was worse in the dialysis cohort than for patients who were not undergoing dialysis, such that the reduction in LDL cholesterol was only 0.60 mmol/L in the dialysis subgroup, whereas it was 0.84 mmol/L in the whole study population. Additionally, dialysis group in fact are larger given the fact that one-third of patients with CKD started dialysis during the study period.

Implications of Studies

In summary, three large randomized, placebo-controlled studies of three different statins have been conducted in the dialysis population, but two of these studies (4D, AURORA) did not demonstrate any benefits of statin therapy, and the third study (SHARP) showed only marginally positive results. The possible reasons for the lack of effectiveness of lipid-lowering therapy are given in Table 16.3. Thus, it is obvious that the basic mechanisms underlying the pathogenesis of dyslipidemia in CKD and ESRD must be critically (re)examined. The characteristics of dyslipidemia in

Table 16.3 Possible factors related to inefficiency of statin treatments in randomized controlled trials

Lack of statistical power
High dropout rate
Low dose of drugs
Advanced stage of disease
Different pathophysiologic mechanisms of dyslipidemia in CKD patients compared to normal population
Predominance of nontraditional cardiovascular risk factors
Ignorance of causes of renal failure and the age of the subjects
Reverse epidemiology

patients with CKD not yet requiring dialysis treatment differ markedly from those of individuals with established ESRD and form the basis for therapeutic recommendations [14]. It was also suggested that in order to detect the effectiveness of statin therapy in dialysis patients, a randomized controlled study should evaluate the causes of renal failure and the age of the subjects at the start of renal replacement therapy. The well-known atherosclerotic vascular damage and extensive vascular calcification of long-term CKD patients could be the cause of competing mortality, thereby reducing the opportunity to show the benefit of statin therapy [24]. It could be possible that the different comorbidities of CKD patients in the different stages of the disease hide the effectiveness of statins on the cardiovascular system.

Conclusion

While preparing the dyslipidemia guidelines in CKD patients, the working group anticipated from the beginning that all guidelines should be updated whenever new, pertinent information becomes available. To anticipate when these guidelines may need to be updated, the Work Group discussed ongoing clinical trials in the general population and in patients with CKD, as those results may be pertinent to some recommendations. They also have reasonable doubts as to whether trial results from the general population are applicable to all patients with CKD. The major trials (4D, AURORA, SHARP) were not completed when these guidelines were published. Thus, in light of these new findings, a new guideline incorporating the data of recent research is necessary. There is no question that new research is strongly warranted regarding the pathophysiology of dyslipidemias in CKD and ESRD patients, with newer treatment options, more patients, and extended follow-up.

References

1. Afsar B, Elsurer R, Akgul A, Sezer S, Ozdemir FN. Factors related to silent myocardial damage in hemodialysis patients. Ren Fail. 2009;31(10):933–41.
2. Kanbay M, Afsar B, Goldsmith D, Covic A. Sudden death in hemodialysis: an update. Blood Purif. 2010;30(2):135–45.

3. Muntner P, He J, Astor BC, Folsom AR, Coresh J. Traditional and nontraditional risk factors predict coronary heart disease in chronic kidney disease: results from the atherosclerosis risk in communities study. J Am Soc Nephrol. 2005;16(2):529–38. Epub 2004 Dec 29.
4. Expert Panel on Detection, Evaluation, and Treatment of High Blood Cholesterol in Adults. Executive summary of the third report of the National Cholesterol Education Program (NCEP) expert panel on detection, evaluation, and treatment of high blood cholesterol in adults (Adult Treatment Panel III). JAMA. 2001;285:2486–97.
5. Grundy SM, Cleeman JI, Merz CN, Brewer Jr HB, Clark LT, Hunninghake DB, et al. Coordinating Committee of the National Cholesterol Education Program. Implications of recent clinical trials for the National Cholesterol Education Program Adult Treatment Panel III guidelines. J Am Coll Cardiol. 2004;44(3):720–32.
6. American Academy of Pediatrics. National Cholesterol Education Program: report of the expert panel on blood cholesterol levels in children and adolescents. Pediatrics. 1992;89(3 Pt 2):525–84.
7. Kidney Disease Outcomes Quality Initiative (K/DOQI) Group. K/DOQI clinical practice guidelines for management of dyslipidemias in patients with kidney disease. Am J Kidney Dis. 2003;41(4 Suppl 3):I–IV, S1–91.
8. Shoji T, Masakane I, Watanabe Y, Iseki K, Tsubakihara Y. Committee of Renal Data Registry, Japanese Society for Dialysis Therapy. Elevated non-high-density lipoprotein cholesterol (non-HDL-C) predicts atherosclerotic cardiovascular events in hemodialysis patients. Clin J Am Soc Nephrol. 2011;6(5):1112–20.
9. Degoulet P, Legrain M, Réach I, Aimé F, Devriés C, Rojas P, et al. Mortality risk factors in patients treated by chronic hemodialysis. Report of the Diaphane collaborative study. Nephron. 1982;31(2):103–10.
10. Iseki K, Yamazato M, Tozawa M, Takishita S. Hypocholesterolemia is a significant predictor of death in a cohort of chronic hemodialysis patients. Kidney Int. 2002;61(5):1887–93.
11. Nishizawa Y, Shoji T, Ishimura E, Inaba M, Morii H. Paradox of risk factors for cardiovascular mortality in uremia: is a higher cholesterol level better for atherosclerosis in uremia? Am J Kidney Dis. 2001;38(4 Suppl 1):S4–7.
12. Kalantar-Zadeh K, Block G, Horwich T, Fonarow GC. Reverse epidemiology of conventional cardiovascular risk factors in patients with chronic heart failure. J Am Coll Cardiol. 2004;43(8):1439–44.
13. Ingram AJ, Parbtani A, Churchill DN. Effects of two low-flux cellulose acetate dialysers on plasma lipids and lipoproteins—a cross-over trial. Nephrol Dial Transplant. 1998;13(6): 1452–7.
14. Epstein M, Vaziri ND. Statins in the management of dyslipidemia associated with chronic kidney disease. Nat Rev Nephrol. 2012;8(4):214–23. doi:10.1038/nrneph.2012.33.
15. Strippoli GF, Navaneethan SD, Johnson DW, Perkovic V, Pellegrini F, Nicolucci A, et al. Effects of statins in patients with chronic kidney disease: meta-analysis and meta-regression of randomised controlled trials. BMJ. 2008;336(7645):645–51. doi:10.1136/bmj.39472.580984.AE. Epub 2008 Feb 25.
16. Collins R, Armitage J, Parish S, Sleigh P, Peto R. Heart Protection Study Collaborative Group. MRC/BHF Heart Protection Study of cholesterol-lowering with simvastatin in 5963 people with diabetes: a randomised placebo-controlled trial. Lancet. 2003;361(9374):2005–16.
17. Colhoun HM, Betteridge DJ, Durrington PN, Hitman GA, Neil HA, Livingstone SJ, et al.; CARDS Investigators. Primary prevention of cardiovascular disease with atorvastatin in type 2 diabetes in the Collaborative Atorvastatin Diabetes Study (CARDS): multicentre randomised placebo-controlled trial. Lancet. 2004;364(9435):685–96.
18. Tonelli M, Keech A, Shepherd J, Sacks F, Tonkin A, Packard C, et al. Effect of pravastatin in people with diabetes and chronic kidney disease. J Am Soc Nephrol. 2005;16(12):3748–54. Epub 2005 Oct 26.
19. Chonchol M, Cook T, Kjekshus J, Pedersen TR, Lindenfeld J. Simvastatin for secondary prevention of all-cause mortality and major coronary events in patients with mild chronic renal insufficiency. Am J Kidney Dis. 2007;49(3):373–82.

20. Shepherd J, Kastelein JJ, Bittner V, Deedwania P, Breazna A, Dobson S, et al. TNT (Treating to New Targets) Investigators. Intensive lipid lowering with atorvastatin in patients with coronary heart disease and chronic kidney disease: the TNT (Treating to New Targets) study. J Am Coll Cardiol. 2008;51(15):1448–54.
21. Slinin Y, Ishani A, Rector T, Fitzgerald P, MacDonald R, Tacklind J, et al. Management of hyperglycemia, dyslipidemia, and albuminuria in patients with diabetes and CKD: a systematic review for a KDOQI clinical practice guideline. Am J Kidney Dis. 2012;60(5):747–69. doi:10.1053/j.ajkd.2012.07.017. Epub 2012 Sep 19.
22. Navaneethan SD, Pansini F, Perkovic V, Manno C, Pellegrini F, Johnson DW, et al. HMG CoA reductase inhibitors (statins) for people with chronic kidney disease not requiring dialysis. Cochrane Database Syst Rev. 2009;(2):CD007784. doi: 10.1002/14651858.CD007784.
23. Kanbay M, Turgut F, Covic A, Goldsmith D. Statin treatment for dyslipidemia in chronic kidney disease and renal transplantation: a review of the evidence. J Nephrol. 2009;22(5): 598–609.
24. Fabbian F, De Giorgi A, Pala M, Tiseo R, Manfredini R, Portaluppi F. Evidence-based statin prescription for cardiovascular protection in renal impairment. Clin Exp Nephrol. 2011;15(4):456–63.
25. Gluba A, Rysz J, Banach M. Statins in patients with chronic kidney disease: why, who and when? Expert Opin Pharmacother. 2010;11(16):2665–74.
26. Inoue T, Ikeda H, Nakamura T, Abe S, Taguchi I, Kikuchi M, et al. Potential benefit of statin therapy for dyslipidemia with chronic kidney disease: Fluvastatin Renal Evaluation Trial (FRET). Intern Med. 2011;50(12):1273–8. Epub 2011 Jun 15.
27. Tonelli M, Collins D, Robins S, Bloomfield H, Curhan GC; Veterans' Affairs High-Density Lipoprotein Intervention Trial (VA-HIT) Investigators. Gemfibrozil for secondary prevention of cardiovascular events in mild to moderate chronic renal insufficiency. Kidney Int. 2004;66(3):1123–30.
28. Davis TM, Ting R, Best JD, Donoghoe MW, Drury PL, Sullivan DR, et al.; Fenofibrate Intervention and Event Lowering in Diabetes Study Investigators. Effects of fenofibrate on renal function in patients with type 2 diabetes mellitus: the Fenofibrate Intervention and Event Lowering in Diabetes (FIELD) study. Diabetologia. 2011;54(2):280–90. doi: 10.1007/s00125-010-1951-1. Epub 2010 Nov 4.
29. Wanner C, Krane V, März W, Olschewski M, Mann JF, Ruf G, et al. German Diabetes and Dialysis Study Investigators. Atorvastatin in patients with type 2 diabetes mellitus undergoing hemodialysis. N Engl J Med. 2005;353(3):238–48.
30. März W, Genser B, Drechsler C, Krane V, Grammer TB, Ritz E, et al.; German Diabetes and Dialysis Study Investigators. Atorvastatin and low-density lipoprotein cholesterol in type 2 diabetes mellitus patients on hemodialysis. Clin J Am Soc Nephrol. 2011;6(6):1316–25. doi: 10.2215/CJN.09121010. Epub 2011 Apr 14.
31. Fellström BC, Jardine AG, Schmieder RE, Holdaas H, Bannister K, Beutler J, et al. AURORA Study Group. Rosuvastatin and cardiovascular events in patients undergoing hemodialysis. N Engl J Med. 2009;360(14):1395–407.
32. Strippoli GF, Craig JC. Sunset for statins after AURORA? N Engl J Med. 2009;360(14): 1455–7.
33. Baigent C, Landray MJ, Reith C, Emberson J, Wheeler DC, Tomson C, et al. SHARP Investigators. The effects of lowering LDL cholesterol with simvastatin plus ezetimibe in patients with chronic kidney disease (Study of Heart and Renal Protection): a randomised placebo-controlled trial. Lancet. 2011;377(9784):2181–92.

Index

A. Covic et al. (eds.), *Dyslipidemias in Kidney Disease*, DOI 10.1007/978-1-4939-0515-7,

E

I

S

T

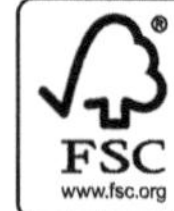

MIX
Papier aus verantwortungsvollen Quellen
Paper from responsible sources
FSC® C105338

If you have any concerns about our products, you can contact us on
ProductSafety@springernature.com

In case Publisher is established outside the EU, the EU authorized representative is:
Springer Nature Customer Service Center GmbH
Europaplatz 3, 69115 Heidelberg, Germany

Printed by Libri Plureos GmbH
in Hamburg, Germany